£3.00

D1356978

Practical Endoscopy

JOIN US ON THE INTERNET VIA WWW, GOPHER, FTP OR EMAIL:

WWW: http://www.thomson.com
GOPHER: gopher.thomson.com
FTP: ftp.thomson.com
EMAIL: findit@kiosk.thomson.com

A service of I(T)P

Practical Endoscopy

Edited by
Mike Shephard
and Jayne Mason

CHAPMAN & HALL MEDICAL

London · Weinheim · New York · Tokyo · Melbourne · Madras

Published by Chapman & Hall, 2–6 Boundary Row, London SE1 8HN, UK

Chapman & Hall, 2–6 Boundary Row, London SE1 8HN, UK

Chapman & Hall GmbH, Pappelallee 3, 69469 Weinheim, Germany

Chapman & Hall USA, 115 Fifth Avenue, New York NY 10003, USA

Chapman & Hall Japan, ITP-Japan, Kyowa Building, 3F, 2–2–1 Hirakawacho, Chiyoda-ku, Tokyo 102, Japan

Chapman & Hall Australia, 102 Dodds Street, South Melbourne, Victoria 3205, Australia

Chapman & Hall India, R. Seshadri, 32 Second Main Road, CIT East, Madras 600 035, India

First edition 1997

© 1997 Chapman & Hall
© 1997 Chapter 2 Brian Taylor, Chapter 7C Samantha Hawkes

Typeset in 10.5/12 Sabon by Photoprint, Torquay, Devon

Printed in Great Britain at the Alden Press, Oxford

ISBN 0 412 54000 2

A catalogue record for this book is available from the British Library

Library of Congress Catalog Card Number: 96–83464

∞ Printed on acid-free text paper, manufactured in accordance with ANSI/NISO Z39, 48–1992 (Permanence of Paper).

Contents

List of contributors

Mr D. Alderson FRCS
Consultant Senior Lecturer,
University Department of
Surgery, Bristol Royal Infirmary,
Bristol, BS2 8HW UK.

**Dr M.F. Bone Bsc Hons
MRCPDCH**
Consultant Chest Physician,
Russells Hall Hospital, Dudley,
West Midlands, DY1 2HQ UK.

Margaret Cox RGN
Springfield Medical Centre, Lawn
Lane, Springfield, Chelmsford,
Essex, CM1 7GU UK.

Dr F. Donald MB BS FRCPath
Public Health Laboratory,
Nottingham City Hospital NHS
Trust, Hucknall Road,
Nottingham, NG5 1PB UK.

Julie D'Silva RGN
Nurse Manager, Endoscopy Unit,
Rotherham District General
Hospital, Rotherham,
South Yorkshire, S60 2UD UK.

**Dr G. Duthie MD(Hons) FRCS
Ed.**
Senior Lecturer/Honorary
Consultant, Department of
Colorectal Surgery, Castle Hill
Hospital, Castle Road,
Cottingham, North Humberside,
HU16 5JQ UK.

Hazel French RGN
Nurse Manager, Medical Day
Unit, Level 4, Bristol Royal
Infirmary, Bristol, BS2 8HW UK.

Jean Harvey RGN M.I.S.M.
Endoscopy Unit Manager, North
Lincolnshire Trust Hospital,
Scartho Road, Grimsby, South
Humberside, DN33 2BA UK.

Samantha Hawkes RGN DPNS
Clinical Nurse Advisor, Pentax
(UK) Ltd, Medical Division,
Pentax House, Heron Drive,
Langley, Slough, Middlesex,
SL3 8PN UK.

Rachel Hodson RGN DN
Nurse Manager, Endoscopy Unit,
Castle Hill Hospital, Castle
Road, Cottingham, North
Humberside, HU16 5JQ UK.

Mark Hughes RGN
Colorectal Nurse Practitioner,
Castle Hill Hospital, Castle
Road, Cottingham, North
Humberside, HU16 5JQ UK.

**Dr Huw R. Jenkins MD FRCP
MCPCH**
Consultant Paediatric
Gastroenterologist, University
Hospital of Wales, Heath Park,
Cardiff, Glamorgan, CF4 4XW
UK.

**Marlene Littlewood
RGN Dip N.**
Clinical Nurse Specialist, G.I.
Unit, Russells Hall Hospital,
Dudley, West Midlands, DY1
2HQ UK.

Jayne Mason RGN Cert.Ed.
Nurse Manager, Endoscopy Unit,
University Hospital of Wales,
Heath Park, Cardiff, Glamorgan,
CF4 4XW UK.

**Mr. Rory McCloy BSc
MD FRCS**
Senior Lecturer/Honorary
Consultant, University Dept of
Surgery, Manchester Royal
Infirmary, Manchester, M13 9WL
UK.

Dr. David A.L. Morgan FRCR
Clinical Director, Oncology,
Nottingham City Hospital NHS
Trust, Hucknall Road,
Nottingham, NG5 1PB UK.

**Dr Suresh Nair MBBS MMED
MRCOG**
Consultant Obstetrician &
Gynaecologist, Dept. of
Reproductive Medicine, KK
Women's & Children's Hospital,
100 Bukit Timah Road,
Singapore 229899.

Miss S.A. Norton FRCS Ed
Surgical Research Registar,
University Department of
Surgery, Bristol Royal Infirmary,
Bristol, BS2 8HW UK.

**Mike Shephard RGN MHSM
Cert MHS**
Gastroenterology Services
Manager, Nottingham City
Hospital NHS Trust, Hucknall
Road, Nottingham, NG5 1PB
UK.

Jenny Smith RGN
Senior Sister, Calcraft Suite,
Royal Gwent Hospital, Cardiff
Road, Newport, Gwent, NP9
2UB UK.

Brian W. Taylor F Inst SMM
Director and General Manager,
Pentax UK Ltd, Medical
Division, Pentax House, Heron
Drive, Langley, Slough, SL3 8PN
UK.

**C. Paul Wicker BSc[Nursing]
RGN RMN**
Education Coordinator, Theatres,
Royal Infirmary of Edinburgh
NHS Trust, Lauriston Road,
Edinburgh EH3 9YW UK.

Jean Wicks RGN
Endoscopy Unit Manager,
Scunthorpe District General
Hospital, South Humberside,
DN15 7BH UK.

Preface

During the past 10 years there have been many changes in the field of flexible endoscopy. The introduction of new procedures and treatments, together with advances in instrument technology, has revolutionized the care of patients suffering from conditions that had previously required, at best, lengthy investigation or, at worst, surgical intervention. In 1984 Ravenscroft and Swan produced a book entitled *Gastrointestinal Endoscopy and Related Procedures*, which was the first book aimed specifically at the endoscopy assistant, and which has been widely used throughout the world. This book aims both to update and to expand on its contents to produce a comprehensive text covering all aspects of flexible endoscopy encountered in the modern endoscopy unit. With the increasingly technical and specialist role demanded of today's endoscopy assistant, together with the introduction in many countries of the concept of multidisciplinary team care, it was evident that a book was required that was suitable not only for the needs of the endoscopy assistant but also for medical practitioners and other health care professionals embarking on a career in this speciality. This book aims to fulfil such a need.

The book covers general issues concerning the provision of an endoscopy service, including endoscopy unit design, staffing, legal issues, documentation and quality assurance, as well as providing an insight into the history of endoscopy nursing and instrumentation.

All aspects of diagnostic and therapeutic upper and lower gastrointestinal endoscopy are covered including ERCP, which is dealt with in great detail because of the complexity of this area. Extensive use of line diagrams, photographs and tables has been made wherever possible both to illustrate points and for easy reference. Other types of flexible endoscopy such as bronchoscopy, thoracoscopy, cystoscopy and hysteroscopy are also covered as many units routinely perform these procedures.

The book also carries chapters on decontamination of instruments, conscious sedation and emergencies, and aspects such as safe use of diathermy (electrosurgery), fluoroscopic screening and laser surgery.

The editors each have over 10 years experience in the field of endoscopy, and Charles Swan is an internationally known gastroenterologist. All authors have been chosen for their experience in their respective fields, and we have attempted to produce a book that is user friendly, and can be used as a source of reference for all personnel working in this specialty.

Michael Shephard
Jayne Mason
Editors

Acknowledgements

Mr. G. Tillett for helping with the proof reading.

Mr. K. Thomas, Senior Registrar, Urology for advice on chapter on flexible cystourethoscopy.

Paula Baran and Mitch Clarke for providing many of the original illustrations.

Leisha Carter for copy typing.

John Tingle, Senior Lecturer in Law, Nottingham Trent University for advice on 'The Endoscopy Assistant and the Law' chapter.

Sasha Andrews and other members of Audio-visual Services, Nottingham City Hospital for photographs and illustrations.

Sally Wood and Jane Boyes, Castle Hill Hospital, Humberside for Standards of Care [Quality Assurance section].

Boston Scientific Ltd, Cook U.K. Ltd and Keymed Ltd for their help in providing many of the photographs, illustrations and diagrams used in the book.

Staff of Endoscopy Units at the University Hospital of Wales and Nottingham City Hospital for help, criticism and advice throughout its preparation.

The history of endoscopy 1

Jenny Smith

1.1 INTRODUCTION

To introduce you to *Practical Endoscopy*, it is necessary to establish what we mean by the word endoscopy. It is derived from the Greek words *endo*, meaning 'within', and *skopeo*, 'to look' or 'to view'. Simply, then, endoscopy techniques allow us to look inside the body (in the medical field) enabling us to form a reliable diagnosis. In the early days of endoscopy this was the only benefit of subjecting patients to a very primitive, uncomfortable and often dangerous procedure. Over the years, improvements in equipment and techniques, together with increased nursing involvement, have allowed endoscopy to develop rapidly into a highly sophisticated procedure allowing both diagnostic and therapeutic benefits to everyone.

The Ancient Greeks at the time of Hippocrates are credited as being the inventors of 'endoscopy'; they used a form of tubing illuminated by an oil lamp. With this equipment they began to explore the interior of the human body centuries ago. Today we are continuing to develop these primitive beginnings.

In 1868, after watching a circus sword swallower, Adolf Kussaiaul used a rigid tube and candle to examine the upper gastrointestinal (GI) tract. Some 11 years later in 1879, Leiter produced both a cystoscope and a gastroscope for Max Nitze. Surprisingly, it was cystoscopy that stimulated the technical improvements. Thomas Edison used a glass bulb, which was made small enough to use inside the endoscopes in 1890; obviously this was a dramatic leap forward but there were concerns for the patient's safety as the bulb would get hot and could damage tissues when in use. A significant improvement came in 1928 when John Logie Baird patented his idea of using glass fibres to carry light.

Practical Endoscopy Edited by M. Shephard and J. Mason. Published in 1997 by Chapman & Hall, London. ISBN 0 412 54000 2

George Wolf made a semiflexible gastroscope in 1932 for Rudolf Schindler, and further development has continued over the years. It is interesting to note that it was at Rudolf Schindler's home, in Chicago, that the first meeting of the American Gastroscopic Club was held. This became the forerunner of the American Society of Gastrointestinal Endoscopy. In 1950 the Olympus Optical Company of Japan produced the gastrocamera. It was swallowed by the patient but remained attached to a tube, which was controlled by the operator. This camera produced the first ever pictures of the stomach interior and was widely used over the next 10 years.

The development of fibreoptic bundles led to the first fibreoptic endoscopy in 1960. The contribution of the fibreoptic bundles and the gastrocamera gave the endoscopist direct vision, improved control and allowed them to photograph chosen areas. A further 10 years of development produced a flexible fibreoptic instrument. This was rapidly acknowledged as a vital instrument for diagnosis of conditions in the GI tract. Originally, the instrument's channels were used simply to take biopsies and to apply suction to clear secretions impeding the vision of the operator; however, it soon became evident that they could be of value in providing a variety of therapeutic procedures. During this period the development of a wide range of accessories allowed further intervention, often negating the need for surgery. Since some patients could not undergo general anaesthesia, such new endoscopic techniques revolutionized the choice of treatments available.

For more than 40 years endoscopic procedures have improved and become more invasive, requiring an increase in nursing involvement. Initially, endoscopy was performed in any available part of the ward environment, very much on an ad hoc basis. This meant that nurses were often required to assist with procedures that were totally unfamiliar to them. It was an exciting and challenging new role for nurses and they soon began to take the initiative in developing appropriate training programmes necessary to care for the expensive equipment. These 'pioneers' soon realized that a dedicated workforce was needed for assessing patients' needs and implementing and evaluating care, as well as for cleaning and disinfecting the endoscopes.

To appreciate the development of endoscopy nursing, it is important to understand what happens to the patient undergoing endoscopic procedures. Patients often arrive expecting to have to 'swallow a camera' – a common explanation given them in clinics or outpatient departments. Many people do not know about endoscopy but have heard about 'the magic eye'.

1.2   THE PROCEDURE

1.2.1   PATIENT SELECTION

Endoscopic examinations are done for many reasons ranging from routine diagnostic procedures for unexplained epigastric discomfort to intensive therapy when a patient is admitted as an emergency with an acute GI bleed. These procedures are usually carried out under sedation, but it is becoming more common for patients undergoing routine endoscopy to choose a throat spray instead of a sedative injection. Obviously this requires the patient to be as informed as possible about the procedure and an expert team of endoscopy assistants to care for them.

Patients may be referred from wards, outpatient clinics or via their general practitioner (GP) and are given appointments to attend the endoscopy unit at the local hospital. The procedure is nowadays usually carried out in a purpose-built endoscopy unit, in contrast to the randomly allocated areas in earlier years. Investigations are carried out by doctors who have an interest either in gastroenterology or in endoscopic procedures. The medical team are assisted by endoscopy nurse assistants who provide highly skilled and trained support.

There are no age limits to endoscopy techniques and procedures may be carried out on both the young and the old. Indeed, those who would not tolerate a general anaesthetic are suitable candidates. It is often the very ill, the frail and the elderly who can benefit the most.

1.2.2   TREATMENT

Day-case procedures are now replacing conventional surgery and offer considerable improvements with minimally invasive techniques, while hospital beds can be freed to accommodate patients requiring high-dependency care. Patients welcome the opportunity to undergo treatment and go home afterwards, rather than undergo admission to hospital. They are more relaxed and the informal atmosphere, encouraged particularly in units of this kind, allows the experience to be less traumatic. Compliance rates are also very high and this is important when lists are carefully planned to maximize resources at each session. This obviously leads to the provision of a quality cost-effective service, with potential financial savings that benefit both patients and staff.

Endoscopy nurses may be employed in units that vary greatly in size and design, but aim to ensure that the patient's care is planned and appropriate to their individual needs. It is important that patients are well informed prior to any procedure, as to what will happen before, during and after their examination. This obviously includes all aspects of their care, including any sedation that may be necessary and what effect it may have. Ideally the patient should receive the minimum amount of sedation to:

1. Allow the procedure to take place comfortably.
2. Ensure that communication is maintained throughout.
3. Produce the preferred amnesic effect when the procedure is complete.
4. Make discharge of the patient possible within 1–2 hours in the majority of cases.

1.3 DEVELOPMENT OF ENDOSCOPY NURSING

1.3.1 GROUP FORMATION

Today, more than 500 000 endoscopies are performed each year in the United Kingdom. The equipment and techniques have improved dramatically and nurses have played an important role in promoting this relatively new area of speciality.

In 1972 Christiane Neumann came to Great Britain from Germany. She attended the British Society of Digestive Endoscopy (BSDE) meetings to find out more about this new field of nursing. Initially, she was the only nurse at these meetings, but as more doctors became involved in endoscopy they began to take their nurses too. Soon, the nurses approached the BSDE for membership; this movement promoted discussion that led to the formation of the first endoscopy nurses' group in 1977. Joy Banks (from Bath) became the first chairman and Christiane Neumann the second. During 1979 the BSDE merged with the British Society of Gastroenterology (BSG). Since then, the number of nurse members has steadily grown (with some 700 to date). They form the BSG Endoscopy Associates Group, which is led by a chairman, elected committee members and the secretary of the endoscopy section of the BSG. This group is responsible for the organization of the Nurses' Study Day at the spring and autumn meetings of the BSG. They are also involved in compiling reports covering such topics as cleaning and disinfection of equipment for gastrointestinal endoscopy, *Interim Recommendations of a Working Party Report* of the BSG (1988) and *Guidelines for Safe Working Practices* (Smith, Mason and Inman, 1989). The committee is also asked to provide two judges for the Irene Cooper Prize, awarded annually for the past seven years; along with two medical gastroenterologists, they judge entries, which should reflect the promotion and development of gastroenterology nursing, and aspects of care. The winner is asked to present their paper at the autumn BSG meeting.

In the United States of America the Society of Gastroenterology Nurses and Associates annually present the Gabrielle Schindler Award. Gabrielle was the wife of Dr Rudolf Schindler and the first gastroenterology assistant: 'The memory of Gabrielle personifies the spirit of professionalism and caring that has become the mark of excellence for today's gastroenterology nurses and associates' (SGNA, 1993).

It was at BSG meetings that nurses established links with others working in similar environments and experiencing the same difficulties. Friendships were formed that have strengthened over the years. Endoscopy nurses began to telephone friends throughout the UK for advice and probably were responsible for setting up the first 'Help-lines' as we know them today. As a direct result of the BSG Endoscopy Associates Group formation, nurses also began to establish local groups, meeting several times a year across the country to support each other and pass on their experiences and knowledge.

In 1986 when nurses from Australia and the USA and Morag Ravenscroft (from Stoke) met in Sao Paulo, Brazil, talks began to formalize the Society of International Gastroenterological Nurse Associates Group (SIGNA). In 1988 a steering group was formed; the constitution was accepted in Sydney, Australia, in 1990, resulting in the formation of the Society of International Gastroenterological Nurses and Endoscopy Associates (SIGNEA). At present the European Society of Gastroenterology and Endoscopy Nurses and Associates (ESGENA) is being formed. A draft of the proposed constitution was presented at a meeting prior to the nurses' conference in Berlin this year. Work is now in progress under the direction of a steering group for formulation of a constitution agreed in Paris during November 1996. It is hoped that the formation of a European group will allow regular annual meetings that will be more easily accessible to its members. It should also ensure EC recognition for endoscopy nurse training programmes. Certainly in some areas, such as Germany, this will be important, as salaries will reflect extra qualifications that carry EC recognition within this speciality. These groups will forge links worldwide and are again a direct result of nurses' commitment and enthusiasm in the field of gastroenterology.

Magazines such as *Gut Feelings* and *Scope* and newsletters maintain communication links around the country. The BSG Endoscopy Associates Committee provides an editor for the Endoscopy Associates Group newsletter, which is published quarterly and is circulated to all its members. These publications rely heavily on articles submitted by nurses and are usually sponsored by equipment manufacturers and/or drug companies.

1.3.2 TRAINING

During 1979, training courses for endoscopy were being established. On 18 July, at Great Portland Street, London W1, the Joint Board of Clinical Nursing Studies Endoscopy Panel met and on the agenda was:

5. Short Course in Nursing Patients Undergoing Endoscopic Examination
    5.1. To discuss the training needs and the courses required.
    5.2. To start planning the agreed course or courses.

Present at this meeting were names we have all become familiar with: Dr C. Swan was elected Chairman of the Endoscopy Panel; the late Dr P. Brown from Shrewsbury was present with Sister A. Lloyd; Christiane Neumann and Morag Ravenscroft were also there alongside Dr C. Williams.

The resulting course was the Joint Board of Clinical Nursing Studies Course 906, entitled a 'Short course in nursing for gastrointestinal endoscopy and related procedures' and it was originally offered in Shrewsbury Hospital. It is now the ENB 906 (gastroenterology and related procedures) course and is available at various sites throughout the country. The increased emphasis on nurse education and the requirements for training and regular updating of knowledge (PREP) has been responsible for a radical rethink in nurse education programmes, with the curriculum and its relevance to the student coming under close scrutiny. The result has been a dramatic increase in the choice of educational programmes on offer. Gastroenterology in particular has benefited enormously as a wide range of courses are now available in endoscopy units throughout the UK. Leading equipment manufacturers are also sponsoring training courses that help to meet the ever-increasing demand as the speciality grows along with the demand for day-case procedures. Endoscopy nurses need no longer feel isolated and are able to provide expert care, meeting the demand that the rapidly growing service requires.

1.4 TOWARDS MULTIDISCIPLINARY CARE

Today there are several exciting new roles for endoscopy nurses to consider. Clinical nurse specialists are involved in training programmes together with their clinical input in the day-to-day management of endoscopy units, combining both theory and practice. The new clinical nurse practitioners are holding clinics, with a defined caseload, selected by consultants. They are working within agreed guidelines to arrange routine investigations and surveillance endoscopies. Many counsel patients about their disease and are able to ensure that patients are aware of any self-help groups that are appropriate. Some nurses are now performing flexible sigmoidoscopy under supervision. The possibilities for endoscopy nurses to undertake challenging new roles are opening up, but we should remember that all of us can enhance patient care. Health education and health promotion are paramount in the philosophy of the National Health Service (NHS) today and we are all participating in this by providing information booklets and advice to our patients. We endeavour to be knowledgeable about self-help and support groups locally, and can arrange 'drop-in' days to allow patients the opportunity to discuss their concerns. Whatever our role, we strive to maintain the enthusiasm of the pioneers to improve patient care.

Many units now have a research team working alongside them, usually with a full-time research sister to co-ordinate the projects and clerical/secretarial support for the vast amount of paperwork that is generated. Many advantages can be attributed to the dedication of such teams. Income generation is important, obviously, for the continued funding of such projects. Nurses are often more motivated and enthusiastic when involved in research trials, and links with other research centres are interesting and prestigious. The potential for positive results from new therapies is always exciting, but probably the most important outcome from research within our units is that we, as nurses, start to look at evidence-based practice.

1.5   INTO THE TWENTY-FIRST CENTURY

Perhaps we should now look to the future and what changes we might expect to see in the twenty-first century. The first point is that 'infection with *Helicobacter pylori* is now considered to be a major aetiological factor in peptic ulcer disease' (Tytgat, Axon and Dixon, 1990). Recent TV programmes have certainly prompted patients to see their GP and request gastroscopy examinations; 90% of patients with duodenal ulcers have this organism present in the gastric antrum. 'A number of studies have demonstrated that the eradication of *H. pylori* prevents relapse of duodenal ulcers and lessens the risk of complications' (Axon, 1991). Is there a changing pattern in GI disease or are we more able to achieve reliable diagnosis with sophisticated endoscopic equipment?

Today colorectal cancer has the second highest cancer mortality in the UK. Screening programmes are therefore important indicators as to the future requirements in the provision of health care. Screening for colorectal neoplasia using faecal occult blood testing and flexible sigmoidoscopy is carried out in certain endoscopy units in the UK. Results are encouraging but the implications, of course, suggest that we should provide screening for colorectal neoplasia as we do for cervical or breast cancer. This would mean considerable financial investment in both manpower and equipment to provide such a programme. However, savings would be made long term as future surgery and lengthy terminal care would be avoided. The Imperial Cancer Research Fund Colorectal Cancer Unit, St Mark's Hospital, Middlesex applied for funding in 1996 for a multicentre randomized trial of 'once only' flexible sigmoidoscopy screening for prevention of bowel cancer morbidity and mortality. This has motivated many centres to meet the selection criteria in order to be part of this exciting project.

1.5.1   USE OF NEW TECHNOLOGY

Computers are used routinely now in endoscopy units to record patient information, for diagnosis and for treatment. Printers produce copies of these reports for inclusion in the patient's notes and to send to their GP. Programmes are limited, at present, but it is likely that they will increase and improve in design. Nurses are also continually revising patient care plan documents. It is important that a comprehensive account of care is recorded, noting individual needs, investigations carried out and drugs administered during the brief stay in these areas. As we look to the future, computers may well provide a reliable tool. They allow easy access to information and also provide statistics; this is a particularly useful aid when nurses require evidence to substantiate change.

Equipment manufacturers are continually improving the design and picture quality of the endoscope. The introduction of videoscopes was the biggest leap forward since 1928. Video endoscopy not only provides clarity of vision, but also allows the nurse assistant and the patient (if they wish) to see clearly what is happening. Images can be recorded on tape for later examination or for teaching purposes. The second-generation videoscopes now being made have significantly better quality pictures. It appears that every 10 years we see a dramatic leap forward in equipment design and technology. The next 10 years will surely see associated technologies merging as they become increasingly electronic, for example, the merging of ultrasound and endoscopy. The range of equipment on offer will expand and improve, allowing more freedom of choice and more competitive prices, a similar revolution to that in the high street where, for instance, the pricing and availability of video cameras and compact disc systems compares very favourably with when they were relatively new on the market.

Accessories are also continually being modified to meet the requirements of new endoscopic procedures. Many accessories are now disposable and it would seem a natural progression eventually to have a disposable endoscope. It would certainly save a lot of cleaning!

In the future, computer simulation, or 'virtual reality', promises to be an excellent method of training in endoscopic procedures. It will provide an alternative method of teaching, requiring no patient involvement. Visual links provided by telecommunication lines could also provide distance learning, allow diagnosis or second opinion, while microchips on smart cards may be used to hold case notes and be worn by the patient, allowing instant retrieval of medical history, endoscopic findings, etc. when required, in an emergency situation or on a routine visit to the GP. There are problems with this, of course; for example, magnetic fields such as those used at airport departure gates would wipe off any information stored.

This is an exciting time as we go into the twenty-first century (when the Western European market for endoscopes is expected to reach 556 million dollars per annum). Despite the many exciting new challenges technology may provide for nurses, we need to embrace such advances whilst continuing to provide a high standard of holistic care, tailored to meet individual patients' needs.

REFERENCES

Axon, A.T.R. (1991) Duodenal ulcer: The villain unmasked? *BMJ*, **302**, 919–20.

BSG Working Party (1988) Interim Recommendations of a Working Party Report. *Gut*, **29**, 1134–51.

SGNA (1993) *Gastroenterology Nursing: A Core Curriculum*. Mosby Year Book, St Louis.

Smith, J., Mason, J. and Inman, P. (1989) *Guidelines for Safe Working Practices*. Astra Pharmaceuticals, Kings Langley, Herts.

Tytgat, G.N.J., Axon, A.T.R. and Dixon, M.F. (1990) *Helicobator pylori*: causal agent in peptic ulcer disease. *Br J Clin Res*, **6**, 163–9.

BIBLIOGRAPHY

Gowland, K. (1995) Gastroenterology specialist nurse practitioner. *Gut Feeling*, 2, 11–12.

Greengrass, S.M. and Cunningham, M. (1993) *Endoscopy*. Key Med Medical and Industrial Equipment, Southend, Essex.

Hughes, M.A.P. (1995) *A new role for the treatment and care of patients with colorectal disease* [newsletter]. The British Society of Gastroenterology.

The development of endoscopy equipment 2

Brian W. Taylor

2.1 INTRODUCTION

The first documented attempts at endoscopy appear to come from Egypt where the court embalmers were able to diagnose ulcers in the stomach of one of the pharaohs using candle light reflected by a mirror down a hollow reed or bamboo cane. However, it would not be surprising if the technique had originated in China at a much earlier date, although no references can be found.

Hippocrates (460–377 BC) is reported to have examined the rectum and lower end of the large bowel using a similar mechanism, but after that date very little progress appears to have been made in this field until near the end of the eighteenth century. In 1795 an Italian physician, Bozzini, performed an examination of the rectum using a rigid sigmoidoscope not dissimilar in design to the present-day instrument.

However, it took almost another hundred years before further advances in endoscopic visualization made the examination of the pelvic and abdominal cavities possible. This was reported by Nitze in 1879, and the technique was later termed 'laparoscopy' by Jacobaeus in 1910. In 1921 the first reported endoscopic examination of a joint (arthroscopy) was performed by Professor Takagi of Toyko on a patient's tuberculous knee joint, and thereafter further development of endoscopic techniques and instrumentation appear to have occurred on an international basis with America and Japan at the forefront of technology. The first endoscopic visualization of the bile duct using a rigid choledochoscope was documented in 1923.

Although not recognized at the time, the discovery of fibreoptics in 1928 by the British inventor John Logie Baird was to have a profound

Practical Endoscopy Edited by M. Shephard and J. Mason. Published in 1997 by Chapman & Hall, London. ISBN 0 412 54000 2

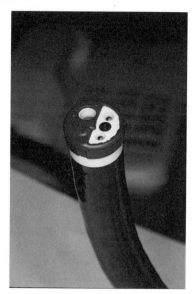

Fig. 2.1   Light guide and image lens

effect on the development of direct vision endoscopy. Fibreoptic technology allowed a beam of light to be passed down a glass tube or fibre (Fig. 2.1) with minimal light loss, and the use of flexible glass fibres made it possible to transmit the light beam around bends or corners, and that the instrument no longer needed to be rigid (Fig. 2.2).

It was several years before this technology was used in the medical arena, and it was probably the Korean War that was responsible for further advances in the use of fibreoptics. Many of the American military personnel returning from Korea were found to have gastrointestinal problems and, as a result of this, the American Government decided to sponsor research into the treatment of gastrointestinal diseases and injuries. This created a demand for more accurate diagnosis and resulted in the development of more sophisticated endoscopic instruments.

Professor Harold Hopkins is accredited with inventing the first coherent fibreoptic bundle to transport an image. In 1953 he, together with Kapany, produced a coherent fibre bundle with the fibres in precisely the same position at both ends; this invention was announced in *Nature* in 1954 (BSG, 1995).

Hirschowitz (USA) reported the use of the first flexible fibreoptic gastroscope in 1957. The controls of this instrument were primitive in comparison with today's instruments; for instance, they used a joystick type of handle to control the distal tip, which only had very limited movement. Rapid and continuous development followed, with in 1965 the first reported use of a flexible choledochoscope allowing direct vision of the common bile duct during surgery.

The Japanese were probably the first to recognize the value of flexible fibreoptic endoscopes in the diagnosis of gastrointestinal disease, and the development of new endoscopic technology advanced rapidly there to meet the demand of the clinicians. The original manufacturer of flexible fibreoptic endoscopes was the American Company ACMI, but it was Japanese optical companies such as Olympus, Fujinon, Pentax and Machida that soon dominated the market. European companies such as Storz and Wolf, who had originally manufactured rigid instruments, also became involved but to a lesser extent, tending to concentrate more on specialized equipment such as flexible cystoscopes, which remained within their areas of interest.

During the 1970s, the technology was still trying to catch up with clinical requirements, where there was a continuing demand for smaller insertion tubes with larger working channels together with improved optics and more flexibility. At this time it was difficult to manufacture high-quality very fine optical fibres, and this in turn restricted the amount of flexibility of the distal tip and dictated the diameter of the insertion tube. It was not until the next decade that new technology allowed the manufacture of fibres less than 8 μm in diameter (half that of a human hair) and this in turn resulted in smaller image bundles giving a clearer, brighter and sharper image. The use of smaller fibre-optic bundles allowed the insertion tube to become thinner, and flexibility of the distal tip was greatly increased, allowing up to 210° of angulation in one direction with a 120° angle of view. This made both diagnostic examination and the performance of therapeutic procedures much easier.

The 1980s also saw other major advances. The first fully immersible fibreoptic endoscope was introduced by Machida in 1982. These were ENT fibrescopes and were the forerunners to the fully immersible upper and lower GI instruments and bronchoscopes introduced in 1983–4. Up to this time the control head of the instrument could not be immersed in fluid during decontamination so the risk of cross-infection was always present.

Advances in technology also started to have a major effect on how procedures were performed and taught. The advent of the video camera allowed all staff in the endoscopy room to see exactly what the clinician saw and did, making teaching much easier. Previously, only one person at a time had been able to see by way of fibreoptic teaching attachment. These early cameras were primitive and converted from industrial use; they were in most cases large and cumbersome, and often required a supporting gantry overhead to help counterbalance the weight of the camera. In addition, the picture quality was not very good as the light sensitivity of the charged coupled device (CCD) was very limited and required a high-powered light source of 300 or 500 watts using a xenon bulb to produce an adequate image. However, advances in electronic technology soon overcame these problems producing smaller, more sensitive and lighter cameras – some no bigger than a matchbox – that easily clipped onto the endoscope without altering its handling characteristics.

The major breakthrough in electronic technology came in the late 1980s with the introduction by Welsh Allen of the video endoscope. This involved the use of a CCD chip at the distal end of the endoscope instead of the conventional optic fibre bundle. It was not long before the major endoscope manufacturers (Olympus, Fujinon and Pentax) were all offering video endoscopy systems. These systems used a number of different types of CCD chip; some used colour chips, whilst others used a monochrome chip with the sequential pickup of red–green–blue (RGB) (colour picture) system. Both systems have many advantages, but currently, although a colour chip is less expensive than its monochrome alternative, it is unfortunately larger and cannot be used in endoscopes with small diameter insertion tubes. For this reason, many systems use a monochrome chip with a strobing red, green and blue light to produce a computer-enhanced colour picture.

Pentax offered the first video Bronchoscope in the late 1980s which used the black and white chip, with the strobing Red, Green and Blue light to produce excellent colour images.

2.2   PRINCIPLES OF FIBREOPTICS

Fibreoptics may be defined as the use of a flexible glass fibre for the transmission of light (Fig. 2.2). Each fibre is between 6 and 15 μm in diameter and, because these have a high refractive index, light at the medial end of a fibre is totally internally reflected along the fibre to its distal end with little or no loss of intensity. In order to achieve this, each fibre is made of two separate layers (Figs 2.2, 2.3): an inner core of glass with a high refractive index, which transmits the light, and an outer sheath of glass with a low refractive index, which reduces any dispersion of light from the core.

There are two types of fibre bundles:

1. The **non-coherent** bundle in which the fibres are bunched together in no particular order (Fig. 2.4a). This is the type used for the light guide of an endoscope, and is used to transmit light from the medial to distal end of the scope. The light guide for a modern endoscope will typically consist of about 80 000 fibres, each of between 8 and 15 μm in thickness.
2. The **coherent** bundle, in which each individual fibre must be in the same position at the ocular and distal ends of the bundle (Fig. 2.4b).

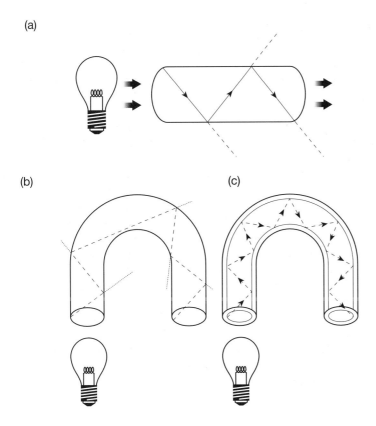

Fig. 2.2 Light travelling down: (a) a rod of glass; (b) a flexible glass rod; (c) a fibreoptic cable

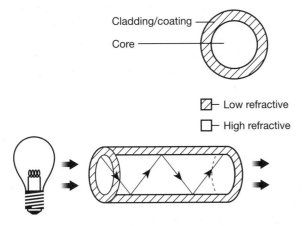

Fig. 2.3 The layers of a fibreoptic cable

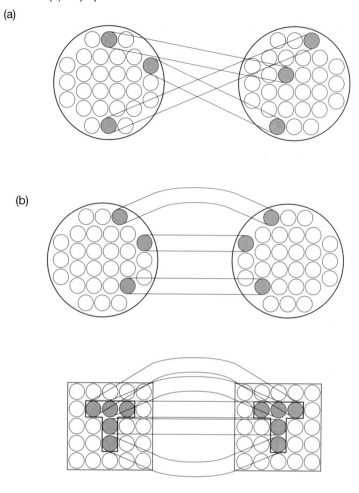

Fig. 2.4 Fibre bundles: (a) non-coherent; (b) coherent

Because of this relationship between the positions of fibres, a coherent fibre bundle (CFB) can transmit an image from one end to the other. This is often referred to as the 'optical bundle'. The average optical bundle will contain between 66 000 and 120 000 fibres, each between 6 and 15 μm in thickness.

2.3   CHARGED COUPLED DEVICES

Throughout the history of the development of endoscopes, the demands of clinicians for improved diagnostic and therapeutic equipment have

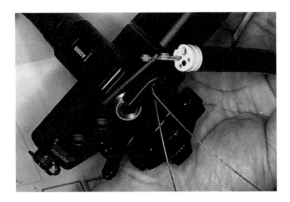

Fig. 2.5   Light guide and image lens

been the driving force behind endoscope design. Many of these demands were met by improvements in the fibreoptics through the use of a greater number of smaller fibres, and computer-designed lens systems. However, there was a limit to the advances possible using this technology, and developments in electronic imaging were seen as an opportunity to meet the increasingly sophisticated demands of the clinician.

By using video endoscopes which have a CCD at the distal end (Fig. 2.5), it is possible to pick up a picture on a matrix of between 48 000 and 480 000 dots (pixels) on a piece of silicone approximately 1.8 mm × 2 mm (CCD) and then transfer this picture down a wire to a processor where the electronic signal is interpreted and relayed to a monitor screen. The type of chip used (colour or monochrome) determines the type of image.

Video systems using a black and white (monochrome) chip (Fig. 2.6) work on the same principle as a television camera, picking up the three separate colours that make up white light, that is, red, green and blue. The processor overlays the three separate tone images to produce a colour picture before transmitting it to the monitor.

In the case of colour chips (Fig. 2.7), there are pixels for each of the three colours, red, green, and blue, which together make up each 'dot' of the picture some of the pixels have to be dedicated to memory. Because of this, a colour chip is larger than its monochrome counterpart, and currently this has restricted its use in endoscopy although future developments may change this.

The major advantage of electronic imaging is that teaching is made far easier, pictures can be captured and hard copies made, and if necessary whole procedures can be recorded on video. The image quality is also excellent and, unlike photographs, does not deteriorate with time. Image management systems have been produced that allow electronic images to be stored on 'floppy', hard or optical disc together

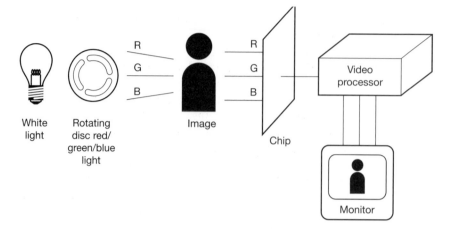

Fig. 2.6   Black-and-white chip video

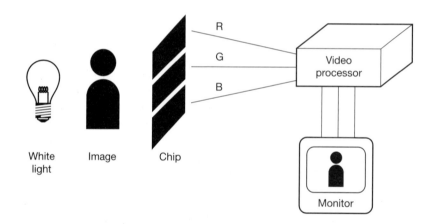

Fig. 2.7   Colour chip video

with patient records so that a visual as well as written record may be kept and recalled as required. These images can also be sent to other areas of the hospital, country or world via telephone line or satellite, allowing a doctor remote from the procedure to give an opinion.

2.4   THE FUTURE

As can be seen from this chapter, the field of endoscopy has developed very rapidly over the last 60 years, and in common with other areas of technology, has jumped from that of the 1930s to the almost Star Wars-like technology of the twenty-first century.

The development of the CCD chip heralded the start of the 'electronic industrial revolution', and future developments in this area will no doubt produce even smaller chips. New methods of capturing images are already being developed that may supersede the CCD: people are experimenting with 3D images and 'virtual reality' endoscopy; advances in endoscopic ultrasound are also helping to advance and augment the development of diagnostic and therapeutic endoscopy, as are experimental techniques such as the 'endoscopic sewing machine', which allows sutures to be placed endoscopically.

Rapid advances in the development of increasingly sensitive cameras may mean that, in the future, a powerful light-source will no longer be required for examinations or even that no light-source will be required at all. Sources of light such as high-intensity neon lights are also being examined as possible alternatives to the traditional halogen or xenon sources, and it may be that future developments in this area use parts of the light spectrum not normally visible to the human eye such as ultraviolet and infrared light, or even microwaves.

Some major breakthroughs with ultrasound endoscopic equipment which work by sending out ultrasonic waves from a small transducer positioned at the distal end of the endoscope, two types are being used; a single element 360 degree mechanical unit primary for diagnostic use, and the more recent curved electronic array using 96 elements in the transducer together, with two wave lengths of ultrasound for both therapeutic and diagnostic use. These scopes allow you to see the area visually, and produce ultrasonic images in colour to show blood flow, depths of growth, ulcers etc., accurately, for diagnostic and therapeutic purposes. Although the pictures are difficult to interpret at this time it could be the way forward for future endoscopy.

Endoscope design continues to improve and become more 'user friendly', with recent advances including the endoscope in which both the air and water channels, as well as the usual suction/biopsy channel, are fully brushable (Pentax) (Figure 2.5). This has greatly improved the ability to decontaminate the instrument and also has reduced maintenance problems associated with blocked air or water channels. Other recent advances have included custom-made controls to fit the operator and revolve around the much sought after disposable scope. A number of companies have come up with disposable sheaths which contain working channels, and air/water channels, which are completely replaced after each use. It may well be possible that the whole of the scope will be disposable in the future. This will depend on how some of the technologies that are becoming available today will be used in the medical field. Where endoscopic technology ends up will no doubt depend on clinical and operator demands. New techniques may reduce or remove the need to endoscope entirely or may continue to increase the demand for this procedure, as at present. However, whatever the final result, the technology and techniques developed in this field have, over the last half century, had an enormous impact on the diagnosis and treatments of a wide variety of conditions.

REFERENCE

BSG (1995) Obituary to Harold Hopkins. *Newsletter*, Winter.

Endoscopy unit design 3

Mike Shephard and Margaret Cox

3.1 INTRODUCTION

This chapter addresses the accommodation requirements of the modern endoscopy unit. It is not the intention to specify the ideal design, but rather the chapter aims to give guidance to the reader who is either seeking to improve or expand their existing facilities or who is lucky enough to be able to plan and design a purpose-built unit right from the start. The chapter draws on information obtained from the excellent NHS Estates document 'Accommodation for day care endoscopy unit' (1994), which provides much useful and relevant information on unit design, and readers actively involved in planning or redesigning a unit are advised to obtain a copy of this document for themselves. The chapter is supplemented by information from equipment suppliers and original papers as well as the extensive experience of many colleagues involved in endoscopy.

3.2 GENERAL CONSIDERATIONS

The modern endoscopy unit needs to be able to cater for a variety of endoscopic procedures carried out either as a day case or during a hospital inpatient stay.

The number of patients seen as day cases in endoscopy has increased greatly over the last 15 years and, with advances in both treatments and medical technology, this number is expected to increase still further. When planning a unit, accommodation should be planned to cope with both present and anticipated demand. It is often better to make plans for a phased increase in facilities to allow for a gradual increase in workload rather than provide a unit which will be underutilized for many years until the demand increases to match capacity. Patients with

Practical Endoscopy Edited by M. Shephard and J. Mason. Published in 1997 by Chapman & Hall, London. ISBN 0 412 54000 2

special needs, such as children, will also need to be considered if they are to be treated on the unit, and this is dealt with in more detail later in the chapter.

Day-care endoscopy has benefits to the patient because the appointment can be fitted in to accommodate their domestic and work commitments, and it is generally perceived to be less threatening than an inpatient stay. Day care is also a cost-effective and efficient use of resources, partly because it can be run independently from other hospital services and is therefore less prone to disruption, and partly because similar procedures can be scheduled at the same time and waiting lists thereby reduced (NHS Estates, 1994).

Endoscopic investigations suitable for the dedicated endoscopy unit are those that do not require a high degree of sterility and include:

upper and lower gastrointestinal endoscopy
bronchoscopy
laryngoscopy
cystoscopy
colposcopy.

If radiodiagnostic facilities are to be available within the unit then endoscopic retrograde cholangio-pancreatography may also be included, but procedures such as laparoscopy, thoracoscopy and hysteroscopy are best performed in the more sterile environment of the operating theatre unless suitable facilities are to be included in the planned accommodation. Colposcopy and hysteroscopy may be linked together and performed in a specific area.

3.3   THE PLANNING TEAM

When undertaking a development of this sort it is usually best to appoint a 'planning team' to oversee the whole project. This will usually consist of:

unit director
nurse manager
capital projects manager
works manager
architect
building contractor.

Other persons may be co-opted onto the group if a particular area of expertise is required, but in general a small team is better.

The planning of an endoscopy unit is a task of some complexity (Notman, 1974), and much work has to be done before even a basic design can be contemplated. The two key questions that need to be answered are:

1. What is the anticipated future demand for the service over (say) the next 10 years?
2. How many endoscopy procedure rooms are needed?

Once these have been determined, then planning can begin in earnest although it will still probably be a minimum of 2 years before the project nears completion (Pethigal, 1992).

3.3.1   ANTICIPATING THE DEMAND

Many factors, such as disease trends, health-screening initiatives, and clinical and technological advances, can affect the anticipated demand for the service. Past and present workload figures form a useful guide, and often show trends. Figures from various professional bodies suggest the annual requirements per head of population for endoscopy in UK to be:

upper gastrointestinal	1 in 100
colonoscopy	1 in 500
flexible sigmoidoscopy	1 in 500
ERCP	1 in 2000
bronchoscopy	1 in 700.

By looking at predicted population trends (demography), together with the other factors mentioned, it is therefore possible to forecast the anticipated endoscopic requirements for a given period in the future, usually 10 years.

3.3.2   HOW MANY ENDOSCOPY ROOMS DO YOU REQUIRE?

To calculate the number of procedure rooms required, it is necessary to calculate the workload capacity of one room. This is dependent on:

1. The average number of cases per day.
2. The length of the working week.
3. The length of the working year.

The daily average can be discovered by studying present use, but if longer lists (perhaps including evenings) are anticipated, then this must be taken into account.

The length of the working week is usually taken to be a minimum of 4.5 days (allowing half a day for cleaning and maintenance) and the working year to be 48–50 weeks to take into account national and other holidays (NHS Estates, 1994).

The number of rooms required can be calculated as:

$$\text{Endoscopy rooms required} = \frac{\text{workload per annum endoscopy rooms}}{\text{workload capacity of room}}$$

This is rarely a whole number, and it may be necessary to look at the influencing factors above to see if they can be altered to bring this equation near to a whole number. For instance, the number of patients seen daily could be increased (be realistic about this) or the holiday allowance could be reduced. Figures just below a whole number are rounded up, thus introducing spare capacity (NHS Estates, 1994).

3.4   THE PATIENT CYCLE

Whether adapting an existing system of patient flow through a unit or starting from new, the whole process should be a simple, compact one that avoids crossover points and retracing of steps. Lengthy walks down corridors should be avoided. Ideally, patients who have had their endoscopy should be in a separate area from those waiting to be seen, although this may not always be possible. A typical flow chart is show in Fig. 3.1.

If patients are required to undress for a particular procedure, then consideration should be given to how their clothing is transferred from the preparation area (where they undress) to the recovery area (where they get dressed). The system adopted should be as simple as possible, and allow secure transfer of clothing and personal effects.

3.5   ACCOMMODATION REQUIREMENTS

In theory, all that is required to carry out an endoscopy is a room to do it, and somewhere for the patient to recover. In practice, the requirements of a modern unit are far more complex.

Requirements cover three main areas:

1. Patient-related accommodation
   – entrance reception
   – preparation
   – treatment rooms
   – recovery areas
   – sanitary facilities
   – special patient needs.

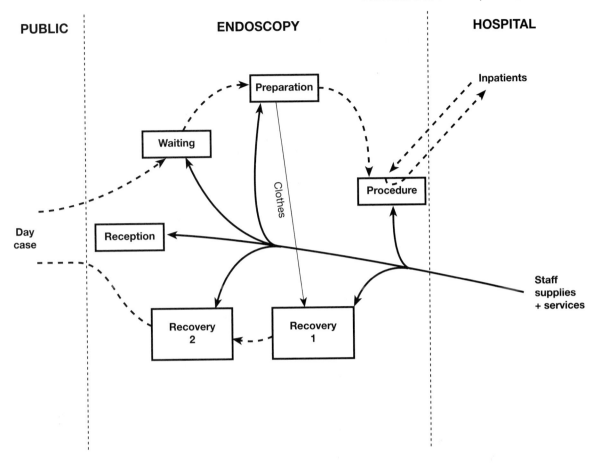

Fig. 3.1   Flow chart of the patient cycle

2. Staff facilities
   – male/female changing
   – rest room/catering
   – office accommodation
   – teaching/training.
3. Support services
   – endoscope cleaning
   – storage space, general and medical
   – clean/dirty utility
   – waste disposal
   – electricity/water, etc.

A full schedule of accommodation, together with 'optional extras', is to be found on p. 39.

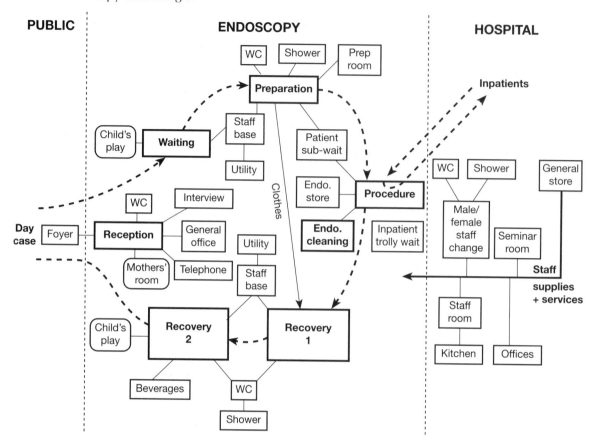

Fig. 3.2   Accommodation: functional relationships diagram (adapted from NHS Estates, 1995)

By drawing a flow chart of the passage of a patient through the unit, it is possible then to relate all areas of accommodation with the aid of a functional relationship diagram (Fig. 3.2).

3.5.1   PATIENT-RELATED AREAS

Patient reception

The type of patient management system used influences the size and design of the reception area. A 'phased admission' system, with patients arriving at intervals, is best as this reduces not only the patient waiting time but also the size of the waiting area (NHS Estates, 1994).

The reception desk should be situated in an obvious, easily accessible part of the reception area, and designed to be both user and patient friendly. It should be the focal point of the area. A low, open-plan design removes communication barriers, and helps make staff appear more approachable. The receptionist should be able to see all patients and their escorts, and should be able to communicate easily with all other areas of the unit. Access for wheelchairs needs to be considered, and the area should also include a public telephone. Low-volume background music has been shown to be of benefit in helping anxious patients relax, as has the use of interior design features such as waterfalls, soft lighting and indoor plants (Cook, 1976).

Patient waiting

The main factor influencing the size of the waiting area is the number of chairs required. In assessing this requirement, it is necessary to decide the average number of patients seen per hour by an endoscopy room. This may be determined by dividing the average length of a list (in hours) by the average number of patients seen per list. Many units carrying out a mixed list of upper and lower GI investigations will average around four patients per hour and, on the assumption that each patient will have an escort, the chair requirement in the waiting area for each room would then be eight chairs. Other investigations, such as flexible cystoscopy, will have a higher throughput and this number would need to be adjusted accordingly. Although it has been assumed all day cases will have an escort, this is not always the case so there will always be some spare capacity.

The area should have a variety of chair designs, suitable for the elderly patient and children, if catered for. Space should be left for wheelchairs. The use of low-level background music and television/video will also be of benefit here, and a child's play area may be included if the unit caters for children. Where possible, the play area should be linked to a secure outside play area.

Patient preparation

This area encompasses a staff base, which should be centrally placed to allow viewing of other areas, patient interview and preparation rooms, and a sub-waiting area for patients awaiting their endoscopy. The staff base needs to be large enough to allow writing, storage of stationery, patient records and telephone/VDU equipment. Similar design principles apply to those of the reception desk in the main waiting area. The interview and preparation rooms should allow privacy for both undressing and confidential discussion and, if pre-endoscopy procedures such as bowel preparation are to be carried out, then these need to be linked to patient toilet facilities. Generally, one preparation room per endoscopy room is sufficient to maintain throughput, but units carrying out large numbers of quick procedures such as flexicystoscopy may need to consider a higher ratio. The use of a sub-waiting area can help to achieve a faster throughput, although this should not be at the expense of loss of privacy (NHS Estates, 1994).

The endoscopy room

The endoscopy room should be of a sufficient size to allow all endoscopic procedures to be carried out with ease. Larson and Ott (1986) have suggested that a small endoscopy room is less stressful for the patient and makes it easier for the endoscopy assistant to reach equipment, so a balance needs to be struck between a cosy environment and adequate space to use all the necessary equipment.

For design purposes, the room may be divided into two areas: that used predominantly by the endoscopist, and that used predominantly by the endoscopy assistant (Fig. 3.3).

The area used by the endoscopist should contain hand-washing facilities, and a desk or writing surface together with VDU if used. A telephone is a distraction, and is probably best located outside this area.

The area used by the endoscopy assistant should include a sink and drainage facilities, storage for endoscopy accessories and sterile supplies and somewhere for the temporary storage of controlled drugs if the main drug cupboard is outside this area. A refrigerator should also be available for drugs and other items such as *H. pylori* tests [Clo-test, HP-fast], which require cool storage conditions. It should have direct access to the endoscope-cleaning room.

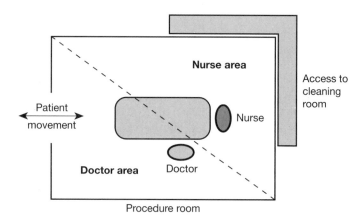

Fig. 3.3 The endoscopy room: working relations (from Key Med (1995) reproduced with permission of Key Med (Medical and Industrial Equipment) Ltd)

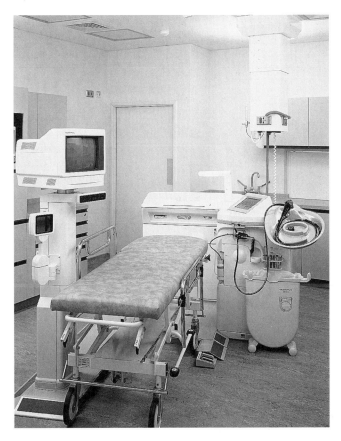

Fig. 3.4   (a) The Cosmos Suite.

Endoscopy equipment such as light-sources and monitor screens are usually located on mobile trolleys for versatility, but may be placed on work surfaces or wall-mounted shelves. Endoscopy room design has now become extremely sophisticated, and the integration of information systems into the running of busy units mean that suppliers are now looking towards custom-built, 'state-of-the-art' endoscopy suites such as the suite illustrated in Fig. 3.4 to provide the unit of the future. This type of system may not be suitable for all endoscopic procedures, but certainly has a place when considering future requirements.

Piped oxygen and a medical vacuum (suction) system should be available in all endoscopy rooms and first-stage recovery. Ideally these services should be provided from ceiling-mounted units above the endoscopy trolley so that views are not obstructed and the floor area is uncluttered. It is also possible to mount monitor screens and, if used, closed-circuit television cameras (CCTV) in this way although this

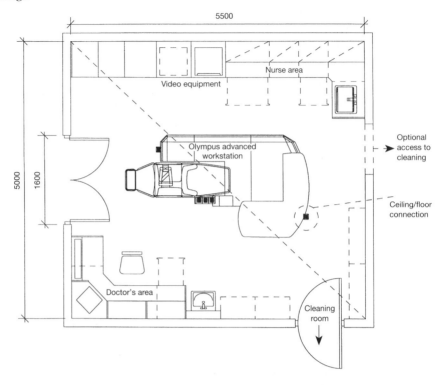

Fig. 3.4   (b) Cosmos room layout (reproduced with permission of Key Med (Medical and Industrial Equipment) Ltd)

restricts the use of monitor screens to that room only. Endoscopy rooms should also be equipped with hand-washing facilities and an emergency call system. Resuscitation equipment should be available either in or close to the endoscopy room.

The ergometric diagrams in Fig. 3.5 show the possible staff and mobile equipment positions for a standard endoscopy room carrying out upper and lower gastrointestinal (UGI and LGI) procedures.

Recovery areas

Most modern endoscopy unit designs incorporate a 'two-stage' recovery system. This comprises a first area, consisting of individual curtained areas where a patient may recover on either a trolley or a reclining chair. Each curtained area requires piped oxygen and suction and pulse oximetry, and should allow adequate privacy for patients to dress. The second area is more informally arranged, with comfortable chairs and occasional tables. Light refreshment facilities should be available and, if children are to be catered for (see following section), then a secure play area may be attached.

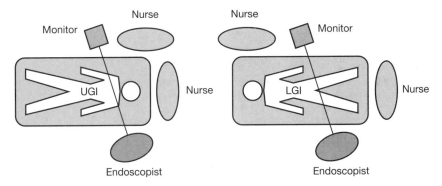

Fig. 3.5 Ergometric diagrams: upper and lower gastrointestinal procedures (reproduced with permission of Key Med (Medical and Industrial Equipment) Ltd)

Both areas need to be overseen by a staff base designed on similar lines to that in the waiting area. Patient toilets and washing facilities should be able to be accessed from both areas, and background music, television and video should be considered for the stage two recovery area. When determining the size of the recovery area it is usual to link this to the throughput of the endoscopy room(s). On the assumption (see section on patient waiting area) that each room sees an average of four patients per hour, and that the average length of stay in recovery is 2 hours (80 minutes in stage one, 40 minutes in stage two), then each endoscopy room will require an average of four stage one and two stage two recovery beds. Units doing large volumes of minor procedures or who use little or no sedation will need to modify this to suit their individual requirements.

Children in the endoscopy unit

The provision of play areas for children within the unit has already been considered. However, if endoscopy is to be performed on child patients then the following principles should be followed:

- Children should not be admitted and treated alongside adults (DoH, 1991).
- Carers should be able to accompany the child for as much as possible of their admission.

This can be achieved in four ways:

1. Dedicated children's endoscopy sessions to allow the temporary conversion of the unit to an appropriate environment for a child.
2. Concurrent adult and children's sessions but with visual and auditory separation of both. This is often hard to achieve.

3. Admission of child to a children's day ward, so that the child visits the unit only for the endoscopy, causing minimal disruption to routine. This is suitable only if a small number of children are to been seen within the working year.
4. Provision of a separate, dedicated children's endoscopy unit. This is viable only in a children's hospital.

3.5.2   STAFF FACILITIES

Unless suitable facilities are available within the hospital which are also close enough to the endoscopy unit to allow access, then the following need to be provided within the unit:

male/female changing rooms
male/female washing/toilet facilities
staff rest room with adjoining kitchen.

Staff numbers dictate the size/number required, and anticipated staffing increases should be considered when designing this area. The staff rest room should be attached to the emergency call system.

Teaching facilities

If teaching of undergraduate or postgraduate medical, nursing and other paramedical staff is to be undertaken, then provision of a seminar room and smaller meeting rooms should be considered. The seminar room should be linked by CCTV and an audio link to the endoscopy room to allow 'live' teaching. To aid versatility of use, many seminar rooms are designed so they can be split into two smaller rooms if required. The CCTV system and audio link can also be extended to link into the office of the medical director and other senior staff.

3.5.3   SUPPORT SERVICES

Endoscope-cleaning room and store

If two endoscopy rooms are to be used (Fig. 3.6), then ideally the cleaning area should be located so as to be accessible from both rooms, and designed in such a way to show distinct 'clean' and 'dirty' areas, to separate the two processes (Schaffner, 1990). A 'dirty' area is used for the reprocessing of equipment, and a 'clean' area for its storage.

The dirty area should at a minimum contain:

automated endoscope disinfector
double sink/drainer
work surface with cupboards under.

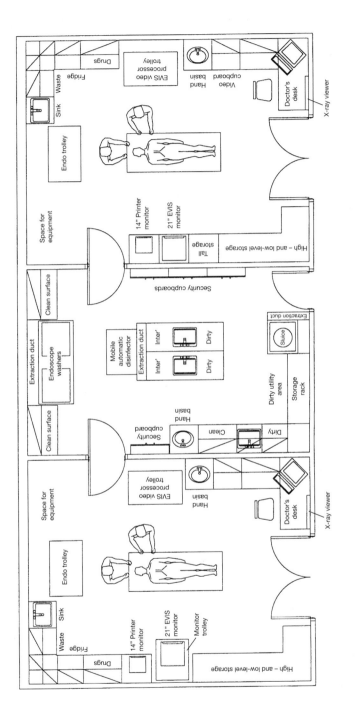

Fig. 3.6 Two procedure rooms linked to common cleaning area (reproduced with permission of Key Med (Medical and Industrial Equipment) Ltd)

Water filtration should be considered if the purity of the water supply is inadequate or if the water piping is old, causing flecks of pipework to contaminate the supply. A filter of 5 or 10 µm is sufficient for removing gross debris from the supply, but one of 0.2 µm is required for microbiological filtration. The 0.2 µm filter is very expensive, and if this is required then a 5 µm and a 1 µm filter should be placed in series before it to prevent frequent blockage. The filters used are normally of the standard 10 inch (25 cm) variety.

If endoscope accessories are to be cleaned and reprocessed on the unit (rather than using the hospital central sterilizing department), then suction should be available for the irrigation of cannulae, and an ultrasonic cleaner and a small autoclave may be required. Leakage testing equipment should also be available (Coghill et al., 1989).

Ideally, modern decontamination methods should be clinically cost effective as well as environmentally safe (Daschner, 1989). Whilst heat is considered to be the best method of disinfection and sterilization, the design of heat-labile fibreoptic endoscopes makes this impractical, and environmentally less friendly chemical disinfection is often the only practical alternative (Babb, 1990).

Chemical disinfectants such as glutaraldehyde can be stored in the cupboard space below the work surface, and many of these disinfectants are covered by specific handling and exposure regulations (COSHH Regulations, 1988). There should therefore be storage facilities for protective clothing such as nitrile gloves and eye protection, and an 'emergency spillage kit' should be kept in a convenient place, close to **but** outside the room. This subject is covered in more detail in Chapter 7.

The 'clean' area should contain storage cupboards for the endoscopes, accessories and spare parts (Fig. 3.7). Hand-washing and waste disposal facilities are also required and a light-source and optical-testing equipment may be incorporated into this area to allow the checking and general maintenance of the endoscopes.

The following should be considered when designing a new or refurbished unit:

1. Dirty utility area. Suitable for the disposal of liquid and solid waste, together with space for storage of waste awaiting disposal.
2. Waiting area for inpatients brought to unit on trolleys or in wheel-chairs.
3. Clothing store for the secure keeping of patients' clothing during transfer from the preparation to recovery area.
4. General storage areas for medical and surgical supplies, mobile medical equipment and trolleys. A separate store is required for equipment used by the unit cleaning staff. This area should not be situated on any of the routes used by patients within the unit to

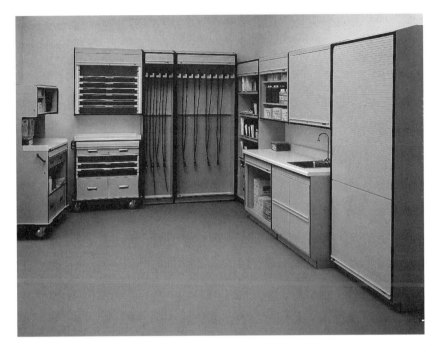

Fig. 3.7   Endoscope and accessory storage (reproduced with permission of Specialist Endoscopy Equipment Ltd)

minimize the disruption caused by the movement of cleaning equipment whilst the unit is open (NHS Estates, 1994).

5. Engineering services access for maintenance and repair of heating, ventilation, electricity, water, piped gases and vacuum, and drainage.

3.6   INFORMATION TECHNOLOGY

The management of information by electronic means is vital to the successful running of an endoscopy unit.

Whilst it is possible to run a small unit with purely manual systems, a large volume of work, together with the requirements of hospital data collection, make the use of electronic information management systems almost mandatory for the larger unit. This may either form part of a larger hospital-wide network or may be a stand-alone microcomputer system within the unit, which may or may not be linked into the main hospital system. The information management functions required by an endoscopy unit, and their interrelation with other hospital departments, are best described by a diagram such as that in Fig. 3.8.

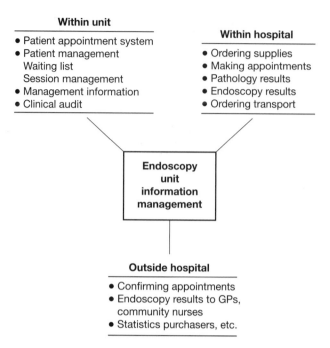

Within unit
- Patient appointment system
- Patient management
  Waiting list
  Session management
- Management information
- Clinical audit

Within hospital
- Ordering supplies
- Making appointments
- Pathology results
- Endoscopy results
- Ordering transport

Endoscopy
unit
information
management

Outside hospital
- Confirming appointments
- Endoscopy results to GPs,
  community nurses
- Statistics purchasers, etc.

Fig. 3.8 Information managment functions

The advantage of an information technology (IT) network (Fig. 3.9) is that it allows swift management of a large variety of functions within the unit, the hospital and the area. The main disadvantages are the expense and the problems caused by breakdown or malfunction of the system. In 1991 Professor M. Classen organized a meeting in Munich on the subject of 'Computers in endoscopy', the outcome of which led to a project identifying minimal standards for a computerized endoscopic database (Crespi *et al.*, 1994). The final results of this project are still awaited.

Patient documentation is considered elsewhere in this book.

3.7 OTHER CONSIDERATIONS

Location/access

If designing a new unit or refurbishing an existing one, consideration needs to be given to location and access. The unit should have easy access for patients, escorts, staff and supplies. The access from outside the hospital should be simple with no need to use lifts or long corridors.

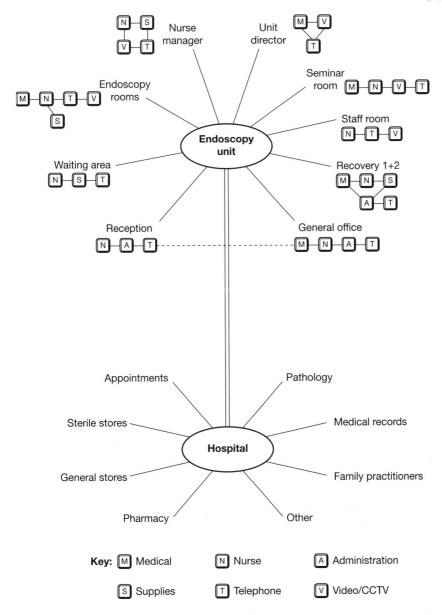

Fig. 3.9 Information technology interrelations between unit and hospital (adapted from NHS Estates, 1995)

It should be situated at ground level with its own road access and parking or set-down/pick-up facilities, and should be linked via a secondary access to the main hospital (NHS Estates, 1994).

Disabled persons

This refers not only to people with physical disabilities who are wheelchair bound, but also to those with sensory disabilities such as visual or auditory impairment. Doors, toilets, and ramp access to areas need to be considered, as do signposting and other visual and audio aids.

Laser

The use of laser surgery via the endoscope requires special design features to be incorporated in the endoscopy room design. These requirements are dealt with in Chapter 19.

X-ray screening

This may be provided in the endoscopy room with the aid of a C-arm (mobile) system or a permanent screening room may be provided. If the former is used, no particular precautions are necessary other than the use of protective lead aprons, gonad shields, etc. If permanent screening facilities are provided with a fixed scanner, then a lead-lined room needs to be provided, as well as warning signs outside the room and the other precautions mentioned. This increases greatly the building costs of the unit, and unless a lot of endoscopy is carried out that involves screening it is doubtful whether the extra cost involved can be justified.

Lighting

Natural lighting provides the best illumination although the need to maintain patient privacy may restrict this. Subdued lighting with a dual dimmer control is useful in the endoscopy rooms particularly if monitor screens are used.

'Pooled' lighting may need to be considered to light specific areas or items of equipment (NHS Estates, 1994).

Communication within unit

In addition to the CCTV/audio system mentioned previously, the provision of an intercom system linking the main areas of the unit provides a quick and easy way of communication within the unit. Outlets should ideally be placed in areas where conversations cannot easily be overheard by patients, although it is appreciated that this is not always possible. Caution should be observed if considering systems using radio frequency transmission as these may interfere with other electronic systems within the unit or hospital.

An emergency call system also needs to be available in all clinical areas, linked to the staff areas/rest room.

Electricity power supply outlets

In general, there can never be enough power outlets in a unit. Changing practices and new technology mean that outlets are often required where none was needed previously, and it is best to add a 50% margin at the planning stage to present requirements in anticipation of these factors. A separate power supply (usually 415 V) is usually required for radiographic screening equipment, and if laser is used then non-reflective socket outlets must be used in treatment room.

Flooring

In general, patient areas should be carpeted, and clinical areas, toilets, showers, etc. should have non-slip floor covering. It is worth considering the provision of a drain in the floor in the endoscope cleaning area(s) in case of leakage of water or disinfectant from the disinfecting machines.

3.8   THE ENDOSCOPY UNIT: A SCHEDULE OF ACCOMMODATION

In summary, a schedule of accommodation (Fig. 3.10) might include the following list:

1. *Entrance and reception*
   entrance
   foyer
   reception
   general office
   records store

   main waiting (including play area if children use unit)
   disabled WC/wash M/F
   visitors' WC/wash M/F

2. *Patient preparation areas*
   staff base/utility
   patient preparation room
   consulting examination room

3. *Patient treatment rooms*
   endoscopy room

4. *Patient recovery areas*
   recovery: stage one
   recovery: stage two
   recovery staff base utility
   resuscitation trolley bay

   beverage bay
   patients' clothing store
   trolley bay
   wheelchair parking bay

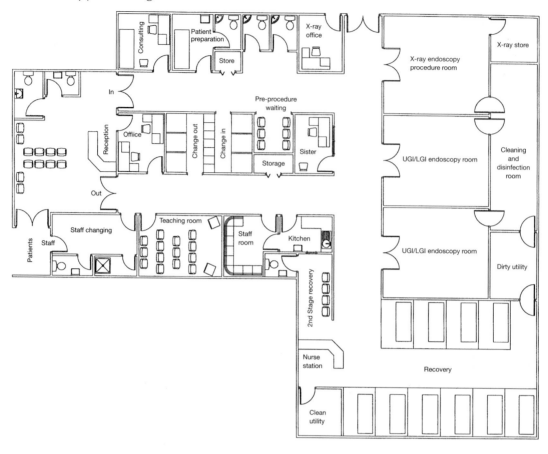

Fig. 3.10 Endoscopy unit (from Key Med, 1995 reproduced with permission of Key Med (Medical and Industrial Equipment) Ltd)

5. *Patients' sanitary facilities*
   patients' WC/wash M/F
   disabled WC/wash M/F
   patients' WC/bidet/wash

6. *Staff facilities*
   male staff change/locker room   staff rest room
   female staff change/locker room   staff kitchen/pantry
   staff wc/wash M/F   unit director's office
   staff shower M/F   nurse manager's office
                                       medical staff office

7. *Teaching facilities*
   seminar room
   clinical teachers' office

8. *Support areas*
   endoscope cleaning and store   unit cleaners' store
   dirty utility   disposal hold
   general store   switch cupboard
   mobile X-ray equipment store

9. *Optional accommodation and services*
   sub-waiting area   recovery play area
   patients' shower   baby feeding and nappy-
   children's reception interview   changing room
   room

REFERENCES

Babb, J. (1990) Disinfection and sterilisation. *Post Graduate Doctor Middle East*, **13**(10), 542–8.

Coghill, S.B., Mason, C.H. and Studley, J. (1989) Endoscopy biopsy forceps and transfer of tissue between cases. *Lancet*, 1 388–9.

Control of Substances Hazardous to Health (COSHH) Regulations (1988) Statutory Instrument No. 1657. HMSO, London.

Cook, H.S. (1976) Interior design sets cheerful calming mood. *Hospitals*, **50**, 117–20.

Crespi, M., Delvaux, M., Schapiro, M. *et al.* (1994) Minimal standards for computerised endoscopic database. *Am J Gastroenterol*, **89**(8), 144–53.

Daschner, J. (1989) Cost-effectiveness in hospital infection control – lessons for the 1990s. *J. Hosp Infect*, **13**(4), 325–36.

Department of Health (1991) *Welfare of Children and Young People in Hospital*. HMSO, London.

Key Med (1995) *Endoscopy Room Design Guide*. Key Med Ltd, Southend, Essex.

Larson, D.E. and Ott, B.J. (1986) The structure and function of the outpatient endoscopy unit. *Gastrointest*, **32**(1) 10–14.

NHS Estates (1994) Accommodation for day care endoscopy unit. *Health Building Note 52*, **2**.

NHS Estates (1995) Accommodation for day care medical investigation and treatment unit. *Health Building Note 52*, **3**.

Notman, E. (1974) Planning an endoscopy room. *Nursing Times*, **6**, 886–9.

Pethigal, P. (1992) Beyond the basics of endoscopy suite design. *Gastroenterol*, **14**(5), 249–51.

Schaffner, M. (1990) Infection control issues in the gastrointestinal unit. *Gastroenterol Nurs*, **12**(4), 279–84.

BIBLIOGRAPHY

British Society of Gastroenterology (1983) *Design of Gastrointestinal Endoscopy Units*. British Society of Gastroenterology, London.

British Society of Gastroenterology (1988) Cleaning and disinfection of equipment for flexible fibreoptic endoscopy. *Gut*, **29**, 1134–51.

British Society of Gastroenterology (1990) *Provision of Gastrointestinal Endoscopy and Related Services for a District General Hospital.* British Society of Gastroenterology, London.

Wayne, J.D. and Rich, M.E. (1990) *Planning an Endoscopy Suite for Office and Hospital.* Igaku-Shoin, New York.

The endoscopy unit staff 4

Mike Shephard

4.1 INTRODUCTION

Although the role of the endoscopy assistant was first recognized in 1941, endoscopy was not carried out in recognized endoscopy units until much later, and it is only over the last 25–30 years (from the early 1970s) that, as a result of both increased demand and improved techniques, these units have become established. Before that, although endoscopy was being carried out in increasing numbers, it tended to be done whenever and wherever necessary (often the side room of a ward) by the doctor involved with the assistance of any person (usually a nurse from that ward) who happened to be available. Specialist training was not thought necessary, and was in some instances discouraged on the grounds that 'any trained nurse' could assist with endoscopy.

With the advent of the endoscopy unit, and with advances both in instrument technology and in the development of new techniques, the need for dedicated and specifically trained staff to assist during endoscopy was recognized. However, this was initially sporadic, and at that time there were no established training courses for endoscopy assistants either nationally or internationally.

Nowadays, endoscopy is accepted as a specialist area of medicine and nurses working in this area are regarded as specialist nurses. The increased value of endoscopy to medicine in general means that today the endoscopy unit is often an extremely busy area, and the number and type of staff, together with the skills they require to do their work, are of vital importance in ensuring the smooth running of that unit. Training is also much improved, and there are thriving regional, national and international societies of endoscopy assistants throughout the world.

Practical Endoscopy Edited by M. Shephard and J. Mason. Published in 1997 by Chapman & Hall, London. ISBN 0 412 54000 2

4.2   STAFFING THE ENDOSCOPY UNIT

There are many factors that affect the number of staff required by a unit. In all cases the number of patients seen, the number of lists, the types of procedure carried out and the financial situation of the unit tend to dictate the number and type of staff required or available, but other factors such as the design of the unit and its geographical location in relation to other hospital facilities may also have a bearing. Also, local policies and nationally accepted guidelines may play a part in determining the final staffing level and mix of the unit, so the following should be used only as broad guidelines when determining the staffing requirements for a unit.

All units should have a person managerially in charge. This is usually, but not necessarily, a registered nurse (RN), who has overall respons- ibility for the unit. Close co-operation between the endoscopy unit manager and the medical director is essential as they will form the nucleus of the management team of the unit. As well as their managerial responsibility, they may also have a clinical role within the unit, and some hospitals have developed this into a specialist clinical role includ- ing performing diagnostic upper and lower GI endoscopy and percutan- eous endoscopic gastrostomy (PEG) insertion. The role, responsibilities and skills required by the holder of this post are addressed in section 4.3. Broadly, though, the endoscopy unit staff can be divided into three distinct groups (Fig. 4.1):

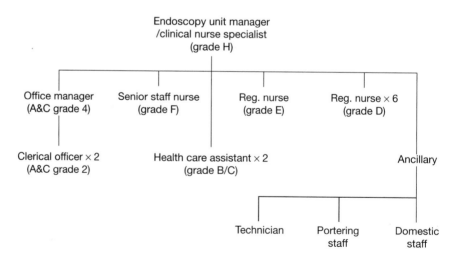

Fig. 4.1   The unit hierarchy

1. The endoscopy assistant who may be an RN, a health care assistant (HCA) or an operating department practitioner (ODP), with specific training in endoscopy and who is involved in patient and equipment care.
2. The clerical/secretarial staff who are responsible for the clerical and administrative side of the unit (patient notes, appointments, etc.).
3. Ancillary staff such as portering and domestic services who have a support role within the unit, and who may or may not come under direct control of the manager.

4.3   ROLES AND RESPONSIBILITIES

One of the main staffing problems that can occur in the endoscopy unit is that the roles of the different grades of endoscopy assistant are broadly the same irrespective of whether the assistant is an RN, HCA or ODP. This can cause conflict as differing pay scales will mean some being paid more than others, and those on lower grades of pay often resent this, feeling that they are being paid less for the same work. It is important, therefore, to remember that although the roles may be similar, it is the **responsibilities** inherent in that post that make it a higher paid post. Because of this potential source of conflict, it is important that these **responsibilities** are itemized in the job description for that post, and that the job description is reviewed regularly to keep it up to date.

4.3.1   THE ENDOSCOPY ASSISTANT

The similarities and differences between the roles and responsibilities of the RN and the HCA/ODP are best seen from Table 4.1. From this it can be seen that the main difference is that the RN has a supervisory role and is able to assess, plan and evaluate patient care, whereas the HCA and ODP each carries out patient and equipment care under supervision, and has little or no input in assessment, planning and evaluation of care. In addition, whilst the RNs will have the same core skills as endoscopy staff who hold no professional qualification, they also need to possess more advanced clinical skills, and have managerial skills appropriate to their level of responsibility. Table 4.2 shows some of the skills required by an endoscopy assistant, and compares those of the RN and the HCA/ODP.

4.3.2   CLERICAL/SECRETARIAL STAFF

This group of staff have a vital role in the smooth running of an endoscopy unit. A small unit may require only one such person whereas

Table 4.1   Roles and responsibilities, RNs versus HCAs and ODPs

Registered Nurse	HCA/ODP
1. Assess, plan, implement and evaluate patient care	Assists RN in delivering patient care
2. Supervision of qualified non-RN staff in the delivery of patient care	
3. Carries out nursing care in accordance with hospital/national policy	Assists RN to carry out nursing care in accordance with hospital/national policy
4. Professionally accountable for his/her actions, and the actions of staff under his/her direction	No professional accountability; responsible to employer
5. Responsibility for control and custody of drugs	
6. Duty to ensure safety of patients, visitors, staff, and their belongings at all times	Duty to ensure safety of patients, visitors, staff, at all times
7. Responsibility to recognize and report change in patient's medical condition to medical and nursing staff	Should recognize and report change in patient's medical condition to RN in charge
8. Responsibility to train and develop staff within the unit; e.g. fire policy, cardiac arrest policy	
9. General and specific management role within unit; e.g. ordering of supplies, pharmacy stock control, duty rota	
10. Duty to keep abreast of developments and ensure other staff are aware	Duty to keep abreast of developments
11. Should participate in research and use results to improve clinical practice	

a larger unit may have three or more members with perhaps an office manager/administrator over them. They have the following key responsibilities:

1. Maintaining an appointments system for all users of the unit, including prioritizing of patients where necessary.
2. Location and preparation of medical records and X-rays.
3. Preparation and dispatch of appointment letters and instructions.
4. Booking of appropriate transport for patients to and from the unit.

Table 4.2. Core skills of endoscopy assistants qualified (RN) and unqualified (HCA or ODP)

	N/A	Essential	Desirable	Specialist
Clinical				
History taking		Q	UQ	
Planning care	UQ	Q		
Evaluating care		Q	UQ	
Discharge planning	UQ	Q		
Drug administration	UQ	Q		
Oxygen therapy		Q	UQ	
Nebulizers		Q	UQ	
Peak flow recording		Q	UQ	
Recording TPR		Q UQ		
Recording BP		Q	UQ	
Escorting patients		Q UQ		
Infection control		Q UQ		
Cleaning and disinfection		Q UQ		
Care of patient during:				
Upper/lower GI endoscopy		Q UQ		
ERCP		Q	UQ	UQ
Bronchoscopy		Q UQ		
Urinalysis		Q UQ		
Blood glucose measurement		Q		
PR examination	UQ	Q		
Enema	UQ	Q		
Specimen collection		Q UQ		
Use of specialized equip.		Q		UQ
Specialist roles				
Intravenous drugs	UQ	Q		
Venepuncture	UQ	Q		
PEG insertion	UQ			Q
Specialized drugs	UQ	Q		
Cannulation	UQ		Q	
Entenox	UQ		Q	
Education				
Teaching:				
Patients		Q	UQ	
Qualified	UQ	Q		
Unqualified		Q	UQ	
Students		Q	UQ	
Relatives		Q	UQ	
Professional updating	UQ	Q		
Training/regular updating		Q UQ		
Assessor/mentorship	UQ	Q		
Link nurse role		Q	UQ	
Dealing with complaints		Q	UQ	

Q = qualified; UQ = unqualified.

5. Reception of patients on arrival at unit.
6. Arranging patient follow-up as required and ensuring reports/notes are available for this.

Other responsibilities vary from unit to unit and may include the training of staff in the use of any computerized endoscopy records system in operation and acting as co-ordinator for clinical research trials.

4.3.3   ANCILLARY STAFF

This group provide support services for the unit, and may be divided into 3 main groups:

1. Endoscopy technicians.
2. Portering services.
3. Hotel (cleaning and catering) services.

Endoscopy technicians

Larger units may employ a technician to look after their endoscopic equipment. This may either be an operating department practitioner who has undergone further training, or someone with a suitable technical background or particular interest in this area. Their main responsibilities may include:

1. Checking and setting up of equipment prior to use.
2. Cleaning and disinfection of endoscopes.
3. Ensuring regular maintenance of endoscopes and other endoscopic equipment.
4. Minor repairs to endoscopes, video systems, etc. (e.g. blockages, worn distal cuffs, etc.).
5. Swabbing of endoscopes, disinfectors, etc. for microbiological study as part of a quality assurance programme.

It is possible to amend/expand these basic responsibilities to suit the individual needs of each unit, and some units may consider developing a 'multiskilled' worker who can not only carry out these responsibilities but may also fulfil a role as a laboratory technician, porter or even cleaner as part of their overall job description. The use of a technician has two main advantages. First, the postholder soon becomes very proficient at the work, with a resultant improvement in the quality of care of the endoscopes and other endoscopic equipment. Second, nursing staff are able to spend more time on direct patient care. The main disadvantage is that it is expensive, and although it can be argued that the savings made on maintenance costs can justify this, for financial reasons it is often only the larger endoscopy units who employ technicians.

Portering services

Twenty to forty per cent of the work of an endoscopy unit is from patients currently admitted to hospital. These patients have to be transported to and from the unit, usually on a trolley or bed, and the organizing of this can cause problems if you have to rely on a general pool of porters. For this reason many units have their own porter attached to the unit. This may either be someone employed directly by the endoscopy unit or a person already employed by the hospital as a porter who is permanently based on the unit. The former has the advantage in that the person becomes part of the 'team' and cannot be removed at short notice; the job description can also be tailor-made to suit the requirements of the unit.

The main responsibilities of a portering assistant attached to the unit are:

1. Transport of patient to and from the unit.
2. Checking of trolleys and attached equipment.
3. Maintenance of trolleys and oxygen/suction equipment.

However, this list is by no means exhaustive and the roles and responsibilities can be changed and developed to suit the individual requirements of the unit.

Hotel services

The cleaning and catering services are often provided by the hospital hotel or domestic services department and it is currently rare in the United Kingdom for the person responsible for this to be employed by the endoscopy unit. Some hospitals now contract these services out to independent companies but the ideal is for the person(s) working in this area to be employed directly by the unit so that adequate managerial control can be exercised and also a 'team spirit' built up.

The services required depend to a large extent on the clinical practices of that unit and this is outside the remit of this book.

4.4 THE MULTISKILLED HEALTH CARE WORKER

Because of changing demands in health care provision, many areas are now looking towards the concept of the 'multiskilled health care worker'. In the context of the endoscopy unit this may mean an individual, or individuals, who are trained for example to carry out portering duties but who also help with cleaning, catering and clerical support on the unit. Often this role can also be expanded to take in basic nursing care and perhaps a role in routine care and maintenance of equipment. The skills required will obviously depend on the duties carried out by that individual.

4.5 STAFFING REQUIREMENTS AND SKILL MIX

Depending on the number of lists and the workload, the requirements for an endoscopy unit are in the following sections.

4.5.1 ENDOSCOPY ASSISTANTS

Generally a staffing ratio suitable for endoscopy is a minimum of:

$$\text{qualified} : \text{trained}$$
$$7 : 3$$

Note: 'Qualified' refers to staff holding a professional qualification (e.g. registered nurse), whilst 'trained' refers to staff who have no professional qualification but who have had specific training in endoscopy.

This is a higher ratio than that required by a general hospital ward (6 : 4) and reflects the specialist knowledge required in this area. Many units work on a higher ratio than 7 : 3 and some units use only qualified staff (RNs). However, economic and other pressures such as a shortage of RNs will inevitably make this harder to achieve in the future. The main advantage of the latter is the versatility brought by an RN-only workforce. All members of staff are, after training, able to perform all duties and are totally interchangeable. This makes it very easy to cover sickness, study or annual leave and makes staff training and development easier as all are starting from a similar knowledge base. The difficulties encountered revolve around those of career progression (or lack of it) and this is addressed in section 4.7.

Requirements per list

Endoscopy room
Minimum two staff, at least one of which should be an RN.

Recovery area
Depending on number of patients to be recovered at any one time:

One–six patients – one RN
seven–12 patients – two RNs or one RN+one HCA
13–18 patients – three RNs or two RNs+one HCA.

The geographical nature of the unit may also influence the numbers required. A method of determining this number is discussed in Chapter 3.

Admissions area

In some units, the endoscopy assistants combine admission and recovery duties because on many older units these areas are combined. Should there be a separate admissions area then, depending on the number of patients to be admitted and the timing of their appointments, one or two RNs are required for this area. It is essential that RNs are employed in this area because of both the knowledge required to assess a patient's medical and psychological condition, and also that needed to answer any questions regarding the patient's endoscopy or medical condition.

4.5.2 RECEPTION/CLERICAL STAFF

On a small unit one receptionist is probably adequate to run the administrative side of the unit. Increases in workload and changes or advances in working practice mean that a larger endoscopy unit needs two or more receptionist/clerical workers.

In addition, if clinical drug trials are carried out by the unit then someone with the required knowledge and skills to co-ordinate these is required. For this reason, many larger units also have an office manager/administrator who is responsible for the administrative side of the unit including the running of these trials. The postholder may also have supervisory responsibility for other clerical or secretarial staff as well as any portering or other ancillary staff attached to the unit.

4.5.3 ANCILLARY STAFF

Portering assistant

All but the smallest of endoscopy units require a dedicated porter to transport patients from other areas of the hospital to the unit. This can help ensure the smooth running of the unit. Larger units with a high inpatient workload require two porters, perhaps working opposite shifts and overlapping at the busiest times, to provide this service.

Endoscopy technicians

The majority of units will only require one such person, and it may be that this role is part of a multiskilled role within the unit. Larger and perhaps geographically isolated units may require two or more such workers.

Catering and hotel services

These are mentioned for completeness, but are outside the remit of this book.

4.6   THE ENDOSCOPY UNIT MANAGER

Although it is usual for a clinician to be in overall charge of an endoscopy unit, the role of manager or head nurse is vital to the everyday smooth running of the unit. He or she is the person who provides the daily continuity required to make a successful unit, and who will be seen as the 'head' by patients, relatives and other members of staff.

The exact roles, responsibilities and skill requirements will vary with the needs of the unit, but all postholders will require excellent professional, communication and management skills. An interest in teaching and clinical research is an advantage. The manager should ideally have considerable endoscopy experience or the ability to learn these skills quickly. The only exception to this is the manager who is employed solely in that capacity and who has no clinical, teaching or research input into the unit. In this situation, it may be that the person concerned has no professional nursing qualification, in which case it is vital that there is a senior grade nurse within the unit who can provide professional and clinical nursing advice.

The problem with the role of the 'pure' manager is the perception of that role. The perception of the manager as someone who sits in an office pushing paper is often hard to break, whilst the **real** responsibility of an endoscopy unit (or any) manager is to provide an environment that enables his or her staff to carry out the job that they have been employed to do. The responsibilities of the endoscopy unit manager are best shown diagrammatically in Fig. 4.2.

The skills required are those common to all managers (Fig 4.3). It is rare for a person to have all these skills, and perhaps the most useful one of the lot is the ability to recognize your own strengths and weaknesses, and being able to build on the weaker areas in order to improve overall performance.

4.7   CAREER PROGRESSION

As mentioned earlier, one of the problems that occurs in endoscopy units is the fact that because people (particularly the senior grades) who

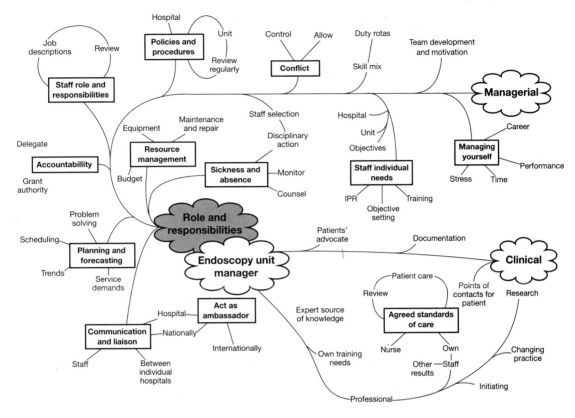

Fig. 4.2   Roles and responsibilities of the endoscopy unit manager

work in endoscopy tend to stay in their posts for a long time, it is not uncommon to have very experienced junior staff who cannot progress their career in endoscopy because no more senior posts are available. Often, they are unable to move to other areas of the country because of family or other commitments so have to rely on what is available locally. Many of these staff have one or more postregistration qualifications and in normal circumstances would be on a more senior grade by virtue of their experience and qualification. This can be an extremely negative situation for junior members of staff, and can lead to them eventually leaving the specialty.

Owning to financial and other constraints, this is often a difficult situation to address. A possible solution is to award a higher grade of pay to junior staff who fulfil previously agreed criteria, for instance:

1. Have a minimum 3 years endoscopy experience.
2. Hold a recognized postregistration qualification in endoscopy nursing.

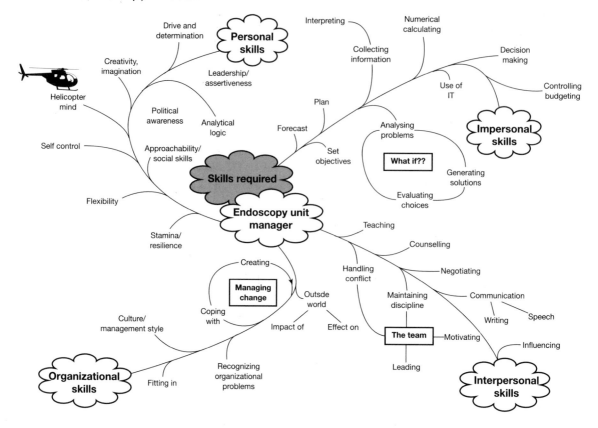

Fig. 4.3   Skills required by the endoscopy unit manager

3. Have undergone further training in, for example:
   (a) teaching and assessing in clinical practice and/or
   (b) counselling and/or
   (c) research and/or
   (d) management.

These staff then become 'clinical nurse trainers' with responsibility for the training of new staff, updating existing staff and monitoring standards of care. The additional cost can be offset against improved quality of care, a reduction in complaints and litigation and reduced sickness and other absence. This would form the basis of a career structure that allows the registered nurse to prepare through diploma or degree level study for their chosen career goal whether this be in a clinical, teaching, research or managerial capacity (Fig. 4.4).

An alternative approach has appeared in the United Kingdom through the introduction in 1992 by the United Kingdom Central

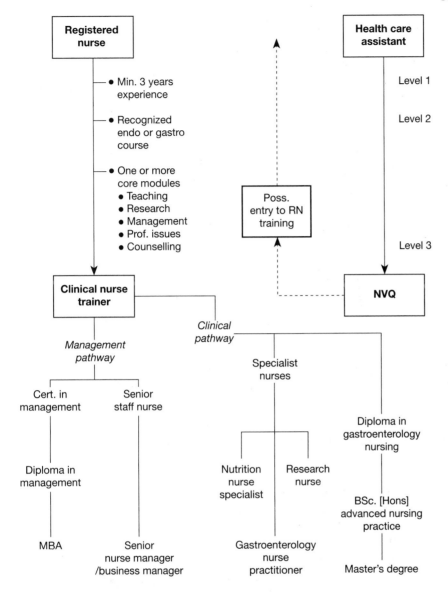

Fig. 4.4   Career pathways

Council for Nursing and Midwifery (UKCC) of the Scope of Professional Practice, which allows the development of new nursing roles.
This puts nurses in the position of being able to choose an expanded
role rather than having no choice but to seek promotion.

If nurses choose to expand their role, it is imperative that they are
relieved of other duties. After all, why should they do the same job as

someone else, plus more, for the same pay? The development of the role of health care assistants and operation department practitioners as persons with specific training in endoscopy makes this possible and allows endoscopy nurses to expand their job roles into one of the following:

1. Nutrition nurse.
2. Research nurse.
3. Gastroenterology nurse.
4. Clinical nurse trainer.

Nurses who choose neither to expand their role not to seek promotion can continue in their present role if this does not hinder the development of the unit, and will still require access to updating study days. In essence, this passes the basic endoscopy skills to the trained helper (HCA or ODP) and allows the RNs to expand their scope of practice. However, it is expensive to implement as extra, although lower paid, staff are required to allow this role expansion. It also assumes that job satisfaction and not money is the prime motivator in the staff concerned.

4.8 THE ROLE OF THE SPECIALIST NURSE PRACTITIONER

Over the past 5 years in the UK, we have seen the development of clinical nurse specialists in endoscopy and more recently the gastro-enterology nurse practitioners who, although still carrying out a number of traditional nursing functions, also carry out duties which have traditionally been the domain of the medical practitioner. An example of this is the training of some nurses to carry out diagnostic upper and lower GI endoscopy. This has evolved partially from the concept of multidisciplinary care and partially through the increasing demand for endoscopy coupled with an increase in endoscopic screening programmes and a lack of suitably trained doctors. In the United Kingdom, the reduction in the working hours of junior medical staff has also had an impact.

At present it is too early to tell how these roles will develop in the future. Some hospitals may be tempted to use nurse endoscopists as a way of reducing labour costs and at the same time increasing patient throughput. However, it could be argued that this was not a nursing role but that of a technician, and it is important when developing these roles to remember that the nurse practitioner role demands a holistic approach to patient care. If designing a job description for a nurse practitioner, apart from the provision of fixed endoscopy sessions, it should ideally include two or more of the following:

1. Monitoring of all patients seen with gastrointestinal conditions against agreed protocols, including alterations to current management and initiating new treatments, and referring to others for further care, treatment and advice.
2. Counselling and preparation of hospital patients undergoing GI investigation or treatment. This would include skills such as venepuncture and intravenous cannulation as well as ensuring informed consent was obtained prior to investigation or treatment.
3. Participation in clinical research.
4. Participation in the teaching of undergraduate and postgraduate medical and nursing staff.

The legal implications of such a role are considered in more detail in Chapter 5.

This combination will give sufficient variety of practice to make the job fulfilling and challenging. It also allows for the further development of the role in the future.

BIBLIOGRAPHY

British Society of Gastroenterology (BSG) (1987) *Staffing of Endoscopy Units*. British Society of Gastroenterology, London.

The endoscopy assistant and the law 5

Mike Shephard

5.1 INTRODUCTION

This chapter addresses the legal issues affecting the endoscopy assistant whilst carrying out his or her duties. It is not meant to be comprehensive, but rather to give an overview of the issues involved. The text is based on current English law and, although not universal, readers in the United States and the Commonwealth countries will see similarities within their own legal systems because English law forms the basis of their systems. There are also broad similarities with the legal systems of countries within the European Community, but there is wider variation within this group owing to the different way in which their legal systems developed.

The term 'endoscopy assistant' is used here in a generic sense to mean a nurse holding a registerable professional qualification (RN) or a person such as a health care assistant (HCA) or operating department practitioner (ODP) who has received specific training in order to fulfil the role of the endoscopy assistant. Throughout the chapter fictitious case histories are used to illustrate various points together with a summary of the key issues in each. These may be used as a basis for discussion with colleagues.

5.2 ACCOUNTABILITY

Whether the endoscopy assistant holds a professional qualification (i.e. is an RN) or not, that person is accountable in law for their actions or

Practical Endoscopy Edited by M. Shephard and J. Mason. Published in 1997 by Chapman & Hall, London. ISBN 0 412 54000 2

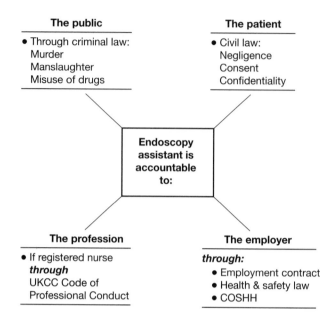

Fig. 5.1   Areas of accountability (adapted from Diamond, 1990)

omissions. A definition of 'accountability' in this sense is: 'being liable, to be called to account, answerable for, accountable for'.

In this context there is no difference between accountability and responsibility as the latter is defined as 'being liable or accountable for'. There is also a moral issue in that, whereas a nurse may have a moral responsibility to tend a person involved, for example, in a road accident, current UK law recognizes no legal liability to do so.

Figure 5.1 shows the areas of accountability relevant to the endoscopy assistant together with the relevant areas of law which apply. It is important to remember that a person may be accountable in law under one or more of the areas shown. The only difference between the endoscopy assistant who is an RN and the endoscopy assistant who is not is that, in addition to the areas of accountability common to both, the RN is additionally accountable in law to his or her professional body.

CASE STUDY 1

A patient with known oesophageal varices is gastroscoped following a haematemesis the previous evening. At gastroscopy a large blood clot is noted close to the gastro-oesophageal junction but no active bleeding is seen.

Shortly afterwards, and whilst still on the endoscopy unit, the patient has another large haematemesis and as a result becomes shocked. Resuscitation procedures are immediately commenced, and owing to the past history and the presumed site of bleeding it is felt that the insertion of a Sengstaken tube would be appropriate. This is inserted by the doctor who carried out the gastroscopy.

As a further precaution RN Smith, an endoscopy assistant who has recently started work on the unit, is asked by the doctor to prepare a vasopressin infusion. RN Smith has had specific training in the giving and preparing of intravenous drugs and infusions but is unfamiliar with the preparation of this form of treatment so asks the doctor how she should do this. The doctor instructs her to put 200 units of vasopressin into 100 ml of dextrose 5%. RN Smith prepares this, and has it checked by the nurse who has escorted the patient from the ward, and who heard the verbal order given by the doctor.

The infusion is started to run over 15 minutes, but shortly after it is commenced the patient has a cardiac arrest, and despite numerous attempts to revive him, he dies. A subsequent post-mortem examination showed 10 times the normal dose of vasopressin in his circulation.

Using Fig. 5.1 as a reference, in what areas of law could RN Smith be held accountable?

Key issues

The case study illustrates the interrelationship between the various areas of accountability.

Because of her action in giving 10 times the recommended dose of vasopressin, which resulted in the death of her patient, RN Smith may:

1. Be charged in the Criminal Courts with 'manslaughter by gross negligence'.

2. Be subject to an action in the Civil Courts by the patient's relatives claiming negligence. This may be an action brought against her as a individual or, more likely her employer would be sued (section 5.4.1). The doctor concerned may also be sued for negligence.
3. Be subject to disciplinary action by her employer for breach of contract (section 5.5).
4. Be called before the Professional Conduct Committee (PCC) of the UKCC to answer charges of professional misconduct.

5.3   CRIMINAL LIABILITY

Following an investigation by the police, the Crown Prosecution Service decides whether or not to bring criminal proceedings against an individual. This is based on the evidence available.

There are two types of criminal offence:

1. *Indictable*; Serious offences such as murder, infanticide and treason, which may only be heard before a judge and jury in the Crown Court.
2. *Summary*; Minor offences such as being drunk and disorderly and minor motoring offences, which may only be heard by magistrates in the Magistrate's Court.

However, there are a large number of criminal offences that fall between these two definitions and may be tried in either court if the defendant agrees. This covers offences such as: theft, handling stolen goods, and assault causing actual bodily harm.

In order to establish guilt, the prosecution must show that the crime was committed 'beyond reasonable doubt'. Defences against a criminal act, apart from the defendant not being responsible for the offence, include: insanity, diminished responsibility, duress, drunkenness, acting on superior orders, and self-defence.

5.4   CIVIL LIABILITY

This area of accountability covers four areas important to the endoscopy assistant.

These are:

1. Negligence.
2. Consent to treatment.
3. Confidentiality.
4. Property.

5.4.1 NEGLIGENCE

Despite all precautions, accidents do happen, and when these occur in a
hospital the person involved or his or her relatives (the plaintiff) may
make a claim for compensation, citing negligence on the part of the
hospital or individual.

For a claim of negligence to succeed, the plaintiff must prove that:

1. There was a 'duty of care' owed to the plaintiff.
2. There was a breach of that duty of care.
3. The breach of care has lead to 'reasonably foreseeable harm'.
4. The breach in duty of care caused the harm suffered.

Duty of care

A duty of care exists if it can be shown that the actions of one person
are reasonably likely to cause harm to another person (*Donoghue* v
Stevenson [1932] AC 562). As a result of the relationship that exists
between the patient and the carer, the endoscopy assistant therefore
owes a duty of care to the patient.

Breach of duty of care

To establish whether there has been a breach of that duty of care it is
necessary to establish the accepted standard of care or practice. The
standard way to determine whether negligence has occurred is to apply
the Bolam test (*Bolam* v *Friern Barnet* [1957] HMC).

The Bolam test

> When you get a situation which involves the use of some special
> skill or competence, then the test as to whether there has been
> negligence or not is . . . the standard of the ordinary skilled man
> exercising and professing to have that special skill
>   (*Whitehouse* v *Jordan* [1981]).

If a person fails to measure up to the above standard then he or she
has been negligent. This is taken to include 'clinical judgement'. In a
claim for negligence, therefore, the standard of care against which the
case would be judged is that of an ordinary skilled endoscopy assistant.
Written procedures, local policies and guidelines from professional

bodies may also be used to assess what the accepted standard of care is in a given situation. Even if there are none of these in existence, a professional would not be considered negligent if what was done was considered reasonable in all the circumstances.

Reasonable foreseeability

A person can take precautions only against a reasonably known risk. In other words, if the event hasn't happened before and there is no reason to suggest such an occurrence might happen, then you cannot be held negligent if it does. However, ignorance is no defence, and a person would be expected to keep their knowledge up to date. This does not mean that not reading every relevant magazine article or research paper would make you negligent, but you would be held negligent if you were not following accepted practice or had not acted on a directive from an official or professional body such as the Committee of the Safety of Medicines or the UKCC.

Causal link

To prove negligence, there has to be a link between the breach of duty of care and the harm done. To succeed, it must be shown that the breach in the duty of care was responsible for the harm suffered.

It is unusual for an endoscopy assistant to be sued directly for negligence as a result of actions (or omissions) carried out as part of their duties as an employee. In this situation the employer is usually held to have vicarious liability for the employee, and the action would be directed against them. However, if the action were successful and the employer had to pay compensation, then **theoretically** the employer could then take action against the employee to recover the money.

Principles of vicarious liability

The employer is liable for the damage or harm (tort) caused by an employee's acts or omissions, regardless of whether the employer has been at fault in any way itself (*Stavely Iron and Chemical Co v Jones* [1956] AC 627; *ICI v Shatwell* [1965] AC 656).

To prove vicarious liability, it must be shown that: **either** the person committing the tort was an employee, and that the tort was committed in course of employment **or** the tort was committed by a person acting as an independent contractor of the employer, and was committed in the course of this work.

CASE STUDY 2

May Jones, aged 75 years, is recovering on a trolley on the endoscopy unit following a gastroscopy. She has been sedated with 2 mg midazolam. The endoscopy assistant in charge of recovery, an RN, has examined Miss Jones after her test and is satisfied that her condition is satisfactory and that she is sleeping peacefully. The trolley she is on has restraining sides, and although they are only 15 cm high, they are in position.

    The nurse goes to see another patient. Suddenly she hears a crash and a cry of pain. She returns to find Miss Jones lying on the floor beside her trolley. Subsequently it is discovered that she has broken her wrist.

Does May Jones have a claim for negligence?

Key issues

Applying the criteria for a claim of negligence to succeed to this case:

1. *Does the nurse have a 'duty of care' to Miss Jones*? **Yes,** a nurse always has this duty to patients under his or her care.
2. *Was there a breach of that duty*? This is debatable. It is unrealistic to expect the nurse to be continuously with the patient, and she had recently checked her and was satisfied with her condition. She would therefore probably not be negligent unless she was breaching any written procedure or protocol or was not following accepted practice.
3. *Could the accident have been 'reasonably foreseeable'*? Again this is debatable. If the trolley had been used before and no similar accident had occurred then this could not be foreseeable. If a similar accident had occurred previously, then this would be 'reasonably foreseeable' and the nurse would be negligent. The hospital and/or the manufacturer may also be negligent for supplying equipment inadequate for its purpose.
4. *Did the breach in duty of care cause the harm suffered*? The answers to points 3 and 4 above determine the answer to this question. The nurse would have to have known the trolley sides were inadequate for the purpose intended or have been aware of a previous accident to have breached her duty of care. The hospital and/or manufacturer may still be negligent.

5.4.2 CONSENT TO TREATMENT

Any adult, mentally competent person has the right in law to consent to, or withhold consent to, the touching of his or her person. A person who touches another without this consent (or without any other legal justification) may be sued in the Civil Court for trespass. Even if consent has been given, then the person requesting the consent may still be in breach of their duty of care (i.e. negligent) if they have given the patient insufficient information to allow an informed decision to be made. Consent may take two forms:

Express – either verbally or in writing.
Implied – where the non-verbal communication by the patient makes it clear that consent is being given. An example of this would be the patient rolling up his sleeve prior to venepuncture.

As far as this relates to an invasive procedure such as endoscopy, it is recommended that written consent is obtained prior to endoscopy. The fact that a patient has attended the unit does **not** imply consent to endoscopy. The patient has the right to be given sufficient information to allow an informed decision to be made. This should include sufficient information to ensure they understand the nature, consequences, and any substantial risks of the proposed treatment or investigation, and what alternatives (if any) are available.

The main purpose of a written consent form (Fig. 5.2) is to provide documented evidence that an explanation of the proposed treatment or investigation has been given, and that consent has been sought and obtained. It is not valid unless sufficient information has been given to allow an informed decision to be made, and even if this is given the patient should be allowed sufficient time to think about it and ask any relevant questions. For this reason some consent forms now outline any significant risks involved, and literature sent to patients provides more information regarding this and other more minor problems relating to the investigation concerned (e.g. sore throat following upper GI endoscopy). Provision of this information may, however, sometimes be detrimental to a patient by frightening them, hence it is sometimes necessary to exercise what is known as 'therapeutic privilege' and withhold information that you feel may be detrimental to a patient.

Examination or treatment without consent

There are only two reasons for an endoscopy to be carried out without the patient's consent:

1. Where it is a potentially life-saving procedure and the patient is unconscious and cannot indicate his or her wishes.

TYPE OF OPERATION INVESTIGATION OR TREATMENT

I confirm that I have explained the operation investigation or treatment, and such appropriate options as are available and the type of anaesthetic, if any (general/regional/sedation) proposed, to the patient in terms which in my judgement are suited to the understanding of the patient and/or to one of the parents or guardians of the patient

Signature..   Date..../...../.....

Name of doctor ....

PATIENT/PARENT/GUARDIAN

1. Please read this form and the notes below very carefully.

2. If there is anything that you don't understand about the explanation, or if you want more information, you should ask the doctor.

3. Please check that all the information on the form is correct. If it is, and you understand the explanation, then sign the form.

I agree	• to what is proposed and confirm that it has been explained to me by the doctor named on this form
	• to the use of the type of anaesthetic that I have been told about.
	• no assurance has been given to me that the procedure will be performed by any particular named surgeon, or that the anaesthetic will be given by any particular named anaesthetist.
I understand	• that any procedure in addition to the investigation or treatment described on this form will only be carried out if it is necessary and in my best interests and can be justified for medical reasons.
I have told	• the doctor about any additional procedures I would not wish to be carried out without my having the opportunity to consider them first.

Signature   ....   Relationship ....
                                                                (if not the patient)
Name   ....
Address   ....
(if not the patient) ....

NOTES TO:

Doctors

A patient has a legal right to grant or withhold consent prior to examination or treatment. Patients should be given sufficient information, in a way they can understand, about the proposed treatment and the possible alternatives. Patients must be allowed to decide whether they will agree to the treatment and they may refuse or withdraw consent to treatment at any time. The patient's consent to treatment should be recorded on this form; further guidance is given in HC(90)22 (*A Guide to Consent for Examination or Treatment*).

Patients

• The doctor is here to help you. He or she will explain the proposed treatment and what the alternatives are. You can ask any questions and seek further information. You can refuse the treatment.

• You may ask for a relative, or friend, or a nurse to be present.

• Training health professionals is essential to the continuation of the health service and improving the quality of care. Your treatment may provide an important opportunity for such training, where necessary under the careful supervision of a senior doctor. You may refuse any involvement in a formal training programme without this adversely affecting your care and treatment.

Fig. 5.2   A written consent form

2. Where the patient is incapable of giving consent by reason of mental disorder or senility, and the investigation or treatment is in the patient's best interest. To be in a patient's best interest, the treatment should be:
   (a) Necessary to preserve the life, health or well-being of the patient.
   (b) In accordance with a responsible body of professional medical opinion.
   (c) Where appropriate, involve the decision being made by all members of an interdisciplinary care team.

CASE STUDY 3

As manager of the endoscopy unit, you are asked to book a gastroscopy for a 95-year-old patient who has been shown by barium meal to have an almost certain gastric carcinoma. The patient would be unfit for surgical treatment of this, owing to her age and to other coexisting medical conditions. In short, this would not normally be a reason for carrying out a gastroscopy as it would not alter the management of the patient. The patient is unable, owing to senility, to consent to the test, but relatives are willing to do this and are pressing the medical staff for a definite diagnosis.

Should you gastroscope this patient?

Key issues

1. As the test will not alter the management of the patient, this cannot be described as being 'in the best interests of the patient'. Endoscopy is known to be a risk, particularly in a patient of this age who has other medical problems, so apart from it not being in their best interest, it probably breaches your duty of care to the patient.
2. The relatives' consent is invalid. Apart from the authority in law given to a parent over a minor under the age of 18 years, there is no situation where consent by a relative is valid. The relatives may be interested in a definite diagnosis not because they feel it is in her best interests, but because they have financial problems and would inherit her money if she dies. They are therefore 'interested parties'.

Note: The Family Law Reform Act 1969 allows a minor (a person under 18 years of age) who has reached the age of 16 years to give consent to surgical, medical or dental treatment. In recent years, provided it can be shown that the person giving consent is able to understand the information given sufficiently to allow them to make an informed decision, then this consent would be considered valid in law even if the person had not reached the age of 16 years.

5.4.3 CONFIDENTIALITY

Every person employed on an endoscopy unit has a duty to ensure the confidentiality of all information held about a patient. This is implied not only in the duty of care to a patient, but also in the contract of employment. If the person is a RN, there is also a duty to maintain confidentiality in the code of professional conduct.

Problems relating to confidentiality usually deal with exceptions to it rather than the question of maintaining confidentiality.

Confidentiality may be broken by an endoscopy assistant:

1. With the consent of the patient.
2. In the interests of the patient.
3. Under court order (subpoena).
4. Under statutory duty (Public Health and Misuse of Drugs Acts).
5. In the public interest.

CASE STUDY 4

Paul Hutting is a 53-year-old lorry driver who has attended the unit for a colonoscopy. He is a tall obese man who by his own admission likes his food, and who regularly consumes 8–15 pints of beer a night. Because of his size and general uncooperative manner, he required a large amount of sedation for the investigation to be successful (midazolam 5 mg and pethidine 50 mg). Following colonoscopy he is very restless, and after 5 minutes he is awake and sitting up on his trolley.

Despite advice from the endoscopy assistant (an RN) responsible for his recovery, he insists on getting off the trolley and getting dressed. He is obviously still greatly affected by the sedation he has received and repeatedly asks the same questions. Shortly afterwards he gets up and announces that he has left his lorry in the hospital car park and that he now intends driving home. Although he is advised both by medical and nursing staff that it is very dangerous to do this because of the sedation he has received he insists he will wait no longer and is going to drive home saying that he is perfectly all right and doesn't know what all the fuss was about. It is suggested that he signs a 'self-discharge' statement but he refuses to do so and leaves the unit.

What should you do?
Should you report this to the police?

Key issues

1. This is often a difficult situation. A person has the right to discharge him- or herself from hospital, and any physical restraint in doing so would be assault.

   However, Paul is under the influence of the sedation and is not in a state to act rationally. He is a danger to himself and the general public. It would therefore be reasonable for confidentiality to be breached on two counts:

   (a) In the patient's interest.
   (b) In the public interest.

   Also, Paul would be committing an offence under the Road Traffic Act by driving or attempting to drive whilst under the influence of drugs, and there is a statutory duty to report this to the police.

2. The 'self-discharge' form is not worth the paper it is printed on because Paul is unable to make a rational decision as a result of the sedation.

5.4.4   PROPERTY

As many endoscopic procedures are carried out as day cases, the care of patients' property whilst they are on the endoscopy unit is of importance.

Whilst instructions sent to patients invariably request that no items of value are brought into the unit, this does occur, and because of the nature of the tests carried out, small items such as dentures may disappear.

In general, a person does not become liable for another person's property unless he or she can be shown to have assumed responsibility for it. Therefore, by asking a patient on admission whether they have any valuables they would like locking away or by looking after their clothing whilst they have their endoscopy, the endoscopy assistant is taking responsibility for these items whilst the patient is on the unit. It could also be argued that, as many patients are sedated for their endoscopy, then a duty of care exists to look after their property whilst they are (temporarily) unable to do so. It is important therefore that any endoscopy unit has an agreed procedure for the handling and safekeeping of patients' property.

If patients are advised not to bring valuables into the endoscopy unit and insist on doing so, they should be advised to have them locked up for safekeeping. If they refuse to do this, they should be asked to sign a disclaimer to this effect.

5.5 EMPLOYMENT LIABILITY

Any employee is accountable to his or her employer. Employees'
responsibilities with regard to their work are laid down in their contract
of employment but there is an implied term in all contracts (unless
stated to the contrary) that is assumed to be there whether it is written
in or not. This is that the employee will 'obey the reasonable instructions of the employer' and will use 'all care and skill'. It follows that an
employee who is negligent has not used 'all care and skill' and is
therefore in breach of the contract of employment. This leaves the
endoscopy assistant open to disciplinary action, which might include a
warning (oral or written), demotion, suspension or dismissal.

Employment law varies greatly from country to country, and a
detailed study of this area is outside the remit of this book. However,
most countries have legislation covering the health and safety aspects of
work, so a brief summary is included here highlighting the points
relevant to endoscopy.

5.5.1 HEALTH AND SAFETY AT WORK

The Health and Safety at Work Act 1974 placed a legal responsibility
on the employer to ensure, so far as is reasonably practicable, the
health, safety and welfare of all employees. This covers aspects such as
regular maintenance of equipment, provisions of training in its use,
adequate protective clothing and generally a safe working environment
for the employee to carry out his or her work. The act also places a
responsibility on employees to ensure both their own and their colleagues' safety at all times, to use any safety equipment provided, and to
report any faulty or damaged equipment to the employer.

Control of Substances Hazardous to Health (COSHH) Regulations 1988

These regulations require the employer to make an assessment of the
risks to the health of the employee posed by potentially hazardous
substances. In the endoscopy unit there are two areas covered:

1. Micro-organisms that may be passed from person to person.
2. Disinfection procedures involving chemical disinfectants such as
   glutaraldehyde.

Ideally the employee should not be exposed to a hazardous substance
and a non-hazardous alternative should be found. This is not always
possible, however, and in this situation measures must be taken to
control and monitor exposure to the hazardous substance. All units

therefore require adequate infection control procedures, and need to control exposure to glutaraldehyde or other chemical disinfectants covered by the regulations by use of fume extraction, protective clothing and equipment. The health of staff should also be monitored regularly (prior to employment, a month after commencing work, and thereafter annually as a minimum) and the concentration of the chemical in the air should be measured to ensure this is below the maximum permitted level. The regulations also place a duty on the employer to inform, instruct and train employees in the risks and control measures appropriate to the hazardous substance. Glutaraldehyde is covered in more detail in Chapter 7.

Product liability

The Consumer Protection Act 1987 places an onus on the supplier of a product to ensure it is suitable for the purpose intended. The importance of this legislation to the endoscopy assistant is that in certain circumstances the assistant or the hospital might become the 'supplier' and could become liable to pay compensation should the product be defective.

This is relevant where equipment is being used more than once and is subject to reprocessing (for example, the redisinfection of an ERCP cannula by the hospital or the endoscopy unit). In this situation the area that reprocesses the equipment becomes the supplier.

If an article is marked 'single use only' it should not be reused although there may be considerable financial pressures to do so. If the product is reused against the manufacturer's instructions, then that hospital or individual becomes liable for any harm caused as a result of its reuse. Items of equipment marked 'reusable' may be reprocessed, but the manufacturer must provide detailed instructions as to how it should be cleaned and reprocessed, and should indicate any inspections or tests required to ensure it is in good working order. Some manufacturers state a maximum or recommended number of times an item of equipment may be reused, and in this case it would be necessary to be able to individually identify that item and to record how many times it had been used. If an item of equipment is marked 'autoclavable' then this means that it may be sterilized prior to use, not that it is reusable (unless this is also indicated). (This area is also discussed in Chapter 7.)

5.6   PROFESSIONAL LIABILITY

If an endoscopy assistant holds a professional qualification such as RN, then he or she is accountable to the governing body of that profession for his or her actions. In the United Kingdom this is the UKCC. This body has a statutory duty to prepare and maintain a register of qualified nurses, midwives and health visitors and set out rules relating to the entry onto, removal from and restoration to the register. The PCC of the UKCC hears evidence of professional misconduct, and can recommend one of the following courses of action:

1. No action.
2. Refer respondent to the Health Committee.
3. Postpone decision.
4. Suspend respondent from register.
5. Strike respondent off the register.

Their concern is to protect the public from the irresponsible nurse, not to punish the nurse.

Professional misconduct is not confined to the workplace, but may be the result of occurrences whilst at home or off duty. The PCC would consider whether the conduct was either unworthy of a nurse or had brought the profession into disrepute.

The UKCC also has a duty to establish and improve standards of education and training, sets conditions for admission to training, and regulates standards of training both before and after admission to the register.

A more detailed discussion of professional liability and the role of a governing body is outside the remit of this book, but the endoscopy assistant with a professional qualification should be aware of their accountability to that body whether enforced by legal statute or not.

5.7   OTHER RELEVANT AREAS OF LAW

5.7.1   DRUGS

The endoscopy assistant handles, prepares and administers a variety of drugs as part of his or her work. The supply, storage and administration of such drugs are controlled by legislation reinforced by local policies and procedures. In the United Kingdom, the two relevant acts are the Medicines Act 1968 and the Misuse of Drugs Act 1971 and the endoscopy assistant should be familiar with their provisions.

Because of the specialist nature of endoscopy, certain procedures involving drugs are carried out by the endoscopy assistant as part of their work that would not normally be undertaken by nurses employed in other areas of the hospital. The injection of sclerosants intravenously or submucosally in the treatment of oesophageal varices is an example of such a procedure. The product concerned is not licensed for this use, and most hospitals require the doctor, not the nurse, to give the first dose if administered intravenously. It is therefore important that the endoscopy unit has a written protocol, signed and agreed by medical and nursing staff as well as the pharmacy manager, which ratifies these procedures as often they are not covered by those used in other areas of the hospital.

5.8 RESEARCH

Many endoscopy units carry out clinical research and the endoscopy assistant is often heavily involved in this, either through their own research project or as part of a larger national trial. It is important therefore that he or she has an understanding of the legal principles involved when carrying out research.

5.8.1 PATIENT CONSENT

Written consent should be obtained from all patients taking part in a clinical research programme. The patient should be given enough information to be able to make an informed decision, as outlined in section 5.4.2, and should be asked to sign a consent form specifically designed for the purpose. In particular they should be advised of their right to withdraw from the research at any time, and that whether or not they take part in the research will not affect the treatment they receive as part of their care.

5.8.2 CONFIDENTIALITY

All information, whether it is used for research purposes or not, is confidential and can be disclosed only on the grounds outlined earlier in this chapter (section 5.4.3). The right to use this information for research purposes is usually included in the consent form, and it should be made clear that the results will be presented in such a way that it would be impossible to identify a particular individual from them. If computerized records are used then these are covered by the Data Protection Act and the fact that the information will be used for research purposes must be registered.

5.8.3 LIABILITY FOR PERSONS TAKING PART IN RESEARCH

Currently there is no automatic compensation for persons harmed as a result of participating in a clinical research programme. It has been recommended that a 'no-fault' compensation system should be implemented, but this has yet to occur. Currently a person harmed as a result of clinical research can make a claim only for negligence as described earlier (section 5.4.1).

5.9 MEDICAL RECORD KEEPING

The endoscopy assistant has a duty to record accurately any information relating to the care and condition of a patient. This is not only to protect the endoscopy assistant, but also to provide an accurate record of the care and condition of that patient whilst in their care, and to assist other health care workers in the care of that patient. Any document requested by a court becomes a legal document, so all records relating to patient care and treatment should be regarded as such.

All such records should be legible, accurate and should be signed and dated. Records by students in training should ideally be countersigned by a trained member of staff who agrees that the record is accurate. If an error is made, it is best to cross this out with a single line and write the amendment above, rather than obliterate it with ink or correction fluid.

5.10 THE NURSE PRACTITIONER/ENDOSCOPIST

Many hospitals are now employing or considering the employment of nurses specifically trained to carry out duties that have traditionally been done by medical practitioners, for instance the siting of enteral and parenteral feeding lines and carrying out of diagnostic upper GI endoscopy and flexible sigmoidoscopy.

The UKCC document *The Scope of Professional Practice* (1992) supports nurses developing the extent of their professional practice as long as the 'nurse concerned is competent for the purpose and mindful of the personal professional accountability they bear for their actions'. The common law of negligence, as discussed earlier in this chapter, requires that a reasonable standard of care is attained at all times, and will judge a person who professes to have specialist skills by the standard expected of a specialist (Bolam test). Thus any nurse carrying out endoscopy will be judged in law at the standard of the reasonably competent endoscopist.

The General Medical Council says the following in its book *Duties of a Doctor* (GMC, 1995).

Paras 28 and 29: 'Delegating care to non-medical staff and students'

28: You may delegate medical care to nurses and other health care staff who are not registered medical practitioners if you believe it is best for the patient. But you must be sure that the person to whom you delegate is competent to undertake the procedure or therapy involved. When delegating care or treatment, you must always pass on enough information about the patient and the treatment needed. You will still be responsible for managing the patient's care.

29: You must not enable anyone who is not registered with the GMC to carry out tasks that require the knowledge and skills of a doctor.

The British Society of Gastroenterology Working Party Report 'The Nurse Endoscopist' published in early 1995 recommended that the nurse should:

1. Follow the same training as a medical endoscopist and have attended a recognized teaching course in endoscopy.
2. Have the employer's support.
3. Have adequate supervision by a competent medical endoscopist who should be immediately available whilst nurse endoscopy was being carried out.
4. Be responsible for obtaining patient consent and discussing the findings with the patient afterwards.
5. Prepare the endoscopy report and have it countersigned by the supervising endoscopist (the interpretation of findings and further patient management remain a medical responsibility).
6. Keep adequate records and periodically audit the work.

Provided the nurse concerned followed these guidelines, was competent, and used 'all care and attention' whilst carrying out the procedure, then it would be very hard to substantiate a claim of negligence. However, the nurse concerned may find that medicolegally, he or she may need further insurance cover as endoscopy may not be covered by the normal professional indemnity insurance offered to nurses or may be inadequate for a full claim of compensation. Furthermore, it should be made clear to the patient that it is a nurse carrying out the endoscopy **not** a doctor, and the patient should be given the choice of having the investigation performed by a doctor instead. Having said that, a patient has the right to expect the same standard of care whether it is provided by a doctor or nurse.

REFERENCES

British Society of Gastroenterology (1995) *The Nurse Endoscopist*, Working Party Report. British Society of Gastroenterology, London.
Diamond, B. (1990) *Legal Aspects of Nursing*, Prentice-Hall, London.
General Medical Council (1995) *Duties of a Doctor*, GMC, London.
UKCC (1992) *The Scope of Professional Practice*, UKCC, London.

BIBLIOGRAPHY

Dept of Health (1993) *A Guide to Consent for Examination or Treatment*, DoH, London.

Howarth, D. (1995) *Textbook on Tort*, Butterworths, London.

The endoscopy assistant, documentation and quality assurance **6**

Jean Harvey, Jayne Mason and Rachel Hodson

6.1 THE ENDOSCOPY ASSISTANT

Anyone entering the specialized field of endoscopy as an endoscopy assistant will find the role complex, fulfilling and demanding. Caring for patients in an area where the length of stay is short, throughput rapid and the level of patient dependency varied requires a highly skilled nurse with good interpersonal skills.

The role of the endoscopy assistant must not be undervalued as it is both complex and demanding. It can be divided into two main areas of responsibility:

1. Management of a patient undergoing an endoscopic procedure.
2. Care and maintenance of endoscopic equipment and accessories.

6.1.1 MANAGEMENT OF THE PATIENT

The primary role of the endoscopy assistant is to ensure the safety of the patient before, during and after the procedure.

Attending the endoscopy unit for investigation or treatment can be a time of extreme anxiety for the patient. It is crucial for the endoscopy assistant to understand that they will require both **physical** and **psychological** preparation and **support** during their stay on the unit. A verbal explanation of the procedure reinforced by written instructions does

Practical Endoscopy Edited by M. Shephard and J. Mason. Published in 1997 by Chapman & Hall, London. ISBN 0 412 54000 2

much to alleviate initial anxiety, as does a friendly and understanding approach to both the patient and their relatives and friends.

The length of time a patient can expect to be in the unit will depend on the procedure, the outcome and whether the patient has been given sedation. The endoscopy assistant must therefore tailor the care to the individual needs of each patient, and base this on the model of care adapted by the unit.

6.1.2   PATIENT ASSESSMENT

Assessment should be carried out by an RN in a room allocated for the purpose, away from the busy working environment of the unit. This allows the patient privacy and dignity in what can be a very stressful situation. The following are mandatory tasks in any pre-endoscopy assessment:

1. Check patient identity is correct; it is surprising how many patients will say 'yes' to any question if they are anxious.
2. Confirm patient details in hospital or records are correct; this ensures your records are accurate and that important information and future appointments are not sent to the wrong person or place.
3. Ensure any specific preparation instructions have been carried out and assess result (e.g. has bowel preparation been effective?).
4. History of current or recent medication especially anticoagulants and antidepressants or sleeping tablets; anticoagulants may prevent biopsy or other therapeutic procedures being performed. Antidepressants and sleeping tables may reduce the sedation effect.
5. History of any allergies (e.g. antibiotics, contrast medium in ERCP).
6. History of endocarditis (antibiotic prophylaxis required).
7. Tolerance of previous endoscopies and/or sedation; this may give an indication of how patient may react. Patients who drink alcohol regularly to excess may react violently to sedation, and are often better investigated using local anaesthesia only.
8. Consent to treatment; has sufficient information been given and understood to allow an informed consent to be made? Does the patient need to be seen by a doctor beforehand?
9. Transport arrangements; are they satisfactory? If sedated, does patient have somebody to collect them? Sedated patients must not drive or operate machinery for 24 hours after endoscopy. Nor should they go back to work in the afternoon.

During endoscopy, the endoscopy assistant is responsible for ensuring that all equipment is prepared before the patient enters the room.

Endoscopes and other equipment required should ideally not be in the patient's direct line of vision.

There should be a minimum of two endoscopy assistants in the procedure room, one of which should be a qualified nurse. One assistant is responsible for reassuring the patient, removing secretions from the mouth (upper GI and bronchoscopy), and monitoring the patient's vital signs. Pulse oximetry has become standard in most units, and is helpful in showing respiratory problems (usually due to over-sedation) before any other physical signs can be noted. The second assistant acts as a technician and takes responsibility for specimen collection, any photographs or other visual records taken, and the endoscope and accessories. Both need to be alert to possible emergencies, and be trained in taking the appropriate action.

Following an endoscopy, the endoscopy assistant is responsible for monitoring the patient's vital signs during recovery, being alert for the complications which may arise as a result of the procedure, and ensuring they are discharged safely from the unit. Whilst carrying out the above roles, the endoscopy assistant should also be aware of the continuing requirement to provide health education and advice, thus allowing the patient to make an informed choice about their health and lifestyle.

6.1.3 CARE AND MAINTENANCE OF ENDOSCOPIC EQUIPMENT AND ACCESSORIES

Much of the equipment and accessories used in endoscopy are both extremely delicate and expensive, and the endoscopy assistant has an important role in ensuring it is correctly used and maintained. Every unit should have written policies on the decontamination of endoscopes and their accessories, and these need to be strictly adhered to. National bodies such as the BSG have produced guidelines to help in this and other areas of instrument and patient care.

Records should also be kept of equipment maintenance and repair, and a stock control system for reusable or disposable accessories should be kept to help minimize overstocking. Endoscopy accessories are expensive and you can suddenly find half your annual budget sitting unused in your store cupboard.

6.2 DOCUMENTATION

The smooth running of any endoscopy unit relies on the use of relevant and concise documentation. Many endoscopy assistants feel that too much paperwork is involved in their work and that this tends to take them away from the direct care of their patients, but correct use of documentation can improve the quality of patient care given and enhance the service provided.

Endoscopy units throughout the country will vary in the documentation used, and the design will depend on the local requirements of the service. However, all units require:

nursing documentation
endoscopy report
patient booking and appointment system
discharge information.

The documentation used in this chapter is an example of that which the author uses. It must be emphasized, however, that whatever documentation is used it is only reliable if it is used correctly.

6.2.1 NURSING DOCUMENTATION

The aim of nursing documentation is to provide a quick and accurate method of recording a patient's care whilst on the unit (Figs 6.1–6.4). At the very minimum this should include:

1. *Patient details*
   - full name
   - address
   - date of birth
   - hospital identification number
   - next of kin/meaningful person
   - transport details (if day case).
2. *Medical risk assessment*
   - significant physical or mental disease
   - ASA classification
   - current medication
   - allergy history.
3. *Admission details*
   - time admitted
   - intended procedure and any specific preparation [e.g. bowel prep.]
   - preprocedure checklist (Fig. 6.2)
   - baseline observations of: oxygen saturation, pulse, respiration and BP.
4. *Procedure record (Fig. 6.3)*
   - consent
   - local anaesthetic/sedation used
   - other medication
   - procedure actually performed
   - record of specimens collected
   - observations during procedure.

ENDOSCOPY UNIT
PATIENT CARE PLAN

Date of admission:

Admitting nurse:

Time of admission:

Type of procedure:

ADDRESSOGRAPH

[pic]   Code: No:

Age: DOB:

Religion:

Occupation:

Preferred name:

General practitioner:

Next of kin:

Address:

[pic]   Code: No:

Person to collect:
Name:
[pic]   Code: No:

Allergies: Yes ☐   No ☐
1.
2.
3.
4.

Medication: Yes ☐   No ☐
1.   5.
2.   6.
3.   7.
4.   8.

MEDICAL HISTORY	YEAR	SURGICAL HISTORY	YEAR

Discharge arrangements / Special information:

Operation / treatment explained: Yes ☐   No ☐

Sedation explained: Required ? :   Yes ☐   Unsure ☐   No ☐

Fig. 6.1   A patient care plan form

PREOPERATIVE

O₂Sats:	P:	R:	BP:

PRE-OPERATIVE CHECKLIST

	✓ / ✗ / N/A	INITIAL
Theatre gown		
Identity bracelet to wrist		
Cover / remove all jewellery		
Wigs / hair pieces / grips		
Remove nail varnish / make-up		
Remove contact lenses / art. eyes		
Remove prosthesis		
Remove dentures - top / bottom / both / in situ		
Check caps / crowns on teeth		
BM stix:		
EMLA:		
Pregnancy / LMP		
Urinalysis		
Patient's notes		
Patient's X-rays		
Fluid balance chart / drugs chart		
Nil by mouth: Time:		

ACTIVITIES OF LIVING	ADDITIONAL INFORMATION
Hearing: Vision: Mobility: Breathing (smoker ?): Others:	IVI infusion pump:

Fig. 6.2   A preoperative checklist

INTRAOPERATIVE

PREPARATION for PROCEDURE

XYLOCAINE SPRAY GIVEN:	Yes ☐ No ☐

CONSENT FORM:	Yes ☐ No ☐

DRUG USED	TIME	DOSAGE GIVEN
Hypnovel		
Diazemuls		
Pethidine		
Buscopan		
Other		

FURTHER DRUG USED	TIME	DOSAGE GIVEN
STD		
Alcohol		
Others		

PROCEDURE PERFORMED

Gastroscopy	☐	Colonoscopy	☐
Inj. varices	☐	Polypectomy	☐
Oes dilation	☐	Sigmoidoscopy	☐
PEG	☐	Banding	☐

Biopsies taken:	Yes ☐ No ☐

Time taken:

H. pylori taken:	Yes ☐ No ☐ Positive ☐ Negative ☐

Nature of biopsies:

OBSERVATIONS IN THEATRE	O$_2$ saturation:
	Pulse:

SPECIAL INSTRUCTIONS / ADDITIONAL INFORMATION

Venflon in situ:

O$_2$ sats on transfer:

Pulse on transfer:

Theatre nurse signature:

Fig. 6.3 An intraoperative checklist

POSTOPERATIVE

TIME IN RECOVERY:

LEVEL OF CONSCIOUSNESS

Fully awake

Easily roused

Unrousable (refer to doctor)

Walking

Trolley

OXYGEN REQUIRED: Yes

No

IV IN SITU   Yes

No

OBSERVATIONS ON RETURN

BP:

Pulse:

O_2 sats:

BM stix:

FURTHER OBSERVATIONS (If necessary)

REVERSAL DRUGS REQUIRED:

FLUIDS GIVEN:

ANY COMPLICATIONS / COMMENTS

Pain score: 0   1   2   3   4   Nausea: 0   1   2   3   4   Signed:

DISCHARGE DETAILS

IV : removed: Yes   No

Instruction sheet given: Yes   No

GP letter given / sent: Yes   No

Spoken to by doctor: Yes   No

Transport home:

Person collecting:

DISCHARGED TO: HOME: WARD / HOSP:

ADDITIONAL INFORMATION

RECOVERY NURSE SIGNATURE:

TIME OF DISCHARGE:

Fig. 6.4   A postoperative checklist

5. *Recovery record(Fig. 6.4)*
   – record of periodic observations
   – level of consciousness
   – oxygen or other medication required
   – complications.
6. *Discharge details*
   – discharge instructions given
   – verbal/written report of results
   – discharge criteria fulfilled
   – time left unit.

All documentation must be signed and dated by the endoscopy assistant responsible for the patient.

A patient's hospital notes must be available, including any relevant X-rays (especially for colonoscopy, ERCP and bronchoscopy) together with the referral letter or form to allow an adequate assessment of the patient to be made. Informed consent should be obtained in all cases prior to endoscopy, and this is dealt with more fully in the chapter on the law. Many units now offer the option of whether to have the procedure carried out with or without sedation, and this should be discussed as part of the admission procedure.

6.2.2 INFORMATION TECHNOLOGY

Recent years have seen the introduction of information technology packages specifically made for endoscopy units. These packages are able to book and schedule appointments, produce appointment letters and information customized to the individual patient, generate endoscopy reports, and store valuable data for clinical, research and management purposes. Some systems are 'free standing' whilst others are linked into or form part of a larger hospital-wide network. Larger units may have their own network of microcomputers enabling data to be entered simultaneously at more than one location. The introduction of the hard disk means that the amount of data stored is no longer a problem, but steps should be taken to ensure adequate backing up of information, and it may be necessary to install emergency power packs to prevent loss of data owing to power failure. Information systems of this type are invaluable for the management of the modern endoscopy unit as they allow trend analysis and projection of workloads together with clinical audit of referral trends, indications, findings and treatments against a wide range of criteria. The workload and requirements of the modern unit dictate that all but the smallest unit will require systems of this sort in the future.

6.2.3   ENDOSCOPY REPORTS

Endoscopy reports, whether handwritten or computer generated, need to be simple and concise. All should contain (Fig. 6.5):

1. Patient details and hospital identification number.
2. Reason for referral.
3. Endoscopist.
4. Instrument used.
5. Medication given and dose.
6. Type of procedure.
7. Extent of examination and findings (including visual records taken).
8. Specimens taken.
9. Conclusion and recommendations for future management.
10. Signature and date.

   Simple line diagrams of the anatomy involved are invaluable for recording findings such as ulcers or polyps, and for indicating the extent of the examination. If handwritten, reports must be legible (including carbon copies). With the advent of video endoscope technology, it is now possible to record visual images as part of the endoscopy record. This can if required be included as part of the endoscopy report or stored for recall at a future date to allow a comparison of past and present endoscopy findings to be made.

6.2.4   BOOKINGS AND APPOINTMENT SYSTEMS

All units need to have an appointment system that allows patients to be placed on an appropriate endoscopy list. Factors that influence this include: degree of urgency, type of endoscopy requested, experience of the endoscopist and time available. Many hospitals run on a 'service' basis with a formal 'endoscopy request form' (Fig. 6.6). Systems need to be versatile enough to cope with patients from a variety of sources, and provision should be made for the emergency patient requiring an immediate endoscopy, and the urgent day case who needs to bypass the normal waiting list.

   In the majority of endoscopy units, most patients are seen as day cases and are referred to the unit either by their own doctor or by another doctor involved in their treatment (Fig. 6.7). Occasionally, established 'endoscopy' patients (e.g. those with known benign oeso-phageal strictures who require periodic dilatation) may be able to refer themselves for treatment whenever symptoms return, and patients with known oesophageal varices may have an emergency admission card that allows them to be admitted immediately to the gastroenterology

ENDOSCOPY REPORT

21/02/96

MR JOHN SMITH   HOSPITAL NO : 000001
1 The Shubbery,   SEX   : Male
Near End,   DoB   : 28/02/01
Westshire.

HISTORY   : Dyspepsia
                          Dysphagia
                          Heartburn/reflux
CURRENT DRUGS   : Antacids, as required dosage,
                          Omeprazole, therapeutic dosage, 20 mg daily
BARIUM MEAL FINDINGS   : Not done

EXAMINATION   : Planned – first diagnostic OGD on 21/02/96
ENDOSCOPIST   : Dr MT Jones
INSTRUMENT   : GIF Q20
MEDICATION   : Xylocaine spray
                          Hypnovel 1 mg
SPECIMENS TAKEN   : Histology

OESOPHAGUS   : Severe streaking oesophagitis length 5 cm at 35 cm
                          Deep ulceration
                          Stricture (benign) at 40 cm
STOMACH CONTENT   : Empty/normal
STOMACH   : Normal
PYLORUS   : Normal
DUODENUM (1st)   : Normal
DUODENUM (2nd)   : 1 ulcer
                          2 mm superficial chronic anterior duodenal ulcer
PAPILLA   : Not seen
COMPLICATIONS   : None

FURTHER INVESTIGS   : None
FURTHER MANAGEMENT   : Start medical treatment
                          Omeprazole, therapeutic dosage, 20 mg BD
                          Refer for therapeutic endoscopy

Histology report to follow

We will arrange for him to have an oesophageal dilatation in 2 weeks' time.
In the mean time his dose of omeprazole has been increased to BD.

Signed: _____

        Dr MT Jones MRCP
        Registrar

Copies to : Dr. NO Blood
            The Surgery
            Near End,
            Westshire

Fig. 6.5   An example endosopy report

INPATIENT ENDOSCOPY REQUEST FORM

☐ Gastroscopy   ☐ Gastroscopy + duodenal biopsy   ☐ Oesophageal
                                                                        dilatation

☐ PEG insertion   ☐ Colonoscopy

This form must be completed in full, and delivered to the endoscopy unit in order to book cases. All bookings are at the discretion of the nurse manager. Requests for colonscopies must all be discussed with the GI team before they can be accepted.

Hospital No.	....	WARD	....
Patient name	....	CONSULTANT	....
Address	....	GP NAME	....
	....	GP PRACTICE	....
Post code	....	TRANSFER ON	☐ CHAIR
Date of birth	....		☐ BED

Clinical details _____

_____

Other medical problems (Tick if applicable)

☐ Valvular heart disease   ☐ Previous gastric surgery   ☐ MRSA

Diabetes :   ☐ Insulin   ☐ Barium study in past 48 hours   ☐ HIV
              ☐ Tablets
              ☐ Diet   ☐ Warfarin (if yes: INR .... DATE ....)

☐ Severe heart or   ☐ Drug allergy ....
respiratory failure

All patients *must* consent on the ward

Referring doctor ....   Bleep no. .... Date ....
          (Print name)

          Endoscopy use: List ..../ Endoscribe / Ward told /   /

Fig. 6.6   An inpatient endoscopy request form

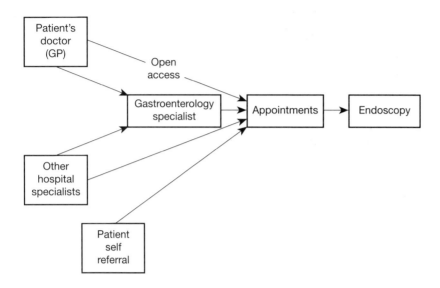

Fig. 6.7 Referral sources

ward of the hospital treating them should they have an acute haemate-mesis. Hospital inpatients are seen either as part of the investigation of their illness or as a planned admission for a particular type of endo-scopy (e.g. ERCP).

Day-case appointments

Most units operate a staggered appointment system whereby day cases arrive at intervals throughout the day. This helps to minimize waiting times and reduces the waiting area requirements of the unit. Because of a variety of local problems or constraints, some units run a block appointment system where all day cases to be seen that session arrive at one time and are seen in rotation. This means that some patients have a long, often anxious wait before being endoscoped. It can also double the waiting area needed, and is more likely to encourage patient complaints.

Patients to be seen as day cases need to be sent a clear appointment, any specific preparation or dietary instructions required, details of how to find the unit, discharge information and information about the endoscopy to be performed (Fig. 6.8). Many companies provide useful information booklets for use in this situation, but it is probably best if these are customized to suit the individual unit. Because of the problems of obtaining informed consent from day cases (Chapter 5), many units also include a copy of the consent form the patient will be asked to sign,

Hospital No / DoB 00001

Dear MR SMITH

Arrangements have been made to admit you as a day case to ward (Annexe one) endoscopy unit of this hospital on 8TH APRIL 1996 under the care of DR . . . . . . and I should be glad if you would come in at 8.15 am.

The examination of your **stomach** will take place at **Annexe one ward (endoscopy unit)** which is situated at the Edwards Lane end of the city hospital and should be approached via gate 4. Take the first turning on your left, then first turning on the right. You will see the sliding doors to the main corridor. Enter through these doors and take the next corridor on the left. You will find the endoscopy unit at the bottom of the corridor.

Please do not eat or drink anything from midnight the previous evening as you will be given a sedative. You will not be able to drive yourself home or return back to work that day, or use public transport. **YOU MUST ARRANGE FOR A FRIEND OR RELATIVE TO COLLECT YOU FROM ANNEXE ONE WARD AND TAKE YOU HOME BY CAR OR TAXI. YOU WILL NOT BE ALLOWED OFF THE WARD WITHOUT AN ESCORT; PLEASE DO NOT MAKE ARRANGEMENTS TO MEET PEOPLE IN THE CAR PARK OR AT THE MAIN ENTRANCE AS YOU WILL NOT BE ALLOWED TO GO AND MEET THEM.**

You will be ready for collection from the unit at 12.30 pm. Bring any medication that you are taking and a dressing gown with you.

If you require an ambulance car or ambulance, please ring the unit on the above number, at least 3 days before your appointment, so we can arrange this for you.

Please leave **ALL** valuables at home. The hospital cannot accept responsibility for patients' money or valuables.

If for any reason you are unable to keep this appointment or if you need further information, please do not hesitate to contact me on the above number between 9.00 am and 12 noon.

Yours sincerely

Fig. 6.8   An example patient notification letter

and information on the risks involved for that type of endoscopy and possible alternative investigations.

Inpatient appointments

Urgent inpatient endoscopy requests should, wherever possible, be scheduled on to the next available list. Non-urgent requests can be scheduled some days in advance as part of the planned investigation of the patient. In some cases it is possible for these patients to be discharged from hospital and seen as an urgent day case.

All inpatients should, wherever possible, be visited by a nurse or doctor from the endoscopy unit to explain the investigation. This can be reinforced by written information. A short while spent with a patient explaining what is going to happen does a lot to relieve anxiety, and helps ensure the patient is able to make an informed decision about their treatment when consent is asked for.

6.2.5   OPEN ACCESS (RAPID ACCESS)

This is a service offered by many endoscopy units that allows a doctor to refer their patient directly to the unit for endoscopy (Fig. 6.9). In effect, the unit carries out the test on behalf of the doctor, and sends them the result. It is popular with GPs as it allows them to manage their patient's treatment without referral to a specialist, and has been shown to reduce the number of patient visits to their doctor over the next year (even if the endoscopy was normal), presumably because the patient is reassured that nothing serious is wrong. However, because the patient is not seen by the endoscopist (or any other member of the unit team) prior to attending the unit, strict referral criteria need to be laid down, and all patients should complete a medical questionnaire (Fig. 6.10) prior to attendance so that the risks of endoscopy can be assessed at time of admission and appropriate action taken. For this reason, the endoscopy assistant will need to spend more time on assessing the 'open access' patient than would normally be required, and due account of this needs to be taken when booking these lists. Open access has been shown to be very successful at the early detection of cancers, particularly oesophageal and gastric, at a stage when they are still treatable and, because of the potential danger of the pathology reports for these patients being 'missed', many hospitals have a system whereby the care of the patient is automatically taken over by a specialist if a cancer is suspected.

It is also important that the system is regularly audited and feedback given to referring doctors about the appropriateness of their requests, number of normal investigations and pathology found.

REFERRAL FOR OPEN ACCESS GASTROSCOPY

PLEASE COMPLETE INFORMATION AS PROMPTED WITH TICK OR CIRCLE.

GUIDELINES:
Referral for open access gastroscopy is appropriate for the following patients:
1. Severe dyspepsia for 2 weeks or more.
2. GI bleeds not requiring admission.
3. Dysphagia.
4. Recurrent GI symptoms after treatment.
5. Recurrent symptoms from known gastric ulcer.

Investigation of cause of ANAEMIA should be referred direct to Dr . . . . consultant gastroenterologist, and will be seen as an outpatient within 2 weeks of referral.

INSULIN-DEPENDENT DIABETICS, patients with INFECTIVE GASTROENTERITIS, and those who have, or are at 'high risk' of HIV/HEPATITIS B are not suitable for open access gastroscopy. A direct referral to a consultant is preferred.

PATIENT DETAILS:

Name ....   Occupation ....

Address ....   Date of birth ....

....   Sex   M/F

.... Postcode ....   Tel: ....

G.P. ....   Surgery ....

Previous hospital contact?	Yes	No
Hospital number	Consultant	

PLEASE RETURN THIS FORM TO: SURGERY STAMP

Open access gastroscopy
Endoscopy unit

FAX NO: ....

REQUESTS MAY ALSO BE SENT BY FAX DIRECT TO THE UNIT ON . . . .

In case of difficulty telephone . . . . between 8.00 am and 3.00 pm Monday–Friday. There is also an 'out-of-hours' answerphone service on either of the above numbers.

[PTO]

Fig. 6.9   (a) An open access referral form

CLINICAL DETAILS OF PATIENT:

1. History of dyspepsia? | Yes | No | 2. Previous gastric surgery? | Yes | No |

   Details: ....

3. Duration of current principal symptoms? | ....yrs | ......wks | ....days |

   Symptoms:

Abdominal pain	Heartburn/reflux	Nausea	
Prev. GU ?	Vomiting	Anorexia	Weight loss
Dysphagia	Melaena	Haematemesis	

   In last week? | Yes | No |

4. Is patient being treated for their symptoms? .... | Yes | No |

   If so what treatment?

H$_2$ blockade	Antacids	Denol
Proton pump inhib.	Motility agents	

   Specify ....
   Dose ....
   Duration ....

   Other medication (other than above) ....

5. Has patient been taking aspirin? | Yes | No | or NSAIDs? | Yes | No |

6. Has patient previously had a barium meal or endoscopy? | Yes | No |

   Result: ....

7. Any other problems? | No | Yes |

e.g. Diabetes	diet control	oral agents	insulin*
Cardiac	angina	valve disease	recent MI	warfarin
Chest	COAD		asthma
Other (specify)	ALLERGY	HIV*	HEPATITIS B*	

*See guidelines

8. Smoking | Yes | No | .... day/week   Alcohol | Yes | No | .... units/wk

9. Any other information e.g. Haemoglobin? ....
   ....

10. Do you want *Helicobacter* status assessed, if appropriate? | Yes | No |

11. Diagnosis expected? ....

I would prefer	Report and brief advice only	Report and follow-up at the discretion of endoscopist

   Signature of GP .... Referral date ....

Fig. 6.9 (b) A clinical record form

PRE-ENDOSCOPY QUESTIONNAIRE

PLEASE COMPLETE THIS FORM AND BRING IT WITH YOU WHEN ATTENDING FOR ENDOSCOPY

Before we carry out this examination, we would be grateful if you would complete the following questionnaire about your health. This is designed to help the doctors and nurses who will be looking after you. If you have any difficulty in answering a question, please either consult your own doctor (GP) or telephone the endoscopy unit between 9.00 am and 3.00 pm Monday–Friday on: . . . .

PERSONAL DETAILS:
Surname .... Date of birth ....
First names ....
Address ....
....
.... Tel: ....

OTHER THAN THE REASON FOR YOUR REFERRAL:
(a) How would you rate your general health? (please tick)

Excellent ☐   Good ☐   Fair ☐   Poor ☐

(b) Has there been a recent change in health?

No ☐   Yes ☐   Comment:

(c) Do you have or have you ever had any of these problems?   (please circle)

Heart attack or heart failure
Stroke
Lung problems (e.g. asthma, pneumonia, emphysema)
Liver problems or hepatitis
High blood pressure
Diabetes
Bleeding problems
Seizures or epilepsy
Rheumatic fever
Other (please specify) ....

(d) Please list any medicines you are taking (include ALL prescription and nonprescription drugs, even asprin and 'the pill').

1 ....   6 ....
2 ....   7 ....
3 ....   8 ....
4 ....   9 ....
5 ....   10 ....

(e) Are you allergic or sensitive to anything e.g. medicines or adhesive tape?

No ☐   Yes ☐   Please list ....
....

(f) Have you, or any close relative, had problems with anaesthetics or sedation?

No ☐   Yes ☐   If 'Yes', what problems? ....
....

(g) Is there any significant possibility of you being infected with hepatitis B or HIV?

No ☐   Yes ☐

(h) Do you have any other health problem at present?

No ☐   Yes ☐   If 'Yes', what problem? ....
....

THANK YOU FOR YOUR CO-OPERATION.

Fig. 6.10   A pre-endoscopy questionnaire form

6.2.6   DISCHARGE INFORMATION

Verbal and written instructions should be given to all patients prior to discharge.

It is usual for written instructions to include details of the procedure performed, what the patient should do or not do and for how long, and relevant details of how the patient may feel and any particular symptoms to report their doctor. Most units also give a contact telephone number where someone is available to give a patient advice should this be required. Written instructions are important as the patient may not otherwise remember what has been said. If possible, it is wise also to give verbal instructions to relatives or friends collecting the patient, being careful not to breach patient confidentiality.

Many patients wish to speak to a doctor after their endoscopy, and this should be granted whenever possible. Again, it is best if a relative or friend is present as the patient may not remember what has been said, and if results are not immediately available then an indication should be given as to when they will be available and how they may be obtained.

It is helpful that if patients are returned to hospital wards to recover then guidelines are given to ward nursing staff on the postprocedure management of their patient. Unfortunately, ward staff often have little knowledge of endoscopy, and written guidelines can at the least help them to provide appropriate care. A longer term aim of all units should be to provide adequate training for ward staff in the management of patients undergoing endoscopic investigation and treatment.

6.3   QUALITY ASSURANCE

6.3.1   THE NEED FOR QUALITY ASSURANCE

Quality assurance is required to protect ourselves and our patients.

Ourselves

Social
Nurses are charged by their professional codes of conduct. Each registered nurse, midwife and health visitor has accountability for his or her practice, and needs to justify both actions and omissions.

Political
This is based on the idea that if you don't do it, someone else will (e.g. commercially produced quality measurement tools, which may not be best for your area).

Personal

Nurses want to improve care and develop best practice, but have not been able to standardize their approach.

Professional

Nurses are accorded high status by the public, and are held up as experts in their field. They have long sought to achieve autonomy from doctors, and quality assurance allows the development of autonomous practice. Quality assurance emphasizes training of nurses, and highlights the need for a sound academic basis for care. By developing specially trained nurses who anticipate and meet the needs of their patients, the possibility for complaints, litigation and complications is reduced.

Patients

Quality assurance allows us to examine our practice in the following areas:

1. *Access to services*; do all patients have fair access to waiting list services, e.g. waiting list analysis?
2. *Relevance to need*; is a service provided that meets the needs of the local population? Are the set targets achieved, e.g. screening figures?
3. *Effectiveness*; does the nursing action achieve the desired result, e.g. comparison of sedation practice with protocols, relapse rates for *H. pylori*-positive patients?
4. *Equity*; what is the fairness of a service and its availability to minority groups: waiting lists, information available in a variety of languages?
5. *Acceptability*; is it acceptable to the community you serve, e.g. do patients have to travel elsewhere for services, what is the timing of services?
6. *Efficiency and economy*; are the resources used relative to an effective service, e.g. patient satisfaction and surveys?

• Quality care and assurance are probably being undertaken in many units, but are not being approached in a structured way. Undertaking quality assurance allows evaluation of care and comparison and change of practice. Documentation of these events provides written evidence of the process.

Examples include:
rewriting an admission form
offering an informed choice on throat spray or sedation to patients

named-nurse approach to care
reviewing care around PEG placements.

Quality assurance can be started by any member of the team.

6.3.2 IMPROVEMENT OF CARE BY QUALITY ASSURANCE

Staff learn and take on new skills as a continuing process. Training
professional endoscopy nurses allows patients to receive research- and
evidence-based care. This reduces the risk of complications and litigation.

Communication systems also improve among patients, nurses and
other health care disciplines. Understanding what is going on breaks
down barriers. By developing a framework from which to practise, the
nurse's position is strengthened. Reference to agreed standards can
provide backing for better facilities and more resources.

It also leads to a shared sense of purpose in the endoscopy unit. Staff
morale increases as what is expected of each team member becomes
clearer. Problem solving becomes easier, as problems are easier to
highlight, and taking action to solve them is more likely. Each team
member feels able to make a difference.

6.3.3 SETTING STANDARDS

A **standard** is an agreed statement of the level at which a service should
be delivered. It is in written form, against which current practice can be
measured. It states what action will occur.

A **criterion** is an element of a standard that can be measured – for
example, admission, discharge, care of valuables, etc. A target should
be included to measure how many times the criterion should be
achieved. Ideas or concern regarding an aspect of care will lead to the
formation of individual standards.

For example, take the following statement: 'each patient shall receive
written information of their endoscopy result and follow-up care on
discharge from the unit'.

Criterion   =   endoscopy result and follow-up care
Target   =   all patients 100%.

All standards use the framework structure–process–outcome as a basis
for working (Fig. 6.11).

- *Structure*; Who and what is needed to make the standard happen?
  This includes resources, time, skills, equipment, etc.
- *Process*; How will it be done? This includes direct care, information
  sheets, patient education, etc. How will data be collected? Where will
  it be found?

STANDARDS OF CARE

TOPIC Admission	APPLICATION TO Endoscopy unit
SUBTOPIC Named nurse	STANDARDS COMPILED BY Endoscopy standard setting group
STANDARD NO. 1	AGREED BY

STANDARD STATEMENT Clients attending the endoscopy unit will be allocated a named nurse.

STRUCTURE
1. DOH The Patient's Charter (a named qualified nurse, midwife or health visitor responsible for each patient)
2. Trained and experienced staff.
3. Assessment forms.
4. Local charter: always have our staff introduce themselves and clearly display name badges.

PROCESS
Named nurse will introduce self to client and document it on the assessment forms.

All staff will wear name badges.

OUTCOME
Clients will be allocated and introduced to their named nurse when attending the endoscopy unit.

Fig. 6.11 Standards of care form

- *Outcome*; What do you hope to achieve? What will be the effect of the care on the patient and the unit? How will the results be measured to establish whether the standard has been met?

This framework allows documentation of ideas in a way that can be measured.

Structure

Nurses need to be aware of patients' results and follow-up care planned. These include:

- Knowledge of health promotion and medical conditions.
- Area available for advice, information and discussion.
- Availability of other professionals, e.g. medical staff/dietitian/support nurse.
- Patient discharge form includes criteria for discharge.
- GP/community support available.

Process

The nurse includes on the patient discharge sheet:

- Brief summary of findings to the patient's level of understanding.
- Info sheets, further information and contacts.
- The nurse then evaluates the patient's level of understanding prior to discharge.

Outcome

- The discharge section of the care plan is completed.
- Patient can explain his results and follow-up care if asked.
- There is a reduction in number of calls from patients related to discharge information given.
- Any contacts/support services are arranged prior to discharge.

  Quality assurance is a continuing process.

6.3.4 MEASURING WHAT HAS BEEN ACHIEVED

Each standard has to be measurable, so that practice can be compared with it. Guidelines used when measuring standards are often referred to as 'RUMBA', as each standard should be:

Relevant – to the aim and objective of the study.
Understandable – simple and clear. Each standard should be one idea.

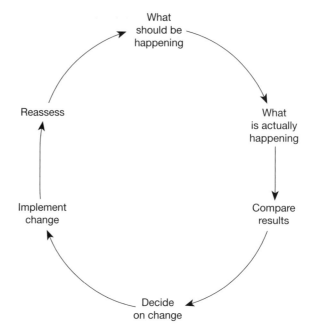

Fig. 6.12   (a) The audit cycle

Measurable – preferably by a simple yes/no answer.
Behaviour/observable – the criterion can be observed, and therefore measured.
Achievable – avoiding unrealistic expectation.

For instance, ideas and standards in endoscopy units could address the following remarks:

1. 'Everyone should have proper training before they work with glutaraldehyde.'
   Each member of the endoscopy unit will receive training on the safe use of glutaraldehyde, in accordance with local and national policies and guidelines.
2. 'Some patients don't get their appointments until the day before – this causes them difficulty.'
   All outpatients will receive at least 48 hours notice of their endoscopy appointment.
3. 'I don't like my patients leaving watches and money on the trolleys.'
   All patients will be offered a safe place to store their valuables.
4. 'The Patient's Charter states each patient should have a named nurse.'
   Each patient will have a named nurse assigned to them in endoscopy, and will meet them within 30 minutes of arrival.

```
+-----------------------------------------------------------------+
|                          AUDIT FORM                             |
|                                                                 |
|                                                                 |
|  STANDARD:                                                      |
|                                                                 |
|  DATE:                                                          |
|                                                                 |
|  AUDITED BY:                                                    |
|                                                                 |
|  CRITERIA ACHIEVED/NOT ACHIEVED:                                |
|                                                                 |
|  % OF COMPLIANCE:                                               |
|                                                                 |
|  COMMENTS:                                                      |
|                                                                 |
|                                                                 |
|  DATE OF REAUDIT:                                               |
|                                                                 |
+-----------------------------------------------------------------+
```

Fig 6.12   (b) An audit form

By keeping the standard simple, it is easy to change each statement into a question, to allow the standard to be audited (Fig. 6.12) to see whether it measures up to what it sets out to do.

To measure the previous standard, a sample of care plans can be examined, and the following questions asked:

- Did you understand what your endoscopy had found?
- Did you receive written instructions for follow-up care?
- Was the discharge section of the care plan completed?

Using these findings, changes can take place leading to improvements in patient care and working systems. Writing standards is challenging. However, nurses find that undertaking quality assurance clarifies everyone's responsibilities and creates a forum for discussing all aspects of care. The experience also helps each nurse to participate fully in various quality assurance programmes developing throughout the country. Most importantly of all, it will equip nurses to provide a quality nursing service.

BIBLIOGRAPHY

Katz, J. and Green, E. (1992) *Managing Quality: a Guide to Monitoring and Evaluating Nursing Services.*

Kitson, A. (1989) *A Framework for Quality: a Patient Centred Approach to Quality Assurance in Health Care*, RCN Scutari Press, London.

Nursing Times (1992) NT Open Learning Package M5 *(1–4)*, 88, 39–42.

Robertson, L. (1992) *Quality Assurance for Nurses*, Longman, Harlow.

Infection control and decontamination of equipment

7

Introduction 7A

Fiona Donald

Flexible endoscopy is now a common clinical procedure and the infection rate following it is thought to be small. An American survey done in 1974 suggested that the infection rate was of the order of one infection per 10 000 cases (Silvis *et al.*, 1976). A similar survey in the UK found that infection was more often associated with ERCP than with other procedures (Colin-Jones, Cocker and Schiller, 1978). Since then there have been no large prospective studies to look at post-endoscopy infections, but it is generally felt that the risk is small as long as recommended guidelines for cleaning and disinfecting equipment are followed (Spach, Silverstein and Stamm, 1993).

Infection may arise after endoscopy by one of three routes (Table 7A.1). During a procedure the endoscope may be contaminated with bacteria or viruses that the patient is either carrying as commensals, or is infected with, in gastrointestinal or respiratory tracts (Plate 1,). If the endoscope is not adequately cleaned and disinfected between patients these organisms will persist on the endoscope and could infect the next patient on the list. Any organisms could be transmitted in this way; the commonest ones that have been reported are *Salmonella* spp., *Mycobacterium tuberculosis*, *Pseudomonas aeruginosa* and hepatitis B virus. There are several reports (Chahal and Armstrong, 1976; O'Connor *et al.*, 1982) of outbreaks of *Salmonella* spp. being transmitted during gastrointestinal endoscopy following the use of contaminated equipment, where it is likely that inadequate cleaning and use of inappropriate disinfectants was the cause. During bronchoscopy there is a risk of transmitting *M. tuberculosis* between patients as it is relatively more resistant to disinfectants, and a longer disinfection time is needed. Cross-infection from patient to patient has been reported following the use of non-glutaraldehyde disinfectants (Nelson *et al.*, 1983). Any type of endoscopic procedure carries a risk of transmitting bloodborne

Practical Endoscopy Edited by M. Shephard and J. Mason. Published in 1997 by Chapman & Hall, London. ISBN 0 412 54000 2

Table 7A.1 Routes of infection and organisms reported to cause infections following endoscopy

Route of infection	Organisms that have been reported
Patient to patient – by inadequately cleaned or disinfected equipment	*Salmonella* spp. *Campylobacter pylori* *Ps. aeruginosa* *M. tuberculosis* Atypical mycobacteria Hepatitis B virus
Environment to patient – contaminated equipment	*P. aeruginosa* *Klebsiella* spp. *M. chelonae*
Autologous infection – patient's own organisms	Examples: Enterococci (endocarditis) *Escherichia coli* (septicaemia)

viruses such as hepatitis B and HIV. The risk is probably small as these viruses are readily killed by many disinfectants, but there has been a documented case of hepatitis B that occurred after gastrointestinal endoscopy (Birnie *et al.*, 1983).

The other source of contamination of instruments is the environment, and this may happen if the instrument is washed or rinsed in contaminated solutions. Some environmental bacteria may be relatively resistant to disinfectants and may persist in the channels and valves of the endoscope, particularly if any material such as blood or faeces remains after washing. Gram-negative bacilli such as *P. aeruginosa* or *Klebsiella* spp. may survive and grow in cleaning solutions, containers and rinse water (Babb, 1993). Once deposited in the channels of the endoscope they may proliferate overnight and hence be inoculated into the patient who may then develop pneumonia or septicaemia. Pseudomonas infections have been reported following ERCP and some patients have died of septicaemia (Earnshaw, Clark and Thom, 1985).

Immunocompromised patients are a group who are more at risk of contracting infections after procedures and are also susceptible to infections with organisms that may not infect a healthy person. Environmental organisms such as *Ps. aeruginosa* and atypical mycobacteria may cause pneumonia in such patients following bronchoscopy (Sammartino, Israel and Magnussen, 1982).

Environmental mycobacteria, or atypical mycobacteria, are widespread in the environment and are often found in tap water. If instruments are rinsed in tap water after disinfection they may become contaminated with these bacteria (Babb, 1993). This could be a problem

for immunocompromised patients, but they can also contaminate micro-
biology specimens taken through the endoscope and lead to a false
diagnosis.

Automatic washing machines and thus the endoscopes may become
contaminated with *Mycobacterium chelonae*, an atypical mycobacterium that is found in water supplies (Fraser *et al.*, 1992). The
bacteria may be difficult to remove from the machines as they form a
biofilm which protects them from the disinfectants.

The third route by which a patient may become infected after
endoscopy is by organisms carried by the patient as commensals. The
respiratory and gastrointestinal tracts are not sterile and autologous
infection such as septicaemia or endocarditis can occur when bacteria
enter the bloodstream during a procedure. This type of infection can be
minimized by good technique and the use of prophylactic antibiotics in
at-risk patients.

REFERENCES

Babb, J.R. (1993) Disinfection and sterilization of endoscopes. *Curr Opin Infect Dis*, **6**, 532–7.

Birnie, G.G., Quigley, E.M., Clements, G.B. *et al.* (1983) Endoscopic transmission of hepatitis B virus. *Gut*, **24**, 171–4.

Chahal, H. and Armstrong, D. (1976) *Salmonella oslo*. A focal outbreak in a hospital. *Am J Med*, **60**, 203–8.

Colin-Jones, D.G., Cocker, R. and Schiller, K.F.R. (1978) Current endoscopic practice in the United Kingdom. *Clin Gastroenterol*, **7**, 775–86.

Earnshaw, J.J., Clark, A.W. and Thom, B.T. (1985) Outbreak of *Pseudomonas aeruginosa* following endoscopic retrograde cholangiopancreatography. *J Hosp Infect*, **6**, 95–7.

Fraser, V.J., Jones, M., Murray, P.R. *et al.* (1992) Contamination of flexible fibreoptic bronchoscopes with *Mycobacterium chelonae* linked to an auto-mated bronchoscope disinfection machine. *Am Rev Respir Dis*, **145**, 853–5.

Nelson, K.E., Larson, P.A., Schraufnagel, D.E. and Jackson, J. (1983) Transmission of tuberculosis by flexible fibrebronchoscopes. *Am Rev Respir Dis*, **127**, 97–100.

O'Connor, B.H., Bennett, J.R., Alexander, J.G. *et al.* (1982) Salmonellosis infection transmitted by fibreoptic endoscopes. *Lancet*, **2**, 864–6.

Sammartino, M.T., Israel, R.H., and Magnussen, C.R. (1982) *Pseudomonas aeruginosa* contamination of fibreoptic bronchoscopes. *J Hosp Infect*, **3**, 65–71.

Silvis, S.E., Nebel, O., Rogers, G. *et al.* (1976) Endoscopic complications. Results of the 1974 American Society for Gastrointestinal Endoscopy survey. *JAMA*, **235**, 928–30.

Spach, D.H., Silverstein, F.E., and Stamm, W.E. (1993) Transmission of infection by gastrointestinal endoscopy and bronchoscopy. *Ann Intern Med*, **118**, 117–28.

Methods of disinfection and sterilization 7B

Julie D'Silva

7B.1 INTRODUCTION

All items of endoscopy equipment and accessories must be decontaminated before use. The process of decontamination involves cleaning (either manually or machine aided), followed by either sterilization or disinfection.

Cleaning is a process by which organic material and micro-organisms are physically removed from the item involved. It may, but does not necessarily, destroy any micro-organisms present.

Sterilization is a process that produces an item free from viable micro-organisms including viruses and spores, and should be considered as the ultimate goal in the decontamination of all items of endoscopic equipment.

The aim of disinfection is to reduce the number of viable micro-organisms present to a level where they are unlikely to initiate infection. Disinfectants may be inactive against certain micro-organisms (e.g. mycobacteria) and are generally not very effective against spores. As far as chemical disinfectants are concerned, whether an item is disinfected or sterilized generally depends on the contact time. (Glutaraldehyde can disinfect an endoscope in 10 minutes, but may take up to 10 hours to sterilize it.)

Endoscopy is generally classified as a non-invasive technique as the endoscope comes into contact only with intact mucous membrane and there is no infiltration into sterile cavities. However, procedures such as ERCP, hysteroscopy and cystoscopy should be considered as invasive as

Practical Endoscopy Edited by M. Shephard and J. Mason. Published in 1997 by Chapman & Hall, London. ISBN 0 412 54000 2

normally sterile body cavities are entered. The choice of decontamination process depends on the heat stability of the item involved. Many accessories are heat stable, and can therefore be sterilized by a heat process such as autoclaving. However, flexible endoscopes are heat sensitive and liable to damage when subjected to temperatures in excess of 60 °C. For this reason, cleaning followed by chemical disinfection is usually the chosen method of decontamination (Table 7B.1). The higher the level of disinfection required, the longer is the immersion time. Other methods such as ethylene oxide sterilization are available, but are not generally used. High-level disinfection eliminates all vegetative organisms, but not all spores.

7B.2   STERILIZATION METHODS

7B.2.1   STEAM STERILIZATION

A bench-top or downward displacement autoclave that sterilizes at 121 °C for 15 minutes or 134 °C for 3 minutes is suitable for sterilizing some flexible endoscopy accessories.

Low-temperature steam and formaldehyde

Low-temperature steam and formaldehyde are suitable for accessories that will not tolerate high temperatures or which may become damaged by repeated autoclaving. This type of sterilization is not readily available in all hospitals and, because of the hazards associated with formaldehydes, strict supervision and specially trained staff must be available for its safe use. If a quick turnaround of accessories is required this method would not be suitable.

Autoclave

Steam autoclaving is the preferred method for sterilizing heat-tolerant endoscopic accessories. This involves the use of steam heated to 134–7 °C at a pressure of 3.2 bar for 3.5 minutes. The process of heating, cooling and drying increases the total cycle time to around 30 minutes.

Endoscopic accessories that are designed to be reprocessed must be supplied by the manufacturers with information concerning the preferred method of decontamination and there may be also restrictions on the number of times a certain accessory may be reused. In these situations a system of individual marking and recording of use is required.

7B.2.2   ETHYLENE OXIDE

Ethylene oxide sterilization is suitable for rigid endoscopes that are not heat tolerant and most flexible endoscopes. The disadvantage of ethylene oxide is that it is a slow process (37 °C or 55 °C for a period of $3\frac{1}{2}$ – 5 hours) and is therefore not viable in situations where rapid turnaround times are required.

Ethylene oxide penetrates materials such as plastic and rubber and an air-venting time of up to 7 hours or longer is required to ensure total removal of the gas. Sterilization is confirmed by testing for spore activity and this can take a further 7 days. However, where sterilization of a flexible endoscope is required then ethylene oxide is an alternative option. Ethylene oxide is not always available and has strict environmental controls because of its toxicity.

7B.2.3   CHEMICAL

It is possible to sterilize an endoscope by chemical means. Immersion times vary from between 3 and 10 hours depending on the chemical used. Shorter periods do not destroy spores and provide high-level disinfection only. Peracetic acid-based products appear to provide sterilization in shorter periods (10 minutes) and are therefore suitable for use in situations where a high degree of sterility is required such as ERCP, cystoscopy and hysteroscopy.

7B.2.4   GAS PLASMA

This is a little-used but alternative method of sterilization. It works by applying energy, in the form of high temperatures and electromagnetic fields, to a gas under vacuum conditions, resulting in the formation of a highly reactive gas plasma. The most commonly known of these systems is 'Sterrad', which produces a low-temperature hydrogen peroxide gas plasma with temperatures of less than 50 °C. The full process takes 75 minutes so it would therefore not be of benefit to endoscopy units with a fast turnaround, but it is said that no toxic emissions or residues result from the cycle.

7B.3   DISINFECTION METHODS

7B.3.1   CHEMICAL DISINFECTION

Chemical disinfection is the most commonly used method in endoscopy. The ideal chemical disinfectant should possess the following qualities:

Table 7B.1   Decontamination of endoscopes and accessories: options in sterilization/disinfection processes

Process	Time/temperature	Comments
Low-temperature steam (disinfectant)	73–80 °C for 20 min	Suitable for accessories only
Low-temperature steam and (sterilant) formaldehyde.	73–80 °C for 2–3 hours	Suitable for accessories only Slow: strict environmental controls
Steam autoclave (sterilant)	134–7 °C for 3.5 min 121–4 °C for 15 min	Preferred method for reusable accessories Ruins (melts) flexible endoscopes
Dry heat (disinfectant)	70–1 °C for 3 min, 80 °C for 1 min, 90 °C for 1 second	Suitable for accessories only Not widely used
Ethylene oxide (sterilant)	37–55 °C for 3–5 hours	Suitable for flexible endoscopes and accessories Slow: subject to strict environmental controls. Total process can take over 1 week
Gas plasma (sterilant)	75 min	Suitable for flexible endoscopes and accessories Slow: not widely used
Glutaraldehyde 2% (disinfectant)	10–60 min immersion at room temp.	Widely used. Flexible endoscopes/accessories Irritant and sensitizer Subject to strict environmental controls
(sterilant)	3–10 hours immersion at room temp.	Slow so not used widely. Comments above apply
Peracetic acid 0.35% (disinfectant)	5 min at room temp.	Suitable for flexible endoscopes/accessories May damage lens cement Flammable Check compatibility with manufacturer
0.2% [Steris] (sterilant)	10 min at room temp. 12 min at 50–6 °C	As above
Chlorine dioxide (sterilant)	10 min at room temp.	Suitable for flexible endoscopes/accessories
(disinfectant)	5 min at room temp.	Check compatibility with manufacturer. Unstable at high temperatures and can give off toxic fumes
Sterox (sterilant)	5 min at room temp.	Suitable for flexible/rigid endoscopes/accessories. Environmentally friendly

Table 7B.1   Continued

Process	Time/temperature	Comments
Alcohol 70% (isopropyl or ethanol) (disinfectant)	5–10 min at room temp.	Suitable for flexible endoscopes/accessories Not widely used; may damage lens cement Not very effective against TB
Quarternary ammonium compounds (disinfectant)	2 min at room temp.	Suitable for flexible endoscopes/accessories Poor activity against viruses, fungi and spores Should be followed by 4 min in 70% alcohol for adequate disinfection in gastrointestinal procedures

1. It should produce rapid disinfection with activity against a wide range of micro-organisms including *M. tuberculosis* and the hepatitis B and HIV viruses.
2. It should have no adverse effects upon lens systems or their cement mounts, and should be compatible with common surgical materials such as carbon, steel, copper, brass, nickel, chrome plate and aluminium, etc., used in endoscopes and automatic disinfectors.
3. It should not be irritant to users.
4. It should not be irritant to tissues.
5. It should not be inactivated by detergents or organic matter such as blood, pus or serum, nor should it coagulate protein.
6. It should not require complicated dilution procedures for different purposes.
7. It should be economical to use.

None of the currently available chemical disinfectants satisfies these criteria. Currently, aldehyde-based disinfectants such as glutaraldehyde probably come closest, although manufacturers are constantly researching new chemical solutions aimed at finding an effective, user-friendly disinfectant.

Although widely used, the main problem with chemical disinfection is that, for a disinfectant to be effective, it has to kill living tissue (micro-organisms) and is therefore also likely to be harmful to humans.

Glutaraldehyde/aldehydes

Aldehydes including glutaraldehyde are the most commonly used chemical disinfectants. In 1992 a survey undertaken to look at the use of aldehydes in endoscopy units proved that 98.6% were using glutaraldehyde; out of the 215 questionnaires returned, 213 were using it (Wickes, 1992). Aldehydes are toxic, irritant and hazardous to health if not used correctly. They are subject to strict environmental controls. Glutaraldehyde is supplied as a 2% aqueous solution, which has to be activated by the addition of sodium bicarbonate. Once activated it has effective fungicidal, sporicidal, bactericidal and viricidal properties. It is not corrosive to most materials and therefore does not erode endoscopes. It is not easily inactivated by organic material but penetrates slowly.

Advantages

1. It produces rapid disinfection to ensure quick turnaround of endoscopes.
2. It does not require complicated dilution procedures for different purposes.
3. It is not inactivated by organic matter such as blood, pus or serum, although the activity is reduced by detergents, and in the presence of a heavy organic load.
4. It does not coagulate protein.
5. It is economical in use.

Disadvantages

Glutaraldehyde solutions are designed to kill micro-organisms and are classified by the Health and Safety Executive as irritants with a threshold limit of 0.2 ppm occupation exposure standard. Regulations relating to the control of substances hazardous to health (COSHH) require employers to assess the risk to the health of employees from using toxic substances of which glutaraldehyde is one (section 7B.4).

The main disadvantages are as follows:

1. Glutaraldehyde is an irritant and sensitizer.
2. The vapour phase may cause conjunctivitis, rhinitis and asthma.
3. The liquid phase may cause dermatitis.
4. Other non-specific symptoms may be headache, nausea, vomiting, dizziness and slowed reactions.
5. Fume extraction may be required when glutaraldehyde is used in order to comply with COSHH regulations. This may not always be feasible (e.g. in the X-ray department), and other methods of disinfection may have to be considered.
6. It reacts violently with oxidizing agents and therefore should be stored alone.

The effectiveness of glutaraldehyde is enhanced by increasing the temperature of the solution.

The Soluscope machine uses a 0.125% solution of glutaraldehyde heated to a temperature of 45 °C with a contact time of 5 minutes. Independent reports have shown this to be a highly effective disinfectant that is more active than the standard 2% solution, particularly with respect to *M. tuberculosis*.

Peracetic acid

Peracetic acid is a peroxygen compound, which has been reported as having bactericidal, tuberculocidal, fungicidal, viricidal and sporicidal qualities. Examples of disinfectants that have peracetic acid as their base are the Steris system and Nu-Cidex.

Peracetic acid in its natural state is highly corrosive, so a corrosion inhibitor is usually included in the formulation.

Advantages

1. Use of peracetic acid results in disinfection in 5 minutes and sterilization in 10 minutes.
2. It is suitable for operating theatre areas where sterility is important or for procedures ideally requiring sterile equipment such as ERCP, cystoscopy and hysteroscopy.

Disadvantages

1. It may damage lens cements with repeated disinfection.
2. It is flammable.
3. It is highly irritant when used at high concentrations. There have been reports of burns to hands or arms with accidental contact.
4. It is corrosive unless a corrosion inhibitor is used in the formulation and should therefore be used with caution with certain metals.
5. When activated to provide the correct concentration it can be used for only 24 hours. Currently available preparations are expensive and could prove to be uneconomical to use in some areas.
6. It is a toxic substance and therefore likely to be hazardous to health although it is not currently subject to the same controls as the aldehyde disinfectants.

The Steris system is probably the best-tried system using peracetic acid and it has many advantages. However, it has precise plumbing requirements, which may restrict use in some areas, and a long cycle time of around 30 minutes, which makes it unsuitable for units with a fast turnaround of patients.

Provided that manufacturers' instructions on usage are followed, peracetic acid-based products would appear to be a safe and effective method of chemical disinfection or sterilization. However, all staff require adequate training in its use, and the effects of exposure. Many staff find the 'vinegar-like' smell unpleasant, and insufficient data is currently available about the long-term effects of exposure to this vapour. For this reason it is probably best used in enclosed systems where adequate mechanical ventilation is provided. It should be remembered that glutaraldehyde was at first thought to be safe, and is now subject to stringent controls because of its effect on health.

Chlorine dioxide

Chlorine dioxide is a powerful oxidizing agent, and has been used for a number of years by both the water authorities (to purify water), and the health care industries (as a sterilant solution or gas). It is a powerful sterilant with a wide range of bactericidal, viricidal, fungicidal and sporicidal activity that will sterilize an endoscope in 10 minutes. An example of a product using chlorine dioxide as its base is Dexit.

Because of its oxidizing properties, it is incompatible with a number of materials used in endoscope, accessory, and disinfector design (stainless steel, copper, silicone rubber, ceramics, PVC and polyethylene), and care should be taken to ensure compatibility with equipment before using any products based on this.

To get over the problem of incompatibility, some commercially available products have had anticorrosive agents added to them, but at the time of writing very few endoscope, accessory or disinfector manufacturers have confirmed compatibility of their products with this group of disinfectants.

Alcohol

Immersion in 70% ethanol or isopropyl alcohol for 5–10 minutes will chemically disinfect an endoscope or accessory. However, the process is subject to control measures similar to glutaraldehyde, and it is not particularly effective against mycobacteria. In addition, alcohol may damage lens cement.

7B.3.2   HEAT DISINFECTION

This is only suitable for use on rigid endoscopes and heat-stable endoscopic accessories. The process requires one of the following:

70–1 °C for 3 minutes
80 °C for 1 minute
90 °C for 1 second.

The equipment necessary for this process is not always available, and it is rarely used in endoscopy.

Low-temperature steam

This requires the item to be surrounded by steam at 73–80 °C for 20 minutes. The process is not always available but it can be an alternative to other methods of disinfection for items such as water bottles and mouthguards.

7B.3.3   STEROX

Sterox is a microbiocidal solution produced by an electrochemical process that contains a mixture of radicals with strong oxidizing properties; chlorine dioxide, hydrogen peroxide and ozone are the main active ingredients.

To be microbiologically effective and non-corrosive, Sterox must have a pH of between 5 and 7, and a redox value in excess of 1000 mV. Once prepared, it is stable for 24 h at normal room temperature. The Sterox solution should be used once and then discarded.

Sterox produces sterilization within 5 minutes, yet is totally benign to human beings. A faint smell of chlorine is evident, but this is no stronger than that encountered in a swimming pool.

The production unit is capable of producing up to 240 litres per hour of the biocide together with an equal quantity of sterile water which can be used for rinsing. The production unit may be connected via a modem to a central monitoring station that continuously monitors production and warns both user and maintenance engineers of any fault.

Sterox has been shown to be a safe alternative to glutaraldehyde, peracetic acid and other chemical disinfectants and sterilants. Although the initial installation costs are high, once installed the costs per litre of solution are considerably less than those of any comparable chemical disinfectant. Sterox is reported to present no health hazards to patients or staff, and to be non-corrosive to endoscopic equipment and accessories. At the time of writing, independent tests by manufacturers have yet to be performed, but the producers of Sterox have agreed to underwrite any equipment damage resulting from the use of the solution.

The Infection Research Laboratory, Birmingham, UK, has shown Sterox to be microbiologically equal to 2% glutaraldehyde against non-sporing bacteria, with a superior sporicidal activity. Unlike glutaraldehyde, Sterox is a surfactant, and does not fix organic material, so is less likely to cause air/water channel blockage. But, in common with all disinfection/sterilization processes, it is dependent on good manual cleaning of equipment beforehand.

7B.3.4   AUTOMATED DISINFECTION MACHINES

Although the use of automated disinfecting machines is to be encouraged, they can themselves potentially become a reservoir of infective micro-organisms, causing contamination of endoscopes and/or accessories with the resultant risk of patient infection. Contamination of pathology specimens by this route can also lead to misdiagnosis.

Sources of endoscope contamination resulting from use of automated disinfection machines

Associated factors

- Inadequate precleaning of endoscope.
- Incorrect cleaning and maintenance of machine.
- Use of static water tanks.
- Water supply of poor microbiological quality.
- Hard water (allows build-up of lime scale).
- Biofilm formation within machine.

Whether the disinfector has a specific self-disinfection cycle programmed into the machine or self-disinfects itself every cycle, it is essential that the disinfectant used comes into contact with all parts of the machine that come into contact with fluid. This includes the water delivery system and, unless isolated, the drainage system.

7B.3.5   DRYING CABINETS

Many countries, particularly the USA, routinely use drying cabinets to store their endoscopes (Fig. 7B.1). After decontamination the endoscope is rinsed with 70% alcohol, which displaces any water present and acts as a drying agent. The endoscope is then placed in the drying cabinet. Drying cabinets have the following features.

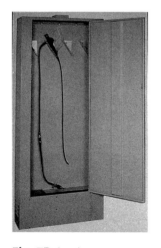

Fig. 7B.1   A drying cabinet

1. A mechanism that pumps dry (microbiologically) filtered air through and around the endoscope. This may be continuous or timed for a fixed or variable time each hour.
2. Absorbent pads (silica gel) to absorb any moisture within the cabinet.

Manufacturers claim that the above provides an environment where bacteria are unable to multiply so that an endoscope can be taken from the cabinet and used immediately, removing the need to disinfect prior to use. There is currently very little published evidence to support this although a recent (unpublished) study has confirmed this for a period of up to 60 hours.

7B.4   HEALTH AND SAFETY

The need to use chemicals to disinfect or sterilize endoscopes and their accessories has had a profound influence on the design and working practices of the modern endoscopy unit. Glutaraldehyde still remains the most commonly used chemical disinfectant (BSG, 1988), although newer and reportedly safer disinfectants and sterilants are increasingly becoming available. Thirty years ago glutaraldehyde was thought to be a safe product, but is now a recognized health hazard with its use governed by strict regulations.

7B.4.1   COSHH

The Health and Safety at Work Act 1974 requires employers to ensure, so far as is reasonable practicable, the health, safety and welfare of all their employees. In 1988 the COSHH Regulations were introduced, requiring employers to assess the risk to health of employees exposed to hazardous chemicals in the course of their work, and either to avoid using such chemicals or to control their use adequately so as to provide a safe working environment for the employee. Failure to do this is an offence under the Health and Safety at Work Act.

The present maximum permitted exposure level in the UK for glutaraldehyde is a 10 minute average exposure level of 0.2 ppm (0.7 mg/m^3). Many countries have a maximum permitted exposure level half of this, and it is likely that in the future the maximum for the UK will be brought into line with this. The odour threshold for glutaraldehyde is reported to be 0.04 ppm (BSG, 1988).

(a)

GLUTARALDEHYDE SPILLAGE

<u>THE 10 COMMANDMENTS</u>

1. Evacuate area.
2. Seal off area to non-essential staff.
3. Put on protective clothing and gear OUTSIDE the affected area (gown, plastic apron, nitrile gloves, RPE, goggles – NOT visors, boots).
4. On entry into affected area – open all available windows (i.e. ventilate area), BUT do not open door into corridor.
5. Dilute glutaraldehyde to reduce evaporation.
6. Mop up with disposables (i.e. inco sheets, tissues, blue paper roll).
7. Put used disposables into yellow bag and seal tightly. Put tightly sealed bag into 2nd yellow bag and seal as before.
8. Clean off boot soles BEFORE leaving the area.
9. Change any clothing that may have come into contact with glutaraldehyde (even vapour contamination can be detected on clothes just like stale cigarette smoke).
10. Wash hands thoroughly and any skin that has been exposed (even to vapour).

7B.4.2   STAFF HEALTH SURVEILLANCE

Routine health screening of staff working in areas where glutaraldehyde is used for disinfecting is mandatory. Occupational health departments are required to perform pre-employment medical checks including a lung function test and enquire whether any problems exist such as asthma, conjunctivitis and rhinitis. Annual health checks are also required to check for the occurrence of any symptoms related to glutaraldehyde exposure. If staff develop any health problems that may be a result of exposure to glutaraldehyde, this must be reported to their line manager and occupational health department immediately. If screening demonstrates occurrence of health problems then further

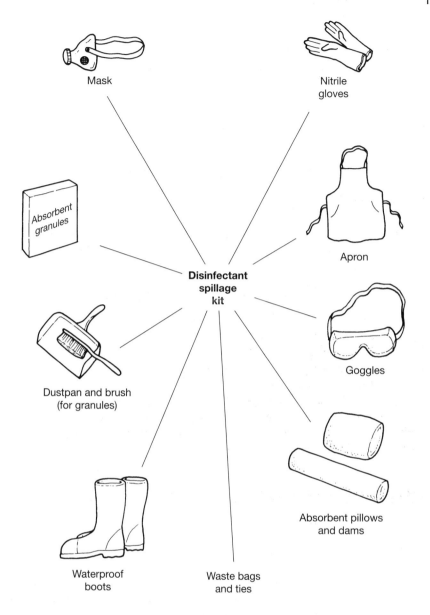

Fig. 7B.2   (a and b) Example of a staff instruction notice on dealing with glutaraldehyde spillage

exposure should be avoided. Education of staff is essential in the safe management of glutaraldehyde. Written procedures for safe working practices should be provided for all members of staff, and these procedures should include instructions regarding use of control measures and spillage procedures.

7B.4.3   DEALING WITH SPILLAGE

Spillage less than 5 litres

1. Secure area where spillage is from non-essential staff.
2. If available use Cidex spillage kit; ensure after use that kit is restocked.
3. Wear protective clothing and suitable mask/respirator before entering area.
4. Follow unit policy for Cidex spillage, ensuring welfare of staff at all times. An example of a staff notice detailing unit policy is given in Fig. 7B.2.

Spillage over 5 litres

1. Seal off the area where spillage has taken place.
2. Depending on unit's policy, raise the fire alarm.
3. Evacuate the unit.
4. Explain toxicity of glutaraldehyde to fire officers, so they are aware what type of substance they are dealing with and can use appropriate equipment.

Disposal of chemical disinfectants/sterilants

Precise instructions for disposal of chemical disinfectants and sterilants may be given by the manufacturer, but more often there are none and the majority of these substances are disposed of via the local drainage system. However, there have been reports, particularly from rural areas, of glutaraldehyde causing problems in water treatment plants by destroying or altering the bacterial colonies used in water purification leading to contamination of water supplies. This does not currently appear to be a problem in urban areas, probably owing to the larger volumes of water processed in such stations diluting the chemicals involved to a level where they are inactivated.

In the absence of special local factors or regulations, it would seem reasonable to continue with this means of disposal for the present although it may be necessary to consider alternative arrangements for these chemicals in the future.

REFERENCES

BSG (1988) Cleaning and disinfection of equipment for gastrointestinal flexible endoscopy. Interim recommendations of a working party (BSG). *Gut*, **29**, 1134–51.

Wickes, J. (1992) *BSG Nursing Associates Newsletter.*

Cleaning and reprocessing of flexible endoscopes and accessories

7C

Samantha Hawkes

7C.1 FLEXIBLE ENDOSCOPES

All patients undergoing endoscopy must be protected from infection. To do this, appropriate cleaning, disinfection and/or sterilization measures must be taken for all endoscopes and accessories.

Flexible endoscopes must be cleaned and disinfected (or sterilized) before each endoscopy list, between patients, and at the end of the list. The only exception to this is if drying cabinets are used for the storage of clean endoscopes, when local policy may enable the prelist process to be omitted.

To decontaminate an endoscope effectively, it is essential to know the anatomy and workings of the instrument. A flexible endoscope consists of three main parts (Fig. 7C.1).

1. The **insertion tube,** consisting of a watertight outer sheath containing the suction/biopsy channel, air and water channel(s), optics (fibre bundles and/or CCD chip), and the control wires (for angulation of distal end).
2. The **control section,** consisting of the angulation control wheels, suction and air/water valves, biopsy port and valve, and eyepiece if fibreoptic endoscope or control buttons if a video endoscope. Many endoscopes also have a connection port for an auxiliary (jet) channel, which allows a pressurized jet of water to be directed from the distal tip of the endoscope to improve visualization.

Practical Endoscopy Edited by M. Shephard and J. Mason. Published in 1997 by Chapman & Hall, London. ISBN 0 412 54000 2

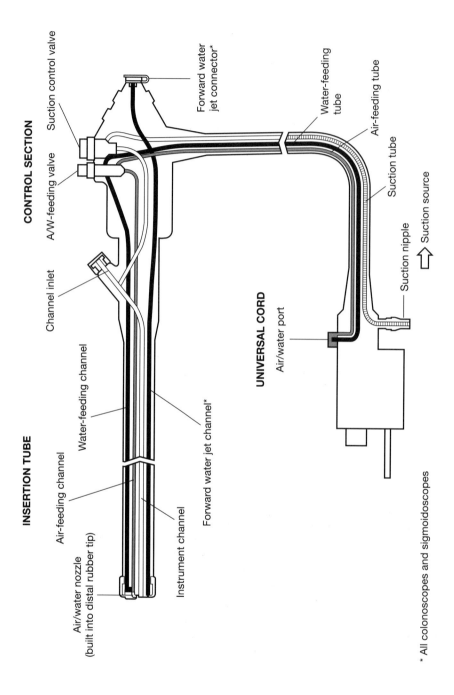
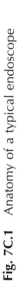

Fig. 7C.1   Anatomy of a typical endoscope

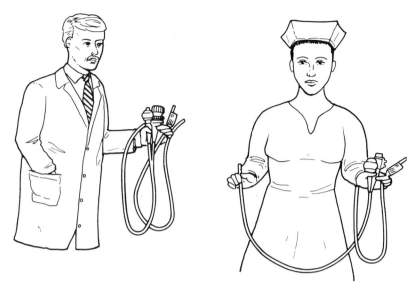

Fig. 7C.2   The correct way to handle an endoscope

3. The **universal cord** (often referred to as the umbilical cord), which connects the endoscope to the light-source and/or video processor, suction, air, and water. There is also a connection for the scope-patient (S-P) cord of a diathermy unit (Chapter 18), and a gas venting cap for ethylene oxide sterilization or leakage testing.

There are variations on this formula, depending on the type of endoscope to be cleaned, and this is referred to in more detail in Chapters 12 and 16–18. The basic principles are, however, the same irrespective of the type of endoscope.

Manual cleaning of the endoscope is of vital importance as this alone removes over 95% of organic debris and micro-organisms present. Any organic debris such as blood and mucus remaining on an instrument will prevent adequate penetration of the disinfectant or sterilant, and it should also be remembered that the most commonly used disinfectant, glutaraldehyde, also acts as a fixative on these materials, causing hardening and making them very difficult to remove. Failure to clean the endoscope adequately prior to disinfection will therefore result in inadequate disinfection and/or blockages to the instrument channels. The instrument should also be held correctly at all times (Fig. 7C.2).

7C.2 CLEANING AND DISINFECTION ROUTINES

7C.2.1 ENDOSCOPES

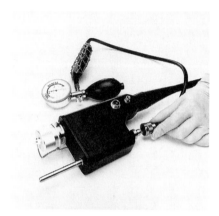

1. First perform a leak test to check the integrity of the endoscope and prevent contamination of its interior with body fluids (Fig. 7C.3).

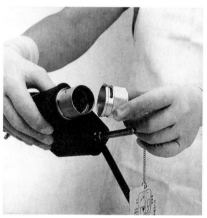

2. Replace the soaking cap to protect electrical contacts and make the endoscope watertight during cleaning/disinfection (Fig. 7C.4).

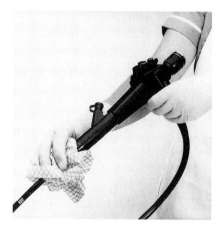

3. Clean the exterior of the endoscope using a soft cloth or sponge and warm soapy water (Fig. 7C.5).

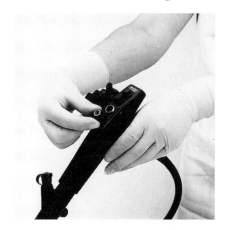

4. Disconnect all valves, distal hoods and other removable parts (Fig. 7C.6).

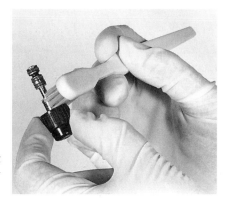

5. Clean all valves using a soft toothbrush and warm soapy water (Fig. 7C.7).

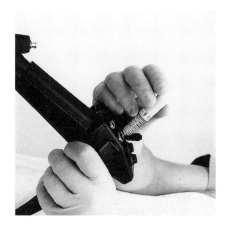

6. Clean valve chambers using a short cylinder brush (Fig. 7C.8).

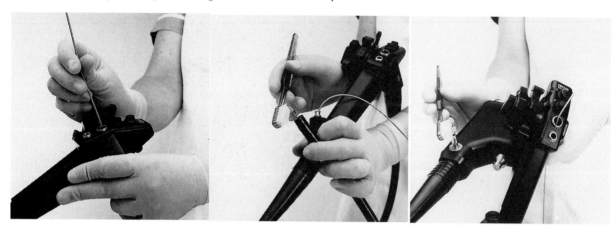

7. Brush the length of the suction/biopsy channel using an appropriately sized cleaning brush (see manufacturer's recommendations) (Fig. 7C.9). Clean the brush bristles with a soft toothbrush each time it emerges from the endoscope to remove accumulated debris from the brush head and prevent debris re-entering the endoscope as the brush is removed. This process should be repeated a **minimum** of three times or until the brush emerges clean when passed through the endoscope.

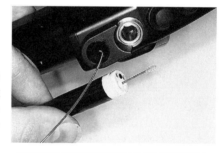

8. Flush or if possible brush the air/water channels following the same procedure, according to the manufacturer's instructions (Fig. 7C.10).

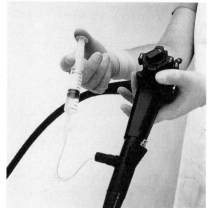

9. Flush or brush the auxiliary (jet) channel (Fig. 7C.11).

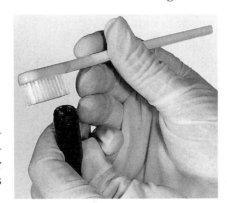

10. Clean the distal tip of the endoscope with a soft toothbrush and warm soapy water to remove debris from optics and nozzles (Fig. 7C.12).

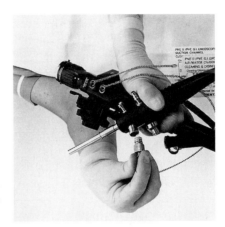

11. Connect the appropriate cleaning adaptors and disinfect according to the agreed policy (Fig. 7C.13), preferably using a fully automated disinfection system or, failing that, manual methods. Whichever method used, the process should include:

   (a) Wash internally and externally using warm water and a neutral detergent. Drain and flush with air.

   (b) Rinse internally and externally using fresh water to remove any remaining detergent (detergent inactivates some chemical disinfectants). Drain and flush with air.

   (c) Disinfect with the chemical disinfectant of choice for the recommended time according to the manufacturer's instructions and/ or the unit policy. Ensure, as far as is possible, that disinfectant is in contact with all exterior and interior surfaces. Drain and flush with air.

   (d) Rinse internally and externally using fresh, sterile or filtered water (according to policy) to remove any traces of disinfectant. Drain and flush with air.

   (e) Many automated systems include a second rinse cycle at this stage as traces of disinfectant have still been found following one rinse only.

   (f) Dry and reassemble the endoscope using a soft dry cloth for the exterior, and 70% isopropyl alcohol followed by forced air for the interior.

Points to note

- Prolonged immersion in chemical disinfectants can damage the integrity of the endoscope.
- Use of alcohol externally has been shown to break the waterproof seals and dissolve the cement surrounding the lenses of some endoscopes. It is, however, a very effective drying agent and a disinfectant in its own right.
- Most countries now recommend the use of sterile or high-quality filtered water for all stages of the disinfection cycle.

Routine maintenance

- Regularly, dependent on usage, lubricate valves with a recommended (endoscopic) silicone oil to help prevent faulty operation.
- Regularly lubricate the exterior of the insertion tube (especially the bending section) with a recommended silicone oil to maintain pliability of the rubber sheath.
- Periodically check and record angulation of the distal tip to check for deterioration of control mechanism. Return for service if this does not meet the manufacturer's specification.
- Periodically check the optics of the fibre bundle for broken fibres. Record the results. Rapid deterioration may indicate poor handling.
- Inspect condition of 'O' rings on all valves for deterioration, and replace as necessary.
- Irrespective of number of emergency repairs required, **all** endoscopes should be included in a regular programme of maintenance.

7C.2.2   ACCESSORIES

Sterilization is the optimum standard requirement for all reusable accessories. If this is not possible then alternatives such as chemical or steam disinfection should be considered, but in this case the risk of possible cross-infection needs to be weighed against the effectiveness of the disinfection method chosen. Single-use accessories may prove a more suitable alternative in high-risk procedures such as ERCP, hysteroscopy or cystoscopy.

Note: Ensure that the accessory has been marked by the manufacturer as 'reusable' before processing. ('Autoclavable' does not necessarily mean that it is reusable.)

All reusable accessories should be inspected for damage prior to reprocessing, and damaged ones discarded or sent for repair (Fig. 7C.14).

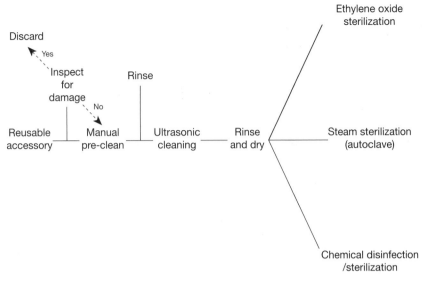

Fig. 7C.14   Decontamination and cleaning of endoscopic accessories

Manual precleaning

Accessories should be cleaned immediately after use to prevent blood, mucous matter or other body fluids drying on the instrument. When dry, these are very hard or impossible to remove, and may cause malfunction of the accessory and/or ineffective chemical disinfection (if used). If immediate cleaning is not possible, the accessory should be placed in a bowl containing warm water and a mild enzymatic detergent until the cleaning process can be commenced.

Process

1. Dismantle the accessory as far as is possible following the manufacturer's instructions.
2. Using a soft cloth, clean all parts in warm water and a mild enzymatic detergent. All hollow lumens should be flushed where possible using either a syringe or pressure gun.
3. Using a soft toothbrush, gently clean any operating mechanisms such as biopsy cups and pivot pins (Fig. 7C.15).

Ultrasonic cleaning

Ultrasonic cleaning is the only effective method of removing organic debris from accessories, particularly those that have a shaft made like a tightly coiled spring (e.g. some biopsy forceps). Accessory manufacturers usually recommend a suitable frequency and time for that particular

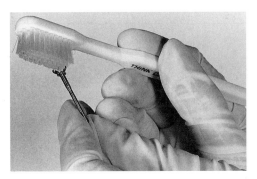

Fig. 7C.15   Manual precleaning of accessory

accessory, but this is usually in the region of 40 kHz for 5–10 minutes. Some automated endoscope disinfectors use ultrasonics for the cleaning part of their cycle, but this is at a lower frequency than that used for accessories. In no circumstances should an endoscope be cleaned using an ultrasonic tank. Prolonged exposure to ultrasonics can cause deterioration or distortion of the accessory.

Most ultrasonic tanks use mild enzymatic detergents similar to that used in the manual precleaning stage, so it is usually not necessary to rinse the accessory between two stages. However, if the same type and brand are not used, then the accessory should be rinsed in between.

Rinsing and drying

All accessories should be rinsed in fresh water to remove any residual detergent. Hollow lumens should be flushed as before. The accessory should then be dried using a soft dry cloth. Interior lumens should be dried using forced air. Industrial drying agents are also available for this purpose, but are not usually necessary and may cause unnecessary health and safety problems.

Preparation for sterilization/disinfection

Whatever method is selected, the accessory should not be tightly coiled or kinked. Ideally this should be placed as straight as is possible to prevent damage and ensure effective sterilization or disinfection. Items for sterilization should be sent to the appropriate department for processing. If chemical disinfection is used, then care should be taken to ensure that all hollow lumens are filled with disinfectant, and that the accessory is thoroughly rinsed afterwards with fresh or sterile water. Accessories should be dried with a soft dry cloth and moving parts such as biopsy cups and pivots lubricated to ensure smooth operation. The accessory should be inspected for damage or malfunction prior to storage.

7C.3 THE FUTURE

Semidisposable endoscopes (Fig. 7C.16) have already been developed using a reusable main body and insertion tube containing optical elements with a disposable outer sheath that includes the air/water and suction biopsy channels. This removes the need for expensive disinfection equipment and has great potential for use in the office or outpatient setting. As minimal disinfection is required (mainly to the controls) the hazards to health associated with chemical disinfection are greatly reduced. Not all types of endoscope are currently available, and thin instruments such as bronchoscopes may not be suitable for this type of

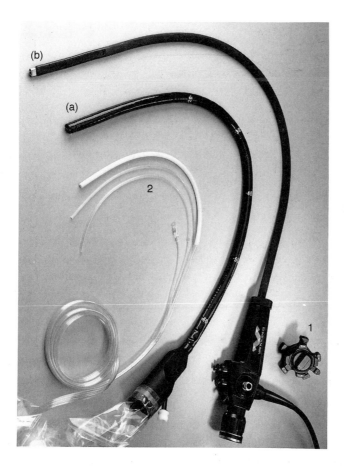

Fig. 7C.16 The semidisposable endoscope. (a) Disposable outer sheath. (b) Reusable inner section with detachable controls (1), and connection tubing (2) (reproduced with permission of Vision Sciences)

design although technological advances may make this possible in the future.

The totally disposable endoscope is a distinct possibility, and some types are already being used by the oil industry, although these are optically inferior to medical endoscopes and too expensive for routine use.

A recent advance is the endoscope that allows manual brush cleaning of the hitherto inaccessible air/water channel (Pentax). This will not only improve the decontamination process, but will also result in the virtual elimination of air/water channel blockages.

Development of new production materials may in future allow the development of an autoclavable endoscope.

Safety, sedation and emergencies in endoscopy 8

RORY McCLOY

8.1 SAFETY AND SEDATION

How safe is endoscopy? Where do the dangers lie? What can be done to prevent and avoid unnecessary morbidity and mortality? These issues are addressed in a critical way since, of all aspects of endoscopy, it is the current practice of sedation that highlights potential differences in interests and priorities for patients, nurses and endoscopists. The patient is anxious, if not scared stiff, but is usually happy to comply with the procedure as long as 'I am not aware of what is going on'. In the United Kingdom the vast majority of patients want some form of sedation, to make an unpleasant procedure more tolerable. The nurse wants a smooth and uneventful rapid transfer of patients through the unit. Often the nursing staff in the endoscopy unit want to avoid the use of sedation, with its implications for recovery of the patient. The endoscopist is primarily concerned with the successful outcome of the procedure, be it diagnostic or therapeutic. Whilst almost no endoscopists have ever received any formal training in sedation or monitoring techniques, they are happy to employ sedation if it ensures improved co-operation from the patient. There is an increasing awareness amongst endoscopists that sedation may not always be safe and can be associated with significant mortality and morbidity. Rather than seeking the appropriate training or education, endoscopists are tending to use sedation techniques less frequently. There is a strange and irrational reluctance for endoscopy units – managers, nurses and endoscopists – to obtain expert input from local anaesthetists concerning the drugs and monitoring systems used on the unit.

Practical Endoscopy Edited by M. Shephard and J. Mason. Published in 1997 by Chapman & Hall, London. ISBN 0 412 54000 2

8.1.1 RISKS OF ENDOSCOPY

Judging by the patients accepted for diagnostic and therapeutic upper gastrointestinal endoscopy including ERCP in many units around the world, there is an implicit assumption that the procedure is safe and applicable to a wide spectrum of patients including those considered to be moribund. With ever-widening indications for endoscopy and the increasing application of therapeutic techniques it is not surprising that there has been a slight increase in overall mortality, although the complication rate of upper gastrointestinal endoscopy has been reported to have decreased by 40% in the last two decades (Hart and Classen, 1990). Instrument perforation and bleeding are rare events in upper gastrointestinal endoscopy but more common in colonoscopy. Guidelines on appropriate indications for upper gastrointestinal endoscopy have recently been published (Axon *et al.*, 1995).

Precise data on the morbidity and mortality of endoscopy are surprisingly difficult to come by and generally suffer from being historic or retrospective. The serious morbidity of upper gastrointestinal endoscopy is about 1 in 1000 (Cotton and Williams, 1990) and mortality is estimated to be between 0.5 and 3 per 10 000 examinations (Carey, 1987; Cotton and Williams, 1990; Hart and Classen, 1990; Keeffe and O'Connor, 1990). The majority of the morbidity appears to be from cardiopulmonary complications (Hart and Classen, 1990; Daneshmend, Bell and Logan, 1991).

A prospective audit of upper gastrointestinal endoscopy was conducted in England during 1991 and, for the first time, included complications and mortality over a 30-day period using appropriately validated techniques (Quine *et al.*, 1995a). The total number of procedures studied was 14 149, of which 92% were diagnostic and the remainder therapeutic. The results for diagnostic gastroscopy alone demonstrated a perforation rate of 1 in 2000 examinations and a procedure-related, cardiovascular and pulmonary 30-day mortality of 1 in 2000.

This data demands a critical examination of procedural safety for endoscopy (Charlton, 1995). However, it is paradoxically the relative safety of endoscopic procedures that lulls the unwary staff of the endoscopy unit into a false sense of security, since serious adverse events or death on the unit are statistically likely to be encountered only once every few years – although the endoscopist and nurses will probably be unaware of the many complications and deaths that occur as a direct consequence of the procedure but well after the patient has left the unit.

There might be many determinants of the outcome of an endoscopic examination (Table 8.1) (Keeffe, 1991a):

- *What procedure is performed*
  - diagnostic versus therapeutic.
- *What conscious sedation or anaesthesia is used*
  - benzodiazepine alone versus with opioid
  - bolus versus titration.
- *What level of monitoring is employed*
  - grade/number of personnel assisting
  - oximetry, electrocardiogram, non-invasive blood pressure
  - resuscitation equipment available.
- *Who undergoes endoscopy*
  - young versus elderly
  - medically fit versus unfit
  - consultation versus checklist.
- *Who performs endoscopy*
  - training and experience
  - competence.
- *Why endoscopy is performed*
  - indicated versus contraindicated (inappropriate).
- *Where endoscopy is performed*
  - fully staffed hospital unit versus clinic or office
  - elective (endoscopy unit) versus emergency (intensive care unit, ward).
- *How the patient is recovered.*
- *How the outpatient is discharged*

Table 8.1   What makes German patients anxious about gastroscopy? (after Schneider-Bandura *et al.*, 1993)

58%	Vomiting
50%	Cancer
36%	Uncertainty
32%	Breathlessness
26%	Pain
16%	The injection
15%	Losing self control
14%	Duration of endoscopy
14%	Being hurt
11%	Drugs injected
11%	Bad past experience
9%	At mercy of others
7%	Infection
6%	Unknown surroundings
4%	Death
3%	The doctor

However, this chapter will focus on sedation and monitoring. The benefits of sedation in terms of better patient tolerance and increased ease of examination for the endoscopists must outweigh the cardio-respiratory morbidity (Froehlich *et al.*, 1995).

8.1.2 ENDOSCOPY WITH OR WITHOUT SEDATION

Anxiety and fear of the unknown, together with an anticipation that private recesses of the body, beyond the back of the throat or up the rectum, will be invaded or violated are understandable in patients about to be endoscoped. In a German study of patients about to undergo a gastroscopy or colonoscopy, 31% were reported to be very or extremely anxious (Gebbensleben and Rohde, 1990) and this was sufficient for 74% of German patients to postpone the appointment for endoscopy as long as possible (Schneider-Bandura *et al.*, 1993), in a country where only a minority of patients undergoing endoscopy receive sedation. Information and reassurance combined with a pleasant relaxed ambience in the endoscopy unit can go a long way to alleviating patients' anxieties, but the causes of anxiety are multiple and complex (Table 8.1), neither are they significantly different between the sexes (Schneider-Bandura *et al.*, 1993). It is anxiolysis, rather than amnesia, that is the main factor for improving patient tolerance for the procedure when using low-dose midazolam (2.5 mg) (Froehlich *et al.*, 1995).

Co-operation from the patient requires descending cortical inhibition to override the basic spinal reflexes encouraging the patient to remove the offending instrument from the hypopharynx or rectum. Intravenous sedation with benzodiazepine drugs, such as diazepam or midazolam, tends to disconnect lower brainstem centres from cortical control and prevent the message from the clinician's verbal encouragement from being translated into physical co-operation from the patient. The oversedated patient thus becomes the unco-operative patient acting with basic survival reflexes (McCloy and Pearson, 1990). Endoscopists and nurses are often unaware that increasing sedation does not necessarily equate with increasing compliance, unless anaesthetic levels of sedation score are achieved.

Of course a skilful endoscopist can perform an adequate endoscopy without premedication or sedation, but the vast majority of patients in the UK will request sedation with a version of the phrase: 'I don't mind what you do doctor, as long as I am asleep' – an unfortunate positive encouragement for the endoscopist to turn 'anaesthetist'. Midazolam (2.5 mg intravenously) has been demonstrated to improve patient tolerance significantly compared with placebo (Froehlich *et al.*, 1995).

Table 8.2 Some questions about sedation asked of German patients (after Landefield *et al.*, 1993)

Gastroscopy (%)	Answer	Colonoscopy (%)
Would patients who have had sedation for gastroscopy or colonoscopy want sedation again?		
86	Yes	86
11	No, other	6
2	Undecided	7
1	Definitely not	1
What did these patients think of the amnesia induced by midazolam?		
47	Amazing/pleasant	51
5	Uncertain	7
3	Unpleasant	2

In the final event, it would be asked whether patients who have had sedation for endoscopy would want sedation again. In a study of German patients undergoing gastroscopy or colonoscopy the majority said 'yes' (Table 8.2) and half the patients found the amnesia induced by midazolam 'amazing or pleasant' (Landefield *et al.*, 1993). In a controlled trial by Froehlich *et al.* (1995), the willingness to undergo a repeat gastroscopy was increased from 74% without midazolam to 95% with low-dose midazolam, irrespective of the use of pharyngeal analgesia.

8.1.3 SEDATION

In the UK, conscious sedation is defined as: 'a technique in which the use of a drug, or drugs, produces a state of depression of the central nervous system enabling treatment to be carried out, but during which communication is maintained such that the patient will respond to command throughout the period of sedation' (Royal College of Surgeons of England, 1993). The drugs and techniques used for sedation should carry a margin of safety that is wide enough to render unintended loss of consciousness unlikely. If contact with the patient is lost then the endoscopist can be judged in a court of law as having given an anaesthetic, with all its attendant consequences and responsibilities.

There are relatively few contraindications to the use of sedation:

- Extremes of age.
- Pregnancy.
- Previous adverse or paradoxical reaction.
- Pre-existing hypoxaemia (oxygen saturation ≤ 90%).
- Clinical shock.

End-points for sedation

Endoscopy units should re-examine their end-points for sedation. All too often the endoscopist reaches for the sedative injection without considering what he is trying to achieve. Successful sedation for endoscopy should achieve anxiolysis and amnesia rather than ptosis and hypnosis (McCloy and Pearson, 1990).

- 'Traditional' end-points
  - ptosis
  - dysarthria
  - drowsiness.
- 'Modern' end-points
  - anxiolysis
  - amnesia
  - co-operation.

The following progressive effects of increasing sedation with benzodiazepines, will be noticed:

Minimum benzodiazepine receptor occupancy
- anxiolysis
- anticonvulsant
- slight sedation
- reduced attention
- amnesia
- intense sedation
- ptosis
- muscle relaxation
- hypnosis
Maximum benzodiazepine receptor occupancy.

The endoscopist and nurse assistant require re-educating to accommodate to the patient lying on the endoscopy table with their eyes open. If the patient is peacefully snoring, then the patient will, in medicolegal terms, have received a general anaesthetic and, unless both the endoscopist has an anaesthetic qualification and the endoscopy nurse is anaesthetic trained, this situation should give rise to serious concern and not the more usual reaction that 'this is a good and co-operative patient'!

Sedative agents

For practical purposes the benzodiazepines are the only class of drug used for sedation during gastroenterological procedures. They are a remarkably safe group of drugs with a wide margin of safety and a high therapeutic index. However, since the majority of deaths following diagnostic endoscopy are related to cardiopulmonary events, this would suggest that use of benzodiazepine-induced sedation may be contributing to this mortality and morbidity, although hard data on this issue are lacking. A corollary might be that endoscopists are unaware of the risks and complications of inappropriate use of benzodiazepines.

Whilst therapeutic endoscopy may be time consuming, diagnostic upper gastrointestinal endoscopy is generally a short procedure that may last only 5–10 minutes. Yet not many endoscopists and nurses realize that diazepam, historically the first benzodiazepine for intravenous sedation and still widely used in the lipid-emulsion formulation (Diazemuls), has a prolonged pharmacokinetic profile with a plasma elimination half-life that can be longer than 40 hours and a desmethyl metabolite with a half-life of about 5 days that has active sedative properties (Greenblatt and Schader, 1978).

In comparison the plasma elimination half-life of the water-soluble benzodiazepine midazolam is 1.5–2.5 hours in both normal subjects (Amerin *et al.*, 1981) and patients with severe concomitant disease (Shelley, Mendel and Park, 1987). Midazolam is well established as the drug of choice for endoscopic procedures in the USA and more recently has become so in areas of the UK (Quine *et al.*, 1995a). However, it is the closer tailoring of the pharmacological profile to the endoscopic procedure that resulted in the decision of the Royal College of Surgeons of England (1993) to recommend the use of midazolam over Diazemuls.

Inhalation agents, in the form of nitrous oxide, are an incredibly safe way of inducing conscious sedation as testified by the extensive use of nitrous oxide in dentistry. It is likely that this agent will find favour with an increasing number of colonoscopists in future years.

Doses of benzodiazepines

Overall, the doses of benzodiazepines used to induce sedation for endoscopy are higher than are necessary and also higher (Quine *et al.*, 1995a) than manufacturers' recommended doses (*ABPI Data Sheet Compendium*, 1996). Doses should be kept to the minimum that are compatible with patient comfort and successful performance of the procedure (Bell *et al.*, 1991b). The reason that some endoscopists may oversedate patients with midazolam is the lack of appreciation of the relative potency compared with diazepam, which was thought to be about 2 : 1 in early reports (Whitwam, Al-Khudhairi and McCloy,

1983); however, midazolam is now thought to be three or four times more potent in terms of sedative effect (Whitwam, 1991). This potential problem is balanced by approximately a twofold increase in achieving amnesia for the procedure over diazepam (Whitwam, Al-Khudhairi and McCloy, 1983). The endoscopist seems to think he or she has a bizarre licence to administer whatever 'is necessary' to achieve unreasonable end-points (see list above); this may reflect both ignorance and lack of adequate training in sedation techniques of the endoscopist, who has usually been taught by the 'apprentice system' by other endoscopists, who in turn were largely self-taught (and rarely instructed by qualified anaesthetists). For further details, a comprehensive review of sedation for endoscopy by Bell (1990) is recommended reading.

Bearing in mind the end-points for sedation discussed above, the author very rarely exceeds a total dose of 5 mg midazolam for any patient undergoing either diagnostic or therapeutic endoscopy, including ERCP, even in young fit patients. With advancing age (biological rather than chronological) and concomitant medical illnesses this total dose must be reduced, so that over the age of 70 years it is unusual to use more than 1 or 2 mg midazolam intravenously.

Influence of the endoscopy nurse on drug usage

The endoscopy nurse can play a crucial role in this potentially unhappy scenario. Many nurses are feeling increasingly unhappy at the sedation practice of their more senior endoscopists and are frustrated at the prospect of being unable to alter their outdated and possibly lethal use of sedative drugs. In fact, the nurse can directly influence both the initial as well as the total dose of sedative drug that is administered, since the endoscopist tends only to use the drugs set out for the procedure and handed to him.

Unfortunately, in the UK midazolam (Hypnovel, Roche UK Ltd, Welwyn) is presented in ampoules with a total dose of 10 mg in 2 ml or 5 ml preparations (the latter is preferred for endoscopic use). (In other countries the more preferable 5 mg/5 ml preparation is available.) This means that if the entire 10 mg/5 ml dose is drawn up into a single syringe, then the dose handed to the (probably ignorant) endoscopist is equivalent to about 20–40 mg Diazemuls and is likely to be two to four times too large for almost every patient. A far safer practice would be for the nurse to split the ampoule into two 2 ml syringes and hand the endoscopist 5 mg/2.5 ml. Furthermore, the nurse should be very reluctant to hand over any additional doses – how this is achieved is left to the nurse's imagination! Gradually, the errant endoscopist finds that he can achieve excellent conditions for endoscopy with smaller doses of midazolam and shorter recovery times and cheaper drug costs are to the benefit of the unit, with probably fewer complications for the patients.

Techniques of drug administration: bolus versus titration

The technique of intravenous administration, bolus or slow incremental titration can influence the effect on the patient (Bell *et al.*, 1990; Swain, Ellis and Bradby, 1990). Bolus titration has advantages of speed of onset and co-operation but may lead to more marked reduction in oxygen saturation and respiratory depression. Conversely, titration of the benzodiazepine will often lead to a larger total dose being employed, with the advantages of possible increase in the number of patients who are amnesic but a more prolonged recovery period.

It is recommended that a careful titration technique is used according to the manufacturer's data sheet. There is, however, a major problem in judging the end-points for sedation (see list above). In the past it was easy to see that the patient was developing drooping of the eyelids (ptosis) and slurred speech, but now that we recognize that these end-points are dangerously close to the induction of anaesthesia, how should amnesia and anxiolysis be assessed? It is not possible to measure amnesia until after the event, but endoscopy staff soon become adept at noticing the gentle relaxation of the patient that is associated with relief of anxiety. The 'white knuckles' begin to unclench, the shoulders are lowered and the patient's facial muscles take on a calmer countenance.

At the present time it has to be recognized that, in the majority of endoscopy units, titration of the benzodiazepine drug is not the practice and if a bolus technique is used then special consideration must be given to the age and sickness of the patient. Supplemental oxygen with pulse oximetry is used (section 8.2.1) and only half to two-thirds of the total dose of the benzodiazepine required for a titration technique is administered (Geller, 1991).

8.1.4 SEDATION AND ANALGESIA

The benzodiazepine drugs such as midazolam that are used for intravenous sedation do not have analgesic properties and it is standard practice for endoscopy to be performed with both sedation and analgesia. The commonest form of analgesia for upper gastrointestinal endoscopy is pharyngeal anaesthesia with a local anaesthetic spray. However, it should be noted that lignocaine is itself a respiratory depressant and it can cause bradycardia, hypotension and cardiac arrest.

Combination of benzodiazepines with opioid drugs

It is surprising that some endoscopists consider it necessary to give an opioid in combination with a benzodiazepine for routine diagnostic upper gastrointestinal endoscopy. In England pethidine is most commonly used and opioids are given in combination with benzodiazepines in 5% of upper gastrointestinal procedures overall, but in 20–40% of therapeutic endoscopies (Quine *et al.*, 1995a).

It is likely that the majority of endoscopists are unaware of the major drug interaction that occurs between opioids and benzodiazepines. This is borne out by the English audit, which revealed that no reduction in doses of either drug was made when the combination was administered and often higher doses of the benzodiazepine were used with pethidine than when used alone. There is up to an eightfold synergy between the drugs that could have major implications for morbidity and mortality from adverse and cardiopulmonary events (Whitwam, 1991). For those patients who require systemic analgesia, possibly during therapeutic endoscopy or colonoscopy, it is not advisable to give the opioid during the procedure and after the benzodiazepine. A safer and more effective regimen has been suggested by Geller (1991) in which a small dose of the opioid (25–30% of the usual dose) is administered, perhaps intramuscularly, 20–30 minutes prior to the procedure. If an intravenous route is used, allow up to 5 minutes for the opioid to take effect. Then the benzodiazepine dose should be titrated carefully again using only 25% of the dose that would be required if the drug was used on its own.

In UK surveys (Daneshmend, Bell and Logan, 1991; Quine *et al.*, 1995a) adverse events were more common in patients who received a combination of pethidine and a benzodiazepine (irrespective of whether it was diazepam or midazolam) than the latter alone.

8.1.5   THE BENZODIAZEPINE ANTAGONIST FLUMAZENIL

Flumazenil (Anexate, Roche UK Ltd, Welwyn), the specific benzodiazepine antagonist, should always be available as an emergency drug in any area where intravenous benzodiazepines are being used (Whitwam, 1991; Royal College of Surgeons of England, 1993). However, the potential for flumazenil to be used as a drug to reverse benzodiazepine-induced sedation routinely and selectively has yet to be realized. Elective reversal at the end of the endoscopic procedure can provide an immediate 'window' of alertness, without reversing the amnesia for the preceding endoscopy, when information can be imparted to the patient and immediate discharge can take place (McCloy and Pearson, 1990; Pearson *et al.*, 1991). The obvious economic advantages of this, with increased turnover through the endoscopy suite and the avoidance of recovery area facilities and staff, have to be balanced against the high cost of flumazenil. Resedation, which should be more appropriately termed 'residual sedation', is a theoretical possibility that could occur owing to the shorter terminal elimination half-life of flumazenil (just under 1 hour) compared with the benzodiazepines. However, this has never been reported to be a problem in routine clinical practices employing sedative, as opposed to anaesthetic, doses of the benzodiazepine.

Paradoxical reactions to benzodiazepines

Rarely, paradoxical reactions can occur during benzodiazepine-induced sedation. On occasions this may be due to a drug idiosyncrasy and can be disturbing. The unco-operative and restless behaviour of the patient is more usually a problem with oversedation and/or hypoxaemia. In either case intravenous flumazenil is the appropriate therapy (Geller, 1991) and the usual demand of the endoscopist for 'more sedation' should be refused by the nurse. Reversal of the benzodiazepine-induced sedation allows the return of the descending cortical inhibition necessary for the compliance of the patient (section 8.1.2). In addition, supplemental oxygen should be administered in case the reaction is due to hypoxaemia (section 8.3.2).

8.1.6 ANTIPERISTALTIC DRUGS

The use of anticholinergic drugs to inhibit gut motility during endoscopic procedures is decreasing. The most commonly used drug is hyoscine-N-butyl-bromide (Buscopan), comprising 20–30% of cases in the Quine *et al.* (1995a) audit, whilst atropine was still used in 0.3–11% of cases. Anticholinergic premedication may not improve the quality of diagnostic endoscopy (Hedenbro, Frederiksen and Lindblom, 1991). Furthermore, Buscopan can cause both tachycardias and hypotension and these are more marked if 40 mg rather than 20 mg is used. Its half-life is short, about 10 minutes, and incremental doses may be needed for longer procedures.

An alternative is to inhibit motility with intravenous glucagon, with the advantages of no physiological adverse effects and a longer duration of action, but it is relatively expensive.

8.2 PROCEDURAL SAFETY AND MONITORING

Recommendations for adequate staffing during endoscopic procedures and the regular training of all staff in cardiopulmonary resuscitation have been made elsewhere (Bell *et al.*, 1991b) and are beyond the scope of this chapter.

8.2.1   OXYGEN SATURATION, OXYGEN SUPPLEMENTATION AND OXIMETRY

The physiological changes that can occur during endoscopy can be profound and have been well reviewed (Fleischer, 1989). They can be various and include marked falls in oxygen saturation during both upper gastrointestinal endoscopy (with or without sedation, but worse with large-diameter instruments) and colonoscopy (with sedation, and particularly if benzodiazepine/opioid combinations are used). However, there is no correlation between the fall in oxygen saturation, the type or dose of sedation used and the age or sex of the patient. In other words, oxygen desaturation cannot be predicted and may occur in otherwise fit patients. Pre-endoscopy checklists and risk assessment may not predict the occurrence of problems.

The use of pre-oxygenation and/or supplemental oxygen during the procedure can prevent significant hypoxaemia during upper gastrointestinal endoscopy (Bell *et al.*, 1987a), ERCP (Griffin *et al.*, 1990) and colonoscopy (Gross and Long, 1990). In England supplemental oxygen is employed in 7–17% of patients classed as ASA (American Society of Anesthesiology) I–II and 15–51% of patients classed ASA III–V (Quine *et al.*, 1995a). Whilst oxygen supplementation has been recommended for 'at-risk' patients (Bell *et al.*, 1991b), surely its routine deployment for every case is more appropriate (Royal College of Surgeons of England, 1993) and can be achieved with minimal expense. If supplemental oxygen is used routinely and prevents significant hypoxaemia then this begs the question as to whether relatively expensive monitoring using pulse oximetry is necessary.

Oxygen can of course be administered by a simple mask during colonoscopy, but during upper gastrointestinal endoscopy the patient may switch from nasal breathing to breathing by mouth when the endoscope touches the soft palate (Bell *et al.*, 1991a). Under these circumstances oxygen is best delivered at 2 l/min via a special endoscope mouthguard (Fig. 8.1) that has apertures to direct the oxygen up the nose and back into the mouth simultaneously (Bell *et al.*, 1992).

Pulse oximetry is normal practice in the USA (Keeffe and O'Connor, 1990) but is variously used in 25–69% of patients in England (Quine *et al.*, 1995a). Again it has been recommended (Bell *et al.*, 1991b) and suggested that it should become standard practice for all (Royal College of Surgeons of England, 1993). However, it is unlikely to be proven that supplemental oxygen and/or pulse oximetry during endoscopy prevents morbidity and mortality, since large enough studies and controlled trials

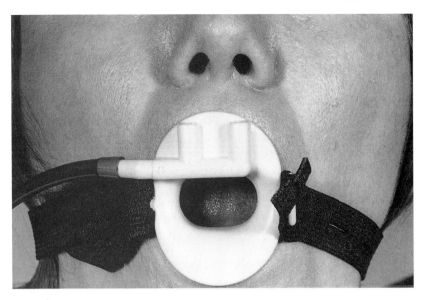

Fig. 8.1 Endoscopic mouthguard showing oxygen attachment and flow directed to nostrils

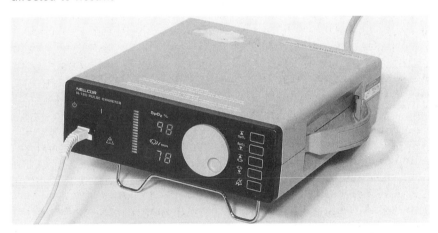

Fig. 8.2 A typical pulse oximeter – the upper figure shows the oxygen saturation (%), and the lower figure the pulse rate

will probably not be performed. A review of 2000 anaesthetic incidents demonstrated that pulse oximetry (Fig. 8.2) detected more incidents than any other monitor and would have alerted the anaesthetist in over 80% of applicable incidents during anaesthesia and recovery (Webb *et al.*, 1993). Anyone who uses monitoring equipment must be aware of its limitations and pulse oximeters are no exception; possible sources of error are as follows:

- *Equipment and environmental factors*
  - faulty equipment
  - poor probe position
  - movement artifact – struggling, shivering, cable
  - diathermy units.
- *Patient factors*
  - carboxyhaemoglobin (recent smoking)
  - thalassaemia
  - drug interaction – phenacetin
  - renal failure
  - jaundice
  - low perfusion states
      local vasoconstriction and tissue hypoxia
      hypothermia
      hypovolaemia (shock)
      hypotension.
- *Social factors*
  - nail varnish
  - nicotine staining (skin pigmentation is irrelevant).

If anaesthetists believe that continuous monitoring from induction to recovery is worthwhile then should this not become the standard for all (Charlton, 1995)?

8.2.2 INTRAVENOUS ACCESS

There are many reasons why adequate, reliable intravenous access throughout the endoscopic procedure is essential:

- *Drug effects immediate and relatively consistent.*
- *Multiple drugs given easily*
  - sedative drug
  - incremental (or top-up) doses
  - opioid analgesics
  - anticholinergics (or glucagon)
  - antibiotics
  - flumazenil (for reversal).
- *Resuscitation – emergency drugs.*
- *Volume expansion – crystalloids, colloids and blood.*

It is surprising therefore that endoscopists in England use continuous intravenous access during the procedure in only 60% of inpatients and 40% of outpatients undergoing gastroscopy (Quine *et al.*, 1995a). Having to place a cannula during an emergency under adverse conditions with a potentially unconscious patient curled up on their side in a semidarkened room is difficult to defend. In the Quine *et al.* (1995a) audit four out of five patients who had a cardiac arrest were without venous access. Intravenous access should be available via a plastic cannula, rather than a 'butterfly' metal needle in all patients until recovery is complete (Royal College of Surgeons of England, 1993). The preferred site of access is the back of the hand or the forearm, but use of the antecubital fossa risks accidental placement in the brachial artery.

8.2.3 RECOVERY AND DISCHARGE

Monitoring and procedural safety extend beyond the endoscopy room into the recovery area, whether this be in the same locale or a remote area, and criteria for safe discharge from the unit following intravenous sedation should be formalized. Those of the Royal College of Surgeons of England (1993) are:

- Stable vital signs.
- Ability to walk without support.
- Toleration of oral fluids.
- Ability to void urine.
- Minimal nausea.
- Adequate analgesia.
- Appropriate aftercare.

They should include appropriate instructions to the patient and escort if discharged home as a day case (Royal College of Surgeons of England, 1993).

8.3 EMERGENCIES

Prevention and early recognition together with appropriate training of the entire endoscopy team should be standard for all units.

8.3.1 LOCAL EMERGENCIES

Aspiration

Theoretically, inhalation is one potential problem when pharyngeal analgesia is combined with sedation. There is little direct evidence but the audit of 14 149 cases by Quine et al. (1995a) did identify 11 cases of pneumonia, of whom 10 had received lignocaine throat spray and eight died, during the 30-day period after gastroscopy. Furthermore, the presence of the endoscope can interfere with glottic closure and swallowing and when pharyngeal analgesia has been used in patients undergoing endoscopy for upper gastrointestinal haemorrhage aspiration there is an association with pulmonary aspiration (Lipper, Simon and Cerrone, 1991). Anaesthetic throat spray should probably be avoided if sedation and upper gastrointestinal endoscopy are being used in patients who may have excess gastric contents (bleeding or gastric outlet obstruction), particularly if they are elderly.

Prevention of aspiration should be attempted by assiduous suction of the oropharynx during upper gastrointestinal endoscopy whenever fluid is apparent in the mouth. Aspiration is rarely recognized during endoscopy unless it is of a significant volume, in which case it represents a potential anaesthetic emergency. The procedure should be discontinued, the sedative reversed with flumazenil, and an urgent chest X-ray and arterial blood gases performed. The duty anaesthetist should be requested to give a clinical opinion, even if the patient appears clinically stable, since deterioration into a full-blown Mendelson's syndrome can be rapid.

Gastrointestinal perforation

The Quine audit (Quine *et al.*, 1995b) identified an upper gastrointestinal perforation rate of 0.05% during diagnostic gastroscopy and 2.6% following oesophageal intubation or dilatation. There are numerous risk factors but inexperience increases the likelihood of perforation. Perforation of the duodenum during ERCP and the colon during colonoscopy are similarly well recognized and not uncommon complications.

If the perforation is recognized at the time of endoscopy the procedure should be discontinued, the sedation reversed with flumazenil, and an immediate appropriate X-ray taken to identify extraluminal free gas (or a pneumothorax for upper gastrointestinal procedures). The patient should be put on a nil-by-mouth regimen and an intravenous infusion set up with molar (i.e. 1 mol/l) saline. A blood sample should be sent to the transfusion laboratory for 'group and save'. The patient should be told the exact nature of the injury and this should be recorded in the medical records. Appropriate antibiotics, such as Augmentin or cefuroxime and metronidazole, should be given intravenously and the patient admitted as an inpatient, with clear instructions on close monitoring of vital signs. A surgical opinion should be sought as a matter of urgency.

Gastrointestinal bleeding

This is likely to be recognized at the time that it occurs and local endoscopic manoeuvres such as injection sclerotherapy, balloon tamponade, electrocautery or laser therapy may variously be appropriate depending on the type of endoscopy being performed, the experience of the endoscopist and local resources. If it is deemed significant the patient should be kept fasted, blood taken for transfusion serology and molar saline set up intravenously. The patient should be sent to the ward for appropriate monitoring of vital signs and the duty surgical team informed.

8.3.2 SYSTEMIC EMERGENCIES

Hypoxaemia

If the pulse oximeter alarm goes off (usually indicating that the oxygen saturation has fallen below 94% or 90% – depending on the instrument settings) the following progressive actions can immediately be taken since the patient should be conscious and responding to commands, if the appropriate sedation technique has been used (the patient should already be receiving supplemental oxygen):

1. Ask the patient to take deep breaths.
2. Increase the supplemental oxygen from 2 to 4 l/min.
3. Remove the endoscope (especially if via mouth).
4. Administer flumazenil.

Respiratory arrest

In the event of a respiratory arrest, the procedure should be discontinued immediately and any oral endoscope removed. The sedation is then reversed by flumazenil 0.5 mg as an intravenous bolus (not slow titration as in the drug information sheet), whilst ventilation is assisted with a Brook's airway and an Ambubag. The resuscitation team should be called. Be aware that within about 30 seconds of administering flumazenil the patient may appear fully alert but full voluntary spontaneous respiration may not be apparent for 2–3 minutes, so continued manual-assisted respiration may be required during this period. If the patient has received an opioid drug in combination with the sedation then this should be reversed using the opioid antagonist naloxone.

8.3 CONCLUSIONS

Gastrointestinal endoscopic procedures are invasive and carry a significant morbidity and mortality, even for diagnostic procedures. The commonest causes of death are cardiopulmonary complications, which may in part be related to sedative techniques. The clinical end-points for sedation need to be reappraised and should aim to induce anxiolysis and amnesia rather than hypnosis. Endoscopists need to be familiar with the pharmacodynamic and pharmacokinetic properties of the benzodiazepines employed for sedation, in particular the protracted half-lives of some benzodiazepines and the major drug interaction with significant synergy that occurs if opioids are used in combination with benzodiazepines, so that appropriate doses of these drugs are administered. The use of supplemental oxygen and pulse oximetry, combined with continuous intravenous access during the procedure, should be standard practice. The endoscopy staff should be aware of national guidelines for safe endoscopic practice and be well versed in and practise the management for dealing with related emergencies. In the event of a collapse or a severe adverse reaction the following difficult questions will have to be answered (Poswillo, 1991):

- What went wrong and why?
- Had an adequate medical history been taken?
- Was the sedative technique justifiable and necessary?
- Was the sedative agent used a correct one in the circumstances?
- Were sufficient properly trained persons present at all times throughout the preparation, the procedure and the recovery period?
- Were adequate resuscitation equipment and drugs available?
- Were those present adequately trained in methods of resuscitation and was each member of the team immediately aware of his or her duties?
- Was the order of the procedure of resuscitation correct?
- Was there any failing, on anyone's part, during or after the sedative technique that contributed to the collapse or failure to resuscitate the patient?

These should act as a timely reminder to all the staff on the endoscopy team to maintain the highest possible standards of vigilance and practice in every case.

REFERENCES

ABPI Data Sheet Compendium (1996) London: Datapharm Publications.

Amerin, R., Cano, J.P., Eckert, M. and Coassolo, Ph. (1981) Pharmakokinetic von midazolam nach intravenoser verabreichung. *Arneim-Forsch/Drug Res*, **31**, 2202–5.

Axon, A.T.R., Bell, G.D., Jones, R.H., Quine, M.A. and McCloy, R.F. (1995) Guidelines on appropriate indications for upper gastrointestinal endoscopy. *BMJ*, **310**, 853–6.

Bell, G.D. (1990) Review article: premedication and intravenous sedation for upper gastrointestinal endoscopy. *Aliment Pharmacol Ther*, **4**, 103–22.

Bell, G.D., Brown, N.S., Morden, A., Coady, T. and Logan, R.F.A. (1987a) Prevention of hypoxaemia during upper gastrointestinal endoscopy by means of oxygen via nasal cannulae. *Lancet*, **i**, 1022–4.

Bell, G.D., Spickett, G.P., Reeve, P.A., Morden, A. and Logan, R.F.A. (1987b) Intravenous midazolam for upper gastrointestinal endoscopy: a study of 800 consecutive cases relating dose to age and sex of patient. *Br J Pharmacol*, **23**, 241–4.

Bell, G.D., Antrobus, J.H.L., Lee, J., Coady, T. and Morden, A. (1990) Bolus or slow injection of midazolam prior to upper gastrointestinal endoscopy? Relative effect on oxygen saturation and prophylactic value of supplemental oxygen. *Aliment Pharmacol Ther*, **4**, 393–410.

Bell, G.D., Antrobus, J.H.L., Lee, J., Coady, T. and Morden, A. (1991a) Pattern of breathing during upper gastrointestinal endoscopy – implications for administration of supplemental oxygen. *Aliment Pharmacol Ther*, **5**, 399–404.

Bell, G.D., McCloy, R.F., Charlton, J.E., Campbell, D., Dent, N.A., Gear, M.W.L., Logan, R.F.A. and Swan, C.H.J. (1991b) Recommendations for standards of sedation and patient monitoring during gastrointestial endoscopy. *Gut*, **32**, 823–7.

Bell, G.D., Quine, A., Antrobus, J.H.L., Morden, A., Burridge, S.M., Lee, J. and Coady, T. (1992) Upper gastrointestinal endoscopy: a prospective randomised study comparing the efficacy of continuous supplemental oxygen given either via the nasal or oral route. *Gastrointest Endosc*, **38**, 319–25.

Carey, W.D. (1987) Indications, contraindications, and complications of upper gastrointestinal endoscopy, in *Gastroenterologic Endoscopy* (ed. M.V. Sivak), W.B. Saunders, Philadelphia, p. 301.

Charlton, J.E. (1995) Monitoring and supplental oxygen during endoscopy. One death per 2000 procedures demands action. *BMJ*, **310**, 886–7.

Cotton, P.B. and Williams, C.B. (1990) *Practical Gastrointestinal Endoscopy*, 3rd edn, Blackwell, Oxford, p. 52.

Daneshmend, T.K., Bell, G.D. and Logan, R.F.A. (1991) Sedation for upper gastrointestinal endoscopy: results of a nationwide survey. *Gut*, **32**, 12–15.

Fleischer, D. (1989) Monitoring the patient receiving conscious sedation for gastrointestinal endoscopy: issues and guidelines. *Gastrointest Endosc*, **35**, 262–6.

Froehlich, F., Schwizer, W., Thorens, J., Köhler, M., Convers, J.-J. and Fried, M. (1995) Concious sedation for gastroscopy: patient tolerance and cardio-respiratory parameters. *Gastroenterology*, **108**, 697–704.

Gebbensleben, B. and Rohde, H. (1990) Anxiety before gastrointestinal endoscopy – is it a significant problem? *Dtsch Med Wschr*, **115**, 1539–44.

Geller, E. (1991) Report of workshop on drugs for sedation, in *Quality Control in Endoscopy* (ed. R. McCloy), Springer-Verlag, Berlin, pp. 22–9.

Greenblatt, D.J. and Schader, R.I. (1978) Pharmacokinetic understanding of antianxiety drug therapy. *Southern Med J*, **71** (suppl 2), 2–9.

Griffin, S.M., Chung, S.C.S., Leung, J.W.C. and Li, A.K.C. (1990) Effect of intranasal oxygen on hypoxemia and tachycardia during endoscopic cholangiopancreatography. *BMJ*, **300**, 84–4.

Gross, J.B. and Long, W.B. (1990) Nasal oxygen alleviates hypoxemia in colonoscopy patients with midazolam and meperidine. *Gastrointest Endosc*, **36**, 26–9.

Hart, R. and Classen, M. (1990) Complications of diagnostic gastrointestinal endoscopy. *Endoscopy*, **22**, 229–33.

Hedenbro, J.L., Frederiksen, S.G. and Lindblom, A. (1991) Anticholingeric medication in diagnostic endoscopy of the upper gastrointestinal tract. *Endoscopy*, **23**, 199–212.

Keeffe, E.B. (1991a) Endoscopic procedural safety, in *Quality Control in Endoscopy* (ed. R. McCloy), Springer-Verlag, Berlin, pp. 33–45.

Keeffe, E.B. (1991b) Sedation and analgesia for endoscopy. *Gastroenterology*, **108**, 932–3.

Keeffe, E.B. and O'Connor, K.W. (1990) 1989 A/S/G/E survey of endoscopic sedation and monitoring practices. *Gastrointest Endosc*, **36**, S13–S18.

Landefield, K., Rohde, H., Müller, J. and Eisebitt, R. (1993) Acceptance, reactivity and side effects in 519 gastroscopy and 506 colonoscopy patients with and without midazolam premedication. *Med Klin*, **88**, 691–8.

Lipper, B., Simon, D. and Cerrone, F. (1991) Pulmonary aspiration during emergency endoscopy in patients with upper gastrointestinal haemorrhage. *Crit Care Med*, **19**, 330–3.

McCloy, R.F. and Pearson, R.C. (1990) Which agent and how to deliver it. A review of benzodiazepine sedation and its reversal in endoscopy. *Scand J Gastroenterol*, **25** (suppl 179), 7–11.

Pearson, R.C., McCloy, R.F., Bardhan, K.D., Jackson, V. and Morris, P. (1991) The use of flumazenil to reverse sedation induced by bolus low dose midazolam or diazepam in upper gastrointestinal endoscopy. *Europ J Gastroenterol Hepatol*, **3**, 829–33.

Poswillo, D.E. (1991) Medico-legal aspects of sedation in endoscopy, in *Towards Safer Sedation: Endoscopy* (ed. R. McCloy), Meditext, London, pp. 1–4.

Quine, M.A., Bell, G.D., McCloy, R.F., Charlton, J.E., Devlin, H.B and Hopkins, A. (1995a) A prospective audit of upper gastrointestinal endoscopy in two regions of England: safety, staffing and sedation methods. *Gut*, **36**, 462–7.

Quine, M.A., Bell, G.D., McCloy, R.F. and Matthews, H.R. (1995b) Prospective audit of perforation rates following upper gastrointestinal endoscopy in two regions of England. *Br J Surg*, **82**, 530–3.

Royal College of Surgeons of England (1993) *Report of the Working Party on Guidelines for Sedation by Non-anaesthetists*. Commission on the Provision of Surgical Services, London.

Schneider-Bandura, M., Vormann, Th., Fischer, M. and Rohde, H. (1993) Fear of outpatient gastroscopy. Influences and consequences for anxiolytic premedication. *Münch Med Wschr*, **135**, 35–41.

Shelley, M.P., Mendel, L. and Park, G.R. (1987) Failure of critically ill patients to metabolise midazolam. *Anaesthesia*, **42**, 619–26.

Swain, D.G., Ellis, D.J. and Bradby, H. (1990) Rapid intravenous low-dose diazepam as sedation for upper gastrointestinal endoscopy. *Aliment Pharmacol Ther*, **4**, 43–8

Webb, R.K., Van der Walt, J., Runciman, W.B. *et al.* (1993) Which monitor? A review of 2,000 anaesthetic incidents. *Anaesth Intensive Care*, **21**, 529–42.

Whitwam, J.G. (1991) Drugs for sedation, in *Quality Control in Endoscopy* (ed. R. McCloy), Springer-Verlag, Berlin, pp.3–21.

Whitwam, J.G., Al-Khudhairi, D. and McCloy, R.F. (1983) Comparison of midazolam and diazepam of comparable potency during gastroscopy. *Br J Anaesth*, **55**, 773–7.

Diagnostic upper gastrointestinal endoscopy 9

Julie D'Silva

9.1 INTRODUCTION

Diagnostic upper gastrointestinal endoscopy is the most common endoscopic examination performed in gastroenterology, accounting for approximately 70% of all investigations of the gastrointestinal tract. The technique forms the basis of all therapeutic endoscopic interventions in this area including dilation, stenting, haemostasis, tumour ablation and ERCP.

There are two procedures:

1. Oesophagogastroduodenoscopy (OGD), commonly known as gastroscopy.
2. Enteroscopy.

As with all diagnostic tests, specimen collection is important, and specimens are obtained by either tissue biopsy, brush cytology or aspiration. The majority of specimens are sent for histological examination, although some require microbiological investigation or other special tests.

The endoscopy assistant must therefore be proficient not only in the procedure itself but also in the various methods of specimen collection and their handling.

Practical Endoscopy Edited by M. Shephard and J. Mason. Published in 1997 by Chapman & Hall, London. ISBN 0 412 54000 2

9.2 ANATOMY AND PHYSIOLOGY

9.2.1 DIGESTIVE SYSTEM

The organs of digestion can be separated into two main groups. The first includes the organs of the alimentary canal or gastrointestinal tract: the mouth, pharynx, oesophagus, stomach, small intestine and large intestine, which leads to the anus. The gastrointestinal tract is a continuous, coiled, hollow muscular tube that runs through the ventral body cavity. It is open to the external environment at both ends. Its function is to digest food by breaking it down into small particles, and absorb the digested particles into the bloodstream.

The second group includes the accessory digestive organs: the teeth, tongue and gall bladder, and the large digestive glands comprising the salivary glands, liver and pancreas. The digestive glands and gall bladder lie outside the gastrointestinal tract and connect with it via ducts. The function of the accessory digestive organs is to produce saliva, bile and enzymes, which are essential in the process of breaking down foodstuffs. The walls of all the organs of the gastrointestinal tract, from the oesophagus to the anal canal, are made up of the following four layers, from the lumen outwards (Fig. 9.1).

1. *Mucosa*; moist epithelial membrane lining the lumen or cavity. Its major functions are:
   (a) secretion of mucus, digestive enzymes and hormones;
   (b) absorption of the end-products of digestion into the blood-stream;
   (c) protection against some infectious diseases.

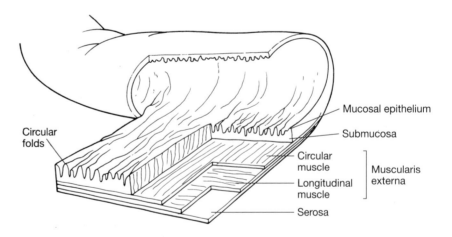

Fig. 9.1   Structure of the gastrointestinal tract

The mucosa consists of a surface epithelium, a small area of connective tissue called the lamina propria and a smooth muscle layer called the muscularis mucosae. The epithelium is a simple columnar epithelium rich in mucus-secreting goblet cells; this slippery mucus protects some organs of digestion from being digested themselves. It also aids in the movement of food throughout the digestive tract. In the stomach and the small intestine the mucosa also contains enzyme- and hormone-secreting cells.

The lamina propria nourishes the epithelium through its capillaries and absorbs digested nutrients. The lymph nodules of the lamina propria are vital in the defence against bacteria and other pathogens that access our digestive tract.

The muscularis mucosae generates local movement of the mucosa; in the small intestine this greatly increases the surface area by forming a series of small folds.

2. *Submucosa*; This is dense connective tissue, external to the mucosa, rich in blood vessels, lymphatic vessels, lymph nodes, nerve fibres and elastic fibres. Its rich vascular network supplies the surrounding tissues of the wall of the gastrointestinal tract. The nerve supply is from the submucosal plexus, which is part of the intrinsic nerve supply of the gastrointestinal tract from the autonomic nervous system.

3. *Muscularis externa*; the muscularis, as it is usually referred to, has two major functions: segmentation and peristalsis, the mixing together and the moving forward of foodstuffs. The muscularis is a thick muscle layer with an inner circular layer and an outer longitudinal layer. The sphincters or valves of the gastrointestinal tract are formed by the thickening of the circular layer. Sphincters prevent back-movement of food and aid in controlling food passing from one organ to the next.

Lying between the circular and longitudinal smooth muscle layers is the myenteric nerve plexus, which provides the major nerve supply to the gastrointestinal tract wall and also controls gastrointestional motility.

4. *Serosa*; this is the protective layer of the intraperitoneal organs, the visceral peritoneum. The oesophagus, which is contained in the thoracic cavity and not the abdominopelvic cavity, is surrounded by adventitia (ordinary fibrous connective tissue binding the oesophagus to surrounding structures).

Oesophagus

The oesophagus (meaning 'to carry food') is a hollow, muscular tube approximately 25 cm long that collapses when not propelling food into the stomach. It runs a straight course through the mediastinum and

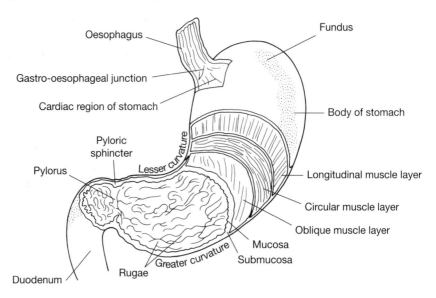

Fig. 9.2   Anatomy of the stomach

joins the stomach at the cardiac orifice. This is surrounded by the gastro-oesophageal sphincter, which acts as a valve. It is formed from circular smooth muscle but as it is only slightly thickened, it is the action of the diaphragm at this point that helps to keep it closed when no food is being swallowed.

The mucosa of the oesophagus changes at the oesophagogastric junction from stratified squamous epithelium to simple columnar epithelium for secretion.

Stomach

The stomach lies between the distal oesophagus and the duodenum, and is situated entirely within the abdomen below the diaphragm. It is a 'J'-shaped dilated portion of the alimentary tract, and is described as having two curvatures (Fig. 9.2). The shorter, lesser curvature lies on the posterior surface of the stomach and is the downwards continuation of the posterior wall of the oesophagus; before the pyloric sphincter it curves upwards to complete the 'J' shape. The greater curvature is where the oesophagus joins the stomach as the anterior part angles acutely upwards towards the pyloric orifice. The gastric glands secrete mucus, pepsinogen, hydrochloric acid, intrinsic factor and the following hormone or hormone-like products that have essential roles in digestion:

- *Gastrin* – a hormone, causes gastric glands to increase secretory activity, producing especially hydrochloric acid. It stimulates gastric emptying and contraction of intestinal muscle in the small intestine, relaxes the ileocaecal valve and stimulates mass movements in the large intestine.
- *Serotonin* – a hormone, causes stomach muscles to contract.
- *Histamine* – a hormone, activates parietal cells and therefore secretion of hydrochloric acid takes place.
- *Somatostatin* – a hormone, inhibits all gastric secretion, gastric motility and emptying. In the small intestine it inhibits blood flow and intestinal absorption. In the gall bladder it inhibits contraction and release of bile, and also secretion in the pancreas.
- *Secretin* – a hormone, inhibits gastric gland secretion and gastric motility.
- *Pepsin* – the most important protein-digesting enzyme.
- *Intrinsic factor* – required for absorption of vitamin B12. This converts foodstuff into chyme.

Small intestine

This is the major digestive organ of the body, the diameter being approximately 2.5 cm, and the average length 6–7 m. It has three divisions: the duodenum, jejunum and the ileum. Most absorption occurs in the proximal part of the small intestine. The plicae circulares, villi and microvilli amplify the absorptive surface tremendously. Plicae circulares are deep folds of mucosa and submucosa. They force chyme through the lumen of the intestine where it mixes with intestinal juice, which slows its movements and allows nutrients to be absorbed. The villi (fingerlike projections) within the core of the lamina propria of each villus are a dense capillary bed and lymphatic capillary called a lacteal. Digested foodstuffs are absorbed through the epithelial cells into the capillary blood and the lacteal. In the duodenum, where most absorption takes place, the villi are large but they gradually become smaller further down the small intestine.

All classes of food are completely chemically digested by the digestive enzymes from the pancreas. Products of carbohydrate, protein and fat that have been broken down are absorbed along with vitamins, water and electrolytes by both active and passive mechanisms.

Cholecystokinin, a hormone released by the small intestine, causes the gall bladder to contract; the sphincter of Oddi then relaxes, releasing bile juice into the duodenum to help in the digestion of fats. Pancreatic juice secretion is controlled by the vagus nerve and cholecystokinin; it is rich in HCO_3-containing enzymes that are involved in the digestion of all foodstuffs.

9.3 OESOPHAGOGASTRODUODENOSCOPY

9.3.1 INDICATIONS

Endoscopy is an excellent method for diagnosis in patients suffering from gastrointestinal symptoms, as it allows the endoscopist to examine the mucosa of the oesophagus, stomach and duodenum to exclude or confirm ulcers, tumours, etc. and then commence appropriate treatment. It is essential that the person responsible for requesting that a patient has an endoscopy is certain that this examination is indicated and there are no major contraindications. Indications for diagnostic OGD include:

- Dysphagia.
- Complicated dyspepsia.
- Oesophageal reflux resistant to therapy.
- Persistent nausea/vomiting.
- Acute or chronic haemorrhage of gastrointestinal origin (haematemesis and melaena).
- Suspected oesophageal or gastric varices.
- Suspected neoplasm.
- Chronic abdominal pain.
- Suspected gastric outlet obstruction.
- Further investigation of lesions shown by barium studies.

Contraindications include:

- Recent myocardial infarction.
- Severe, uncontrolled cardiovascular disease.
- Severe respiratory impairment.
- Symptoms of gastrointestinal perforation.
- Known large aortic aneurysm.

Note: observe caution in patients with:

- Severe cervical arthritis (use a cervical collar).
- Acute oral or pharyngeal inflammation.
- Severe shock.
- Uncontrolled epilepsy.

An emergency endoscopy may be performed in patients presenting with an acute upper gastrointestinal bleed. This procedure must be performed by an experienced endoscopist and is more reliable than barium radiology for confirming diagnosis in this group of patients (Chapter 10).

If an 'out of hours' emergency endoscopy service is provided it is essential that trained endoscopy nurses are available to cover this service.

9.3.2   USE OF SEDATION

Not all patients are suitable candidates for having procedures performed without sedation and some procedures (e.g. therapeutic procedures) require the patient to have some degree of sedation.

The sedation of choice is administered prior to the procedure being performed; the amount of sedation required will depend on the age, weight and physical condition of the patient and also the procedure in question.

Reversal agents should always be available, and the patient should always have an intravenous cannula *in situ*.

9.3.3   TOLERANCE OF THE PATIENT

Every patient has individual needs and some patients will have a higher tolerance level than others. Some patients will request their procedure performed without sedation and other patients will require more sedation than is normally required. Patients undergoing the procedure for the first time will be frightened of what is going to happen to them; reassuring the patient is most important and explaining the procedure and answering any fears the patient may have can be completed whilst admitting the patient to the unit.

9.3.4   PATIENT POSITION/PROCEDURE/DISCHARGE

First of all, patient education is important. This begins when the request for gastroscopy is received. If the patient is not seen for consultation prior to the examination, information leaflets explaining the procedure in patient-friendly terminology should be sent to the patient. Informed consent should be obtained for all endoscopic procedures (Chapter 5).

The patient should be instructed not to eat or drink for 4–6 hours prior to the procedure. If the patient is known to suffer from a gastric outlet obstruction it will be necessary for the period of fasting to be longer and gastric lavage may be required. Dentures, spectacles and contact lenses should be removed prior to the procedure and should be kept somewhere safe, according to unit policy.

If the patient requires sedation for the examination, the endoscopy assistant should ensure first that there is someone to collect them from the unit and look after them once they are discharged home. Sedation should be administered via an intravenous cannula and the appropriate reversal agent should be readily available. All patients should have intravenous access whether sedated or not. Pharyngeal anaesthesia administered via throat spray is beneficial, especially if a small amount or no sedation is requested by the patient.

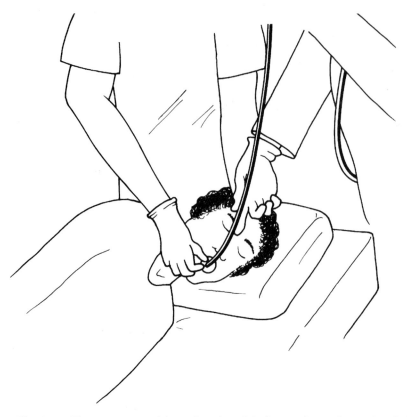

Fig. 9.3   The correct position. One hand is free to keep the patient's head flexed slightly forwards and to administer oral suction, whilst the other holds the mouthguard in position

The patient will then attend the endoscopy unit and the admission procedure is carried out (Chapter 6). For endoscopy, the patient is positioned in the left lateral position, with the head possibly elevated slightly by the use of a pillow, or the head of the trolley may be raised. A disposable towel or similar is placed under the patient's head to catch any secretions. (The head should be flexed forward slightly to enable any regurgitated secretions or saliva to drain from the mouth and to aid intubation.) A mouthguard is then gently placed between the patient's teeth or gums. Extra care should be taken if the patient has crowned or capped teeth as these may become dislodged or broken. The mouthguard also enables the endoscope to run midline during intubation.

The endoscopy assistant stands at the patient's head, ensuring that the airway is maintained and the mouthguard is correctly positioned throughout the procedure (Fig. 9.3). Oral suction must be available to clear the patient's airway if necessary. The assistant should reassure and talk to the patient throughout the procedure. The patient's oxygen saturation levels, pulse and respirations should be monitored throughout the procedure, and recorded in the patient's records

On completion of the procedure, the patient is transferred to the recovery area. If sedation has been administered then the patient will need to rest on a trolley until the effects of the sedation have worn off and should then be instructed to go home and rest and not drive or operate machinery for 24 hours. Unsedated patients are able to leave the unit once they have recovered and the results of the examination and any treatment or further investigations discussed with them.

9.3.5 COMPLICATIONS/PRECAUTIONS

Complications include the following:

1. *Patient distress*; this occurs occasionally, and is more common if the patient has requested that the procedure be performed without sedation. The most common cause for distress is a feeling by patients that they are choking and cannot swallow. The endoscopy assistant can help alleviate this by talking the patient through the test, suggest slow breathing, etc., but, failing this, intravenous sedation may be required.

2. *Food residue*; the gastroscopy should be abandoned in this situation, because of the risk to the patient from aspiration and because the suction channel on the endoscope is not adequate to aspirate food residue. This may be due to incorrect fasting or because of gastric outlet obstruction.

3. *Oversedation*; this can usually be avoided by correct dose titration (Chapter 8). Specific antagonists (reversal agents) must always be readily available.

4. *Hypoxia*; this can be avoided by ensuring patients' oxygen saturation and pulse levels are recorded and by the routine administration of oxygen.

5. *Perforation*; common regions for perforation are in the pharynx and cervical oesophagus where the endoscopist has to pass the endoscope blindly. The risk is higher if therapeutic procedures such as dilation are performed or with an inexperienced endoscopist.

6. *Haemorrhage following endoscopic biopsy*; there is a small risk of haemorrhage, especially if the patient has impaired coagulation or portal hypertension. The risk in the normal healthy patient is almost negligible.

7. *Infection*; this can be transmitted via the endoscope but is now very rare owing to the cleaning and disinfecting procedures routinely carried out in endoscopy units.

8. *Cardiac dysrhythmias*; these can be induced during periods of hypoxia, if a patient suffers from cardiac problems or if there is direct stimulation of the myocardium during intubation of the oesophagus. It is advisable for these patients to have ECG monitoring for the procedure and recovery. (Resuscitation equipment must be always available and checked daily.)

9.3.6 LOCAL PHARYNGEAL ANAESTHESIA

Local pharyngeal anaesthesia is more commonly used in patients who require little or no sedation for the procedure to be performed.

Anaesthesia can take the form of a lozenge that is sucked by the patient prior to endoscopy, but is more often in spray form. The advantage of spray is that the jet can be directed on to the posterior pharyngeal wall, rapidly producing anaesthesia. The effect is to suppress the 'gag' reflex. It is important when this is administered that the patient is **not** asked to say 'aah' as this exposes the vocal cords and larynx which, if anaesthetized will increase the risk of aspiration.

Two main types are available: xylocaine and benzocaine. The effects of the xylocaine spray can last for up to 2 hours, whereas the benzocaine spray wears off within 20 minutes. The latter is therefore useful for lists with a quick turnaround.

Patients should not drink whilst still anaesthetized because swallowing may be affected, the risk of aspiration is increased and if drinks are hot they may burn their mouth. An easy test if the assistant is unsure whether a patient can have a drink is to let them try a sip of cold water. If they can swallow it easily without coughing and it feels cold then the sensation is normal and they can drink. (A small sip of water will not harm the lungs.)

All the sprays available have a bitter taste, although the manufacturers have disguised this to a greater or lesser degree. (Flavours include: banana, wild cherry and pina colada.) It is worth warning the patient that the taste of the spray is 'vile' as they will then find this more acceptable and may even be pleasantly surprised!

9.3.7 OPERATING THEATRES/ITU

It is sometimes necessary for endoscopy to be performed under a general anaesthetic and unless the endoscopy unit is equipped with an anaesthetic room these procedures must be performed in main theatres. This may be a routine or an intraoperative endoscopy.

Patients who need emergency endoscopy for gastrointestinal haemorrhage may have their endoscopy performed in main theatre if the

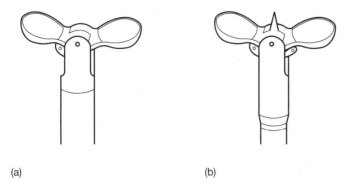

(a)   (b)

Fig. 9.4 Biopsy forceps: (a) non-spiked; (b) spiked

surgeon considers surgery as the outcome. Endoscopy may also have to be performed on intensive care units as the patients here cannot be transferred to the endoscopy unit; in this instance it will be necessary to transfer equipment to the intensive care unit for the procedure.

9.3.8 SPECIMEN COLLECTION

Biopsy

If there appear to be any abnormalities in the mucosal features on endoscopic examination then biopsies of the area in question will be taken. Biopsies can be performed anywhere throughout the gastro-intestinal tract. It is usual to take multiple biopsies of suspicious areas to ensure accurate histopathological results. In some cases it may be necessary for the lesion to be re-biopsied if initial results are not conclusive or the specimen is inadequate.

The methods used for fixing and handling of specimens differ depending on the requirements of the pathology laboratory.

There are many different types of biopsy forceps available for tissue collection (Fig. 9.4):

1. *Non-spiked biopsy forceps*; these are cupped and are available in differing shapes and sizes.
2. *Spiked forceps*; these have a needle in the centre of the cups; this makes it easier to take a biopsy, but care must be taken not to perforate the area.
3. *Alligator jaw forceps*; these have a longer cup than do standard forceps and the edges are serrated, making it easier for the operator to hold the specimen.

4. *Hot biopsy forceps*; these forceps are insulated and can be used with diathermy; they are useful if biopsying a lesion that may bleed following collection.

Procedure
The forceps are passed down the biopsy channel of the endoscope by the endoscopist. Keeping the area to be biopsied under direct vision, the forceps are advanced until they contact the mucosa. The assistant controls the opening and closing of the biopsy forceps by operating the handle and opens and closes them on the instruction of the endoscopist. The biopsy forceps are then withdrawn in the closed position; the assistant removes the biopsy from the cup of the forceps using the fixing and handling procedure of the unit.

Larger and deeper tissue specimens can be obtained by using a diathermic snare loop; this procedure is similar to polypectomy.

Biopsy sites may bleed a little after collection of the specimen, but this is normally insignificant and will stop without any intervention.

Cytology

Cytology is used if biopsy specimens of the lesion are difficult to obtain or if biopsy is contraindicated (e.g. patient is taking anticoagulant therapy). It may be necessary to obtain cytology as well as biopsy specimens for some lesions.

Procedure
A sleeved disposable brush is used for taking the specimen (Fig. 9.5). The brush is passed down the biopsy channel under direct vision, and the endoscopist identifies the area in question. When instructed the assistant opens the brush to allow the brush head to extend out of the plastic sheath. The endoscopist rubs the brush across the surface of the lesion, and the brush is then withdrawn back into the plastic sheath. (This safeguards the brush and prevents the specimen from drying out.) The brush is withdrawn from the endoscope. It is important that the specimen is quickly fixed as this will prevent drying of the cells and specimen damage.

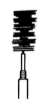

Fig. 9.5   A cytology brush

Aspirate

A suction trap can be fixed on the suction outlet of the endoscope and the suction tubing leading to the suction machine (Fig. 9.6). It has been shown that suction through the channel after a biopsy procedure also produces useful cellular material ('salvage cytology') (Cotton and Williams, 1990).

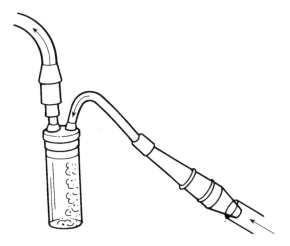

Fig. 9.6 'Trap' specimen collection

This procedure is commonly used in bronchoscopy for the collection of sputum for cytology, but is less common in OGD except in special circumstances.

9.3.9 CLO TEST

This is a test used for the identification of *Helicobacter pylori* in the gastric mucosa. It acts by detecting the urease enzyme of *H. pylori* (previously named *Campylobacter pylori*).

H. pylori has been shown to cause active chronic gastritis and has been implicated as a primary aetiological factor in duodenal ulcer, gastric ulcer and non-ulcer dypepsia by causing chronic inflammation. *H. pylori* is thought to weaken the mucosal defences and allow acid and pepsin to disrupt the epithelium. It can be detected with histology or culture of gastric tissue, but simple tests for the presence of urease enable more rapid and convenient diagnosis.

9.4 ENTEROSCOPY (SMALL-BOWEL ENDOSCOPY)

Enteroscopy is the endoscopic examination of the small bowel from the pylorus to the ileocaecal valve. As with other endoscopic examinations, a complete examination is not always possible because of either physical difficulties (anatomical or procedure tolerance) or the technical ability of the endoscopist.

Enteroscopy is indicated for:

Table 9.1 Pull versus push methods

	Pull (Sonde)	*Push*
Patient preparation	Difficult	Easy
Procedure time	1.5–6.5 hours (mean 4.15 hours)	40 min–1 hour
Patient tolerance	Poor?	Generally good
View of intestine	Limited	Good
Biopsy	No	Yes
Diathermy	No	Yes
Laser	No	Yes

- The investigation of obscure gastrointestinal bleeding. (This may form part of an intraoperative investigation.)
- The investigation of chronic unexplained iron deficiency anaemia (NSAID ingestion, angiodysplasia).
- Evaluation of Crohn's disease in the small bowel.
- Small-bowel obstruction suggestive of:
  (1) Small-bowel tumour (rare).
  (2) Tuberculous lesions (particularly if from Africa or South America).
  (3) Polyps.

Procedure

The patient is prepared for upper gastrointestinal endoscopy.
  There are two methods (Table 9.1):

1. The 'pull' (Sonde) method.
2. The 'push' enteroscope (like upper gastrointestinal endoscopy but using a longer instrument, either a paediatric colonoscope or custom-made instrument).

9.4.1 THE SONDE METHOD

The Sonde endoscope consists of a long, thin endoscope approximately 3 metres in length that has at its distal tip an inflatable balloon and a thread loop. The enteroscope is passed nasally in a manner similar to that of a nasogastric tube so that the tip is placed in the stomach. An upper gastrointestinal endoscope is then passed alongside the entero-scope, the thread loop is grasped with a pair of biopsy forceps (or similar instrument) and the enteroscope pulled through the pylorus. At this stage the balloon is inflated and, if required, medication such as metoclopramide (Maxolon, Reglan), which increases intestinal peristalsis, is administered. This speeds transit of the enteroscope down the small intestine. Progress is assessed radiologically at intervals until the desired position is obtained. The enteroscope is then slowly withdrawn, and possible lesions are documented. It is not possible to perform any therapeutic procedures with this type of enteroscope although the extent of examination is probably better than that obtained with the 'push' version. During withdrawal, a continuous slow infusion of molar (1 mol/l) saline is required to maintain optical clarity. The total procedure can take up to 6.5 hours (the average is 4.15 hours).

9.4.2   THE 'PUSH' METHOD

This method can either be carried out using a paediatric (or adult) colonoscope or there are commercially produced enteroscopes available. The length varies from 1.5 to 2.5 metres and can, if required, be 'made to measure' to suit the endoscopist's requirements. The endoscopic technique is similar to that for colonoscopy, with the tip of the enteroscope being 'hooked' around bends in the small intestine to straighten and advance the scope. For this reason, the flexible distal tip of the instrument is slightly longer than that of the normal gastroscope or colonoscope to make the 'hooking' procedure easier. It is often necessary to change the patient's position on to the back, stomach or side to aid the procedure and, like colonoscopy, judicious abdominal pressure can help with the negotiation of tight bends.

Looping in the stomach can be a problem, so some units have tried using a straight overtube to 'stiffen' the enteroscope. This is inserted over the scope and positioned through the pylorus, eliminating the gastric loop and allowing straight access to the small intestine.

Because of its length, the endoscopist has to hold this type of enteroscope in their hand with it double-looped to maintain control.

The use of this type of enteroscope allows biopsy and other procedures (laser, heat or bipolar probes) to be performed. It is also a considerably shorter procedure (40 min–1 hour) than the above, which can be scheduled as part of a normal endoscopy list.

Procedure

The majority of patients tolerate 'push' enteroscopy very well, and can be prepared in a manner similar to that of a normal upper gastrointestinal endoscopy. No specific bowel preparation is necessary but the patient should remain 'nil orally' for 6 hours before and for the duration of the test. The procedure can be uncomfortable and require sedation and use of analgesia, although the experienced enteroscopist often appreciates the less sedated but co-operative patient who is able to change position easily when asked.

The Sonde type of enteroscopy requires considerable psychological preparation of the patient because of the time involved; it is also very labour intensive, both in nursing and radiology time. It also usually involves an inpatient stay whereas the 'push' type can be performed as an outpatient. Because of the amount of air and/or saline that can be introduced into the bowel, some patients experience diarrhoea that can be difficult to control. This can be immediate or delayed. Honest, factual information, together with provision of padding and/or extra underwear, can do much to help the patient deal with this potentially embarrassing situation.

Enteroscopy is not a common procedure, and it is doubtful whether the cost of a dedicated instrument can be justified unless it is as part of a regional referral or research centre.

REFERENCES

Cotton, P.B. and Williams, C.B. (1990) *Practical Gastrointestinal Endoscopy*, 3rd edn, Blackwell, Oxford, pp. 80–2.

Therapeutic gastrointestinal endoscopy 10

Dilatation, prosthetics and foreign body removal 10A

Julie D'Silva and Mike Shephard

10A.1 OSEOPHAGEAL DILATATION

10A.1.1 INTRODUCTION

The latter half of the century has seen many advances in therapeutic endoscopy. Procedures that were initially performed surgically using rigid instrumentation and open operations are now being performed endoscopically, with a resultant reduction to risk to patients both from the complications of surgery and also from those associated with general anaesthesia.

10A.1.1 INDICATIONS/CONTRAINDICATIONS

Oesophaegeal dilatation is performed on patients suffering from dysphagia due to a stricture of the oesophagus (Plate 2). Strictures may be either benign or malignant. Any patient with a stricture that will not admit an endoscope should be considered for endoscopic dilatation (Bennett, 1981).

Benign strictures

Benign strictures are usually caused by reflex oesophagitis. Acid reflux causes inflammatory and erosive changes to the oesophageal mucosa (Bennett, 1991); in time this results in a firm fibrous stricture being formed. Other causes include achalasia and monilial infection. Gastro-oesophageal reflux disease (GORD) can be defined as symptoms and/or tissue damage caused by the backflow of gastric contents into the

Practical Endoscopy Edited by M. Shephard and J. Mason. Published in 1997 by Chapman & Hall, London. ISBN 0 412 54000 2

oesophagus. The symptoms vary, but the most common presentation is heartburn and regurgitation. The disease is extremely common in the adult population, causes much discomfort and suffering and can lead to serious long-term effects (D'Silva, 1994). Concern about the potentially serious nature of gastrointestinal symptoms appears to be a more pressing reason for many such patients to consult their doctor than do the severity, frequency or duration of symptoms. Many sufferers seem content with self-medication and three-quarters never consult a doctor about their problems; evidence from those who do indicates that they tend to receive inadequate advice, with little emphasis on reduction of alcohol or smoking (Bennett, 1991). Patients may therefore present at endoscopy already suffering from dysphagia and in need of oesophageal dilatation owing to the chronic effects of their illness.

Malignant strictures

Malignant strictures can be dilated but the risk of perforation is high, up to 10%, and improvement is only short term. However, endoscopic dilatation is sometimes the treatment of choice because of advanced disease or the patient's medical condition or surgical management being contraindicated owing to secondary metastases. The return of dysphagia after dilatation can be prevented by the insertion of an oesophageal stent or tube as a palliative measure.

Caustic stricture

Strictures may also be caused by the accidental or attempted suicidal ingestion of tablets or corrosive or caustic substances (e.g. acids, alkalis). Patients who swallow corrosive agents may have chemical burns on the tongue, palate and posterior pharynx but their absence does not exclude oesophageal and gastric injury. Patients who have suffered corrosive injury to the upper gastrointestinal tract are at risk of stricture formation and gastric outlet obstruction, and require close supervision (Baillie, 1992).

Other causes

Schatzki ring
An uncommon cause of oesophageal stricture is the Schatzki ring – bands of connective tissue occurring in the lower oesophagus and covered by a bundle of smooth muscle fibres. Patients remain symptom free, but dysphagia may occur if large pieces of meat are swallowed quickly.

Achalasia
Achalasia of the cardia is a unique type of oesophageal stricture. The Greek root of achalasia means 'without relaxation'. The condition was

originally named 'cardiospasm' but was renamed achalasia by Hurst who proved that no actual spasm existed. Achalasia is a neuromuscular disorder involving the entire oesophagus and is caused by degenerate changes in the ganglion cells. Abnormal motility patterns or a complete absence of peristalsis can be shown. Failure of the cardia to open is due to the lack of the necessary stimulus of a peristaltic wave. There is hypertrophy of the muscular wall and dilatation above the obstruction. Oesophagitis from stasis of food is frequent and it is sometimes followed by fibrous contraction or, rarely, malignant change (Hawkins, 1985).

10A.1.3   ROLE OF THE ENDOSCOPIC ASSISTANT

On admission to the endoscopy unit patients may be extremely distressed and frightened because of their inability to swallow. Dysphagia can be so severe in some circumstances that patients may not even be able to swallow their own saliva, often because of a bolus obstruction of food. The endoscopy assistant can help in alleviating patients' fears by reassuring them and explaining exactly what is going to happen to them.

The endoscopy assistant plays an important role throughout the procedure. One assistant takes care of the patient's head, ensuring that the mouthguard is positioned correctly and does not move, so that no damage occurs to the patient's lips, tongue or teeth during the procedure. The second assistant aids the endoscopist and assembles the dilators of choice (D'Silva, 1994).

10A.1.4   PROCEDURE

Great care is required by the endoscopist when performing oesophageal dilatation and the procedure should not be performed by inexperienced staff, unless under strict supervision.

The endoscopist advances the gastroscope until the stricture is reached, and in some cases it may be possible to dilate the stricture using the gastroscope as a dilator (Plate 3). The rule in dilatation is to start small and increase slowly; dilators should never be forced against major resistance as the impressive radial and axial forces generated can result in a mucosal tear, bleeding or perforation.

Many endoscopists adhere to the 'rule of threes'. **From the time resistance is first encountered, no more than three dilators of increasing diameter should be passed.** This technique minimizes the risk of perforation (Baillie, 1992).

If a wire-guided technique is used it is important that the second assistant supports the guide wire at all times and does not allow it to migrate up or downwards.

Oral suction must be available to remove any secretions from the patient's mouth during the procedure. Radiological control is not always necessary, but may be beneficial in some cases where the stricture is extremely tight (Ravenscroft and Swan, 1984).

Individual techniques are described in more detail in later sections of this chapter.

10A.1.5   POSTPROCEDURE

Postprocedure, the patient should remain in the recovery area and be observed by the nurse for any possible complications resulting from the dilatation or sedation.

Complications

1. *Perforation*; the recovery nurse should observe the patient for any signs of perforation, such as chest pain, breathlessness or surgical emphysema.
2. *Sedation*; drugs such as flumazenil should be available to reverse the effects of any sedation given.

Once the effects of the sedation have worn off, the patient is returned to the ward or discharged home.

Note: In some hospitals patients are admitted to hospital for 24 hours postprocedure care and their care is given over to ward staff. However, hospital admission is becoming less common and many units now allow patients to go home once the effects of the sedation have worn off and they are able to take fluids without any problems (D'Silva, 1994).

10A.1.6   TYPES OF DILATOR AND PROCEDURE

Eder–Puestow dilators

Eder–Puestow dilators (Fig. 10A.1) were initially popular, but have been superseded by other designs. They are made up of a series of metal olives (increasing in size), which are screwed on to a flexible metal wand and a flexible distal tip is then screwed into the end of the olive; the guide wire passes up the middle of the shaft.

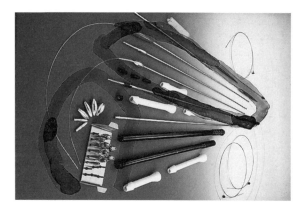

Fig. 10A.1   Eder–Puestow dilators and Atkinson tube introducer set

Eder–Puestow dilators range from 21 to 54 French (Charrière gauge 6.5–17 mm)

Tridilators

Tridilators (Fig. 10A.2) superseded the Eder–Peustow dilators and, as their name suggests, they are made up of three metal olives increasing in size on a flexible metal wand, with a screw-in flexible metal tip. The endoscopist is able to dilate the oesophagus using fewer stages, therefore the procedure is performed more quickly and is less traumatic for the patient. It is also easier for the nurse preparing the dilators.

Dilator system

The Keymed Advanced Dilator System (KADS) (Fig. 10A.3) are the most common type of dilators used. They have a flexible metal wand or shaft with a tapered plastic screw-in flexible end and so do not require a metal leader. The guide wire passes through the tapered plastic end. This is less traumatic to the patient and when dilating the oesophagus they are not as hazardous because of the flexibility of the plastic end.

Procedure
The endoscopist introduces the gastroscope until the stricture is reached. (A standard or paediatric gastroscope is the instrument of choice.) A flexible-tipped guide wire is then passed down the biopsy channel of the gastroscope. (Guide wires are now available with markings at determined intervals, enabling the endoscopist to see that they are at the exact position at all times during the dilatation.) The second assistant supports the guide wire whilst the endoscopist obtains the correct position. The guide wire is passed under direct vision

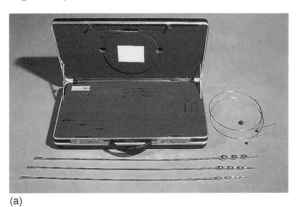

(a)

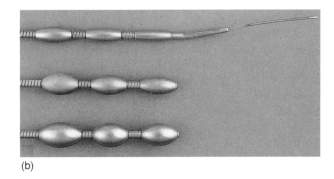

(b)

Fig. 10A.2   (a) 'Tridil' tridilators; (b) the tips

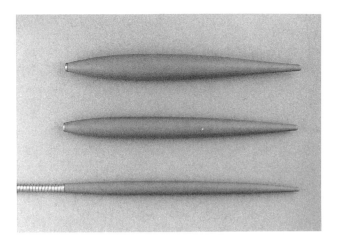

Fig. 10A.3   Keymed Advanced Dilator System (KADS)

through the stricture. This must be done with great care to ensure the stricture is not perforated.

When the guide wire is in the correct position, X-rays are taken to give confirmation. The gastroscope is then removed. The assistant holding the patient's head also holds the guide wire firmly at the mouth, maintaining its position.

The endoscopist then passes a lubricated dilator through the stricture, repeating the procedure with successively larger dilators until the desired degree of dilatation is achieved.

The guide wire is removed with the last dilator, taking great care to minimize risk of perforation of the pharynx, oesophagus or stomach (D'Silva, 1994).

At the end of the dilattion it is usually wise to check its effect by repeating the endoscopy; biopsy and cytology can also be taken (Cotton and Williams, 1990). This also allows the endoscopist to examine the stomach and duodenum and gives a retroverted look at the cardia.

Celestin/Savary dilators

Celestin and Savary dilators are an alternative to the above techniques. Both types of dilators are passed over a guide wire previously positioned endoscopically through the stricture.

Celestin dilators (Fig. 10A.4) are plastic with a tapered end and have a series of short steps. The advantage of using a stepped dilator is that only two insertions are required and the stricture can be dilated by gradual progression of the increasing-sized steps through the oesophageal stricture. The disadvantage of a stepped system is that it can be difficult for the endoscopist to determine which step they have accomplished. There is also a long length of bougie within the stomach when the highest steps of a Celestin dilator are reached, which makes their use potentially hazardous in patients who have had gastric resection (Cotton and Williams, 1990).

Savary-Gilliard dilators (Fig. 10A.5) are more popular. They are soft plastic wands with a long tapered end and are less traumatic than metal olives to the patient. They come in a range of different sizes with an external diameter ranging from 5 mm to 20 mm. They have a radio-opaque band at the top and bottom of the taper, which is advantageous when dilating tight strictures under X-ray control as the endoscopist can determine the exact position of the bougie.

Procedure

The guide wire is positioned as discussed previously. The endoscopist will decide which size bougie to commence with depending on how constricted the stricture is on visual examination; a bougie should first be chosen that will pass easily through the stricture. The assistant will

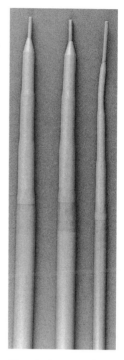

Fig. 10A.4 Celestin dilators

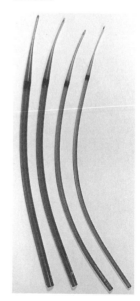

Fig. 10A.5 Savary dilators

lubricate the tapered end when it is positioned over the guide wire near to the patient's mouth (lubricating the guide wire in this position prevents the lubricant getting onto the endoscopist's gloves, making it difficult for them to manoeuvre the bougie). The endoscopist then advances the bougie; the assistant will apply counter-traction on the end of the guide wire. It is important at this stage that the endoscopist does not apply too much pressure when advancing the bougie, so as not to cause distal perforation. The stricture is dilated in stages, ensuring between each that the guide wire is in the exact position.

Hydrostatic balloons

Oesophageal
Alternatively, 'through the scope' balloon dilators (Fig. 10A.6) can be used. It is not necessary for the endoscopist to pass a guide wire through the stricture. Balloons are cylindrical, made of non-distensible polyethylene and can be passed under direct vision. The endoscopist can therefore observe the dilatation taking place. To ensure correct position of the balloon, instead of filling the balloon with air a contrast medium can be used and the procedure controlled using fluoroscopy.

Wire-guided balloons can also be used; in these the guide wire is positioned and the balloon sited over the wire into the correct position before inflation.

Balloons are 3–8 cm in length and vary in diameter. The most commonly used are 10, 15 and 18 mm diameter, and 5 cm length.

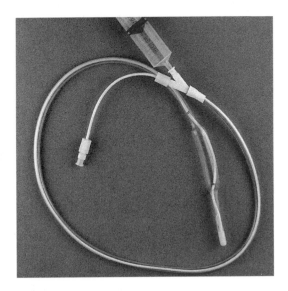

Fig. 10A.6 Oesophageal balloon

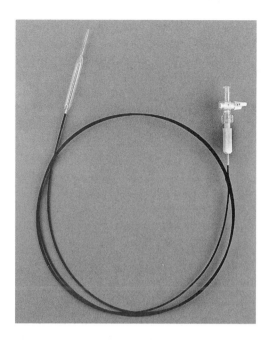

Fig. 10A.7   Pyloric balloon

These are easier than longer balloons to pass and less likely to 'pop out' of the stricture than shorter ones.

Treatment by balloon dilatation may be beneficial to patients with pyloric stenosis. The dilator is shown in Fig. 10A.7. Pyloric dilatation must never be performed where there is active peptic ulceration, as perforation of the duodenum may occur.

Biliary

Biliary balloon dilatation was adapted from the technique used for angioplasty. Common bile duct structures can now be dilated using this relatively uncomplicated procedure. Biliary strictures are most commonly due to operative accidents and sclerosing cholangitis (Cotton and Williams, 1990.) The procedure is performed therapeutically at endoscopic retrograde cholangio-pancreatography (ERCP) and is dealt with more fully in Chapter 11.

Colonic

Colonic balloon dilatation is not performed routinely. Colonic strictures are usually short and occur postoperatively at anastomosis sites.

Procedure

The balloon is passed through the biopsy channel of a standard endoscope. The passage of the balloon is uncomplicated if it is well lubricated. This can be accomplished either by lubricating the balloon with silicone spray or oil or by injecting 2 ml of silicone oil down the biopsy channel, followed by 10 ml of air; this will ensure that all the biopsy channel is lubricated, allowing easy passage of the balloon. If suction is applied to the balloon during passage the balloon will glide through the channel effortlessly.

The endoscopist will examine the stricture under direct vision and the soft plastic tip of the correct-sized balloon is passed through the stricture. The balloons are fairly translucent, so that it is possible to observe the waist of the balloon endoscopically during the procedure, and to note the extent of the dilatation (Cotton and Williams, 1990). Upon dilating the stricture, the waist on the balloon disperses.

The balloon can be inflated with air or water, but water is used for optimum dilatation of tight strictures. If water is preferred for inflation the balloon must be primed with fluid and all the air withdrawn from the balloon prior to insertion down the biopsy channel. Manufacturers advise a fixed pressure for inflation to prevent balloons from bursting during dilatation.

The advantage of balloon dilatation is that the results can be checked instantly by the endoscopist who then can go on and complete the examination. The disadvantages of using balloon dilatation are that the balloons are expensive, must be handled with care and maintained correctly; also, it is sometimes difficult to ensure the degree of dilatation achieved.

Pneumatic balloons

Pneumatic balloons are used for dilatation of strictures caused by achalasia of the oesophagus. The tight stricture at the end of the distal oesophagus is dilated with a balloon dilator that exerts high pressures of up to 300 mmHg. The reason that high pressures are used is to ensure rupturing of the smooth circular muscle.

Diagnosis of achalasia (Fig 10A.8) should always be confirmed by oesophageal manometry before the patient receives any treatment. Endoscopy is also required to rule out pseudoachalasia, a small tumour of the cardia that mimics achalasia.

The types of balloons that are used for achalasia dilatation are guide wire-placed balloons (Rigiflex), which have diameters of 30–40 mm, or the Witzel-type balloons (Fig. 10A.9) that are positioned using an over-the-scope technique.

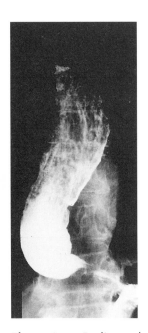

Fig. 10A.8 Radiograph showing hugely dilated distal oesophagus and tight cardia characteristic of achalasia

Procedure

If oesophageal stasis is present the patient may have to take a liquid diet for several days prior to the dilatation being performed to ensure that

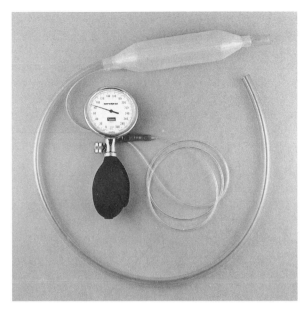

Fig. 10A.9   Witzel achalasia dilatation balloon

any food debris is cleared from the oesophagus and to minimize the risk of aspiration during the procedure. In some circumstances naso-oesophageal suction or oesophageal lavage may be necessary to ensure that no food residue is present prior to dilatation. It is sometimes necessary to perform 'stomach washouts' prior to the procedure.

The endoscopist begins dilatation with the smallest balloon. There are no set guidelines for how long the balloon should be inflated. Many endoscopists inflate for a period of 1–2 minutes, which can be repeated up to three times during one treatment. Nevertheless patients can become very agitated during the procedure because of the pain when the balloon is inflated and most endoscopists will either terminate the procedure or use shorter inflation periods. On removal it is common to observe some blood on the balloon, showing that the dilatation has been effective.

The Witzel dilator is placed over a paediatric gastroscope. The outer surface of the gastroscope is lubricated using silicone oil or spray, to make it easier for the assistant to mount the balloon on the gastroscope. The dilator is introduced with the gastroscope and when the gastric fundus is reached the tip of the endoscope is retroflexed through 180° and the middle of the dilator placed in the narrow segment of the oesophagus under direct vision. Fluoroscopy is not required for this procedure.

The endoscopist will keep the dilator in view whilst the balloon is inflated to a pressure of 200 mmHg. This can be maintained for a period of 2 minutes without causing the patient too much discomfort.

It is sometimes necessary for the dilatation to be repeated if symptoms reoccur; in some cases several dilatations are required.

Traces of blood will be observed on removal of the balloon. Some endoscopists prefer to carry out this procedure under general anaesthesia.

10A.1.7   COMPLICATIONS AND PRECAUTIONS OF DILATATIONS

Complications are as for routine gastroscopy, plus the following.

Perforation

Perforation of the pharynx, oesophagus or stomach occurs most commonly from the dilatation itself or a poorly placed guide wire. The endoscopy assistant should always check the guide wire prior to use to ensure that it is not kinked and that the tip is not bent. If the endoscopist passes too much guide wire into the stomach there is a risk of the wire perforating the abdominal wall or becoming knotted. Guide wires with graduated markings are useful as the endoscopist can assess the length of wire introduced.

If the patient becomes distressed or is in pain the dilatation should be abandoned. This can be avoided if the dilatation is taken step by step and not attempted by the inexperienced unless under close supervision. Dilatation should not be taken to the largest balloon or dilator simply because they are available and each stricture should be assessed before dilatation is performed. Perforation occurs in less than 1% of cases of benign stricture. Pain and surgical emphysema usually develop within hours. A chest X-ray and a barium swallow should be performed to confirm the diagnosis.

Surgical intervention or the placement of a covered metal stent is indicated where there is an obvious midoesophageal perforation. In the case of minor perforations, where the pain is less severe and there is no sign of a leak on a barium swallow, conservative treatment (consisting of naso-oesophageal suction, intravenous fluids and antibiotics) may be considered.

With malignant strictures the risk of perforation is higher than with dilatation of simple strictures of the oesophagus. It is essential to observe the patient for at least 4 hours postprocedure. In some cases it is necessary to admit the patient for overnight observation, especially following a difficult procedure or if there is reason to suspect perforation.

10A.1.8   DISCHARGE INSTRUCTIONS

1. The patient recovers on the endoscopy unit until the effects of sedation have subsided and no obvious complications have occurred. The patient must be able to take a drink of water without any problems developing.
2. On discharge they must be accompanied by a relative or friend and someone must stay with them overnight if they live alone. A contact telephone number should be available in case any problems occur once at home.
3. The patient will be given an outpatient appointment to see the consultant following dilatation; this is to assess whether further dilatation is necessary and what significant relief, if any, the dilatation has had on the patient's swallowing.

   If the stricture was caused because of the effects of reflux oesophagitis then lifestyle advice should be given to prevent further damage. An example 'patient advice sheet' is shown in Fig. 10A.10.
4. Patients must also be aware that their swallowing may not appear to be improved or may seem worse for 2–3 days owing to swelling of the tissues.

---

1. Overweight patients will benefit from going on a weight-reducing diet, as weight loss will improve symptoms.
2. Smoking should be stopped, as smoking increases lower oesophageal sphincter pressure and increases salivation and mucosal resistance to acid.
3. Food and drink that cause symptoms should be avoided; in particular, spicy foods, fat chocolate, peppermint, coffee and alcohol are known to provoke reflux by reducing lower oesophageal sphincter tone or by directly irritating already damaged mucosa.
4. Eating late at night should be avoided as this increases nocturnal gastric secretion.
5. Patients who suffer from nocturnal reflux should be advised to raise the head of the bed.
6. Tight clothing should not be worn as this will raise intra-abdominal pressure, which tends to promote reflux.
7. Bending, lifting and stooping can bring on reflux symptoms in some patients and advice should be given on how to perform these correctly.

Fig. 10A.10   Lifestyle advice for patients with reflux oesophagitis

10A.2   PROSTHETICS

10A.2.1   INTRODUCTION

The introduction of oesophageal prostheses through malignant oeso-phageal tumours has become common practice to relieve dysphagia in patients with advanced disease. It is a palliative procedure performed on patients who are either unsuitable for surgery because of the nature of the disease or because of established metastases. In some cases the patient's general condition is such that they would not survive a major operation or general anaesthetic and the placement of an oesophageal prosthesis is the only alternative to relieve symptoms.

Patients with benign strictures of the oesophagus can also be treated by the insertion of expandable stents but the number treated is few as a new stenosis tends to develop at the stent edges. In these patients, stent insertion may be advisable only as an aid to preoperative nutritional support or in selected elderly patients.

10A.2.2   INDICATIONS/CONTRAINDICATIONS

Ultrasonography is proving useful in detecting the degree of tumour spread outside the mucosa and into nearby nodes. Barium studies are necessary in narrow strictures to document their length (Cotton and Williams, 1990).

Patients presenting with midoesophageal tumours with a life ex-pectancy of only a few months are the best candidates for stent insertion.

The insertion of stents in patients presenting with a malignant tracheo-oesophageal fistula is particularly useful if the tumour extends near to the cricopharyngeus. Stent placement is difficult in the case of tumours at, or near, the cardia, as the effectiveness of the stent is less certain because it may lie against the oesophageal wall causing a partial blockage. Before stent placement the stricture must be assessed endo-scopically and radiologically. This enables the endoscopist to establish the nature of the stricture and decide what treatment is best for the patient. This can then be discussed with the patient to ensure they understand the aims and risks of the procedure to be undertaken, and also discuss any alternative therapy that may be available.

10A.2.3   SPECIFIC NURSING CARE

Patients presenting with inoperable malignant disease are often fright-ened and angry and will need specific counselling to be able to come to terms with and understand the disease and treatment they are going to undertake. Nurse specialists along with the endoscopy staff will be of great assistance in helping the patient understand and accept the illness. It is also very important that the family are also included so they will understand what is going to happen and what aftercare will be necessary for the patient.

10A.2.4   EQUIPMENT: TYPES OF PROSTHESIS

Two types of self-expanding metal stent are available – covered and uncovered. The stricture is dilated as previously described to the diameter recommended by the manufacturer. If the patient has undergone a course of radiotherapy the dilatation may be difficult owing to scar tissue, and the risk of perforation is increased because the tissue involved becomes friable. Tube prostheses are available in various forms but their basic design is similar. They all consist of a lumen of at least 10 mm diameter, and have flanges at each end to prevent migration of the tube once it is positioned. They should be suitably flexible so that they do not collapse but will fit accurately into the oesophagus. They vary in length and diameter to fit all types of stricture, with a cuffed tube being available to fit malignant tracheo-oesophageal fistulae. Some self-expanding metal stents are reinforced with metal rings or springs to help prevent tumour overgrowth.

Atkinson tube

The Atkinson tube (Fig. 10A.11) is so named after Professor Atkinson of Nottingham who pioneered prosthetic tube insertion in the 1980s and designed the tube and the 'Nottingham' introducer in collaboration with Keymed/Olympus. The Nottingham introducer consists of a flexible metal shaft with an expanding plastic olive, which grips the interior of the stent. It is inserted over a guide wire, which is left in position

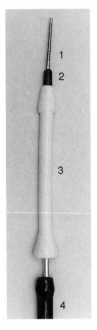

Fig. 10A.11 (a) Distal end of Nottingham introducer showing flexible tip (1), expanding olive (2) grasping Atkinson tube (3), and pusher tube (4)

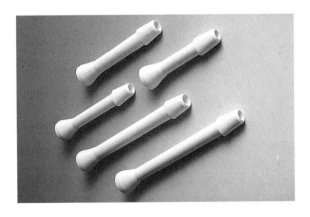

Fig 10A.11 (b) The Atkinson tube range

after dilatation. Once the endoscopist is certain the stent is correctly positioned using fluoroscopy, the tube is released and the insertion assembly and the guide wire are removed.

Different endoscopists use variations on the technique to suit their requirements. Some use an overtube to maintain position whilst removing the insertion assembly. This allows an endoscope to be passed through the overtube on completion so that the position can be observed endoscopically as well as radiologically.

Savary

The Savary stent system (section 10A.1.6) is produced commercially by Wilson Cook. The dilator, stent and pusher are passed as a complete unit over the previously placed guide wire. With this system it is possible to lock the pusher tube on to the dilator, so they advance together over the guide wire, making stent insertion quicker. Position is determined radiologically. If the stent position needs adjusting slightly, it can be carried out by using the pusher over the endoscope.

Celestin tubes

The stricture is dilated using a Celestin dilator (section 10A.1.6) which is left in position whilst the stent is introduced over it using fluoroscopic screening. Once positioned correctly the inner dilator and guide wire are removed. The pusher tube remains in place allowing the endoscopist to examine the final placement and judge whether any adjustment is necessary.

Metal stents

Metal stents are becoming more frequently used for patients with malignant oesophageal strictures. The most commonly used at the moment are the self-expanding wall stent and the Strecker stents but new designs are being introduced periodically. There are two types of stents: mesh and covered; both are made of knitted titanium wire.

The Ultraflex oesophageal stent (produced by Boston Scientific Corp.) is composed of nitionol, which adapts itself to oesophageal peristalsis and permits normal swallowing. It has remarkable elasticity and therefore is gentle and reliable once positioned. The delivery system is compact, reducing predilatation, and can be used for both endoscopic and fluoroscopic delivery. The delivery system includes a 95 cm long (2 mm diameter) Teflon catheter with a distal olive-shaped widening, a soft 4 cm long tip (to simplify insertion) and a covering sheath to minimize the diameter of the stent. Unexpanded, it is stretched, compressed, and encased in gelatine (Wojciech, 1995).

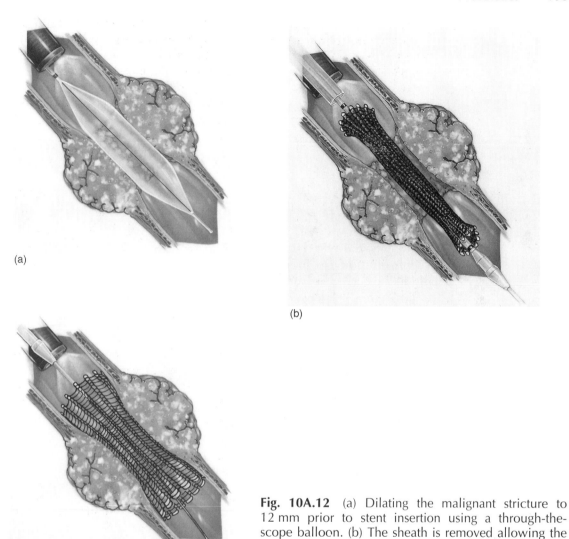

(a)

(b)

(c)

Fig. 10A.12 (a) Dilating the malignant stricture to 12 mm prior to stent insertion using a through-the-scope balloon. (b) The sheath is removed allowing the stent to gradually expand whilst the introducer is still in position. (c) Removal of introducer and guide wire (reproduced with permission of Boston Scientific).

Prior to insertion the stricture is assessed endoscopically and radiologically, and if necessary the stricture is dilated to 12 mm diameter (Fig. 10A.12a), but because of the compact delivery system the dilatation is not always required. A standard 0.035 inch (0.89 mm) guide wire is passed through the stricture. The delivery system is then placed over the guide wire, the Teflon sheath preventing fluid within the oesophagus contacting the stent during positioning. Once the correct position is achieved, the Teflon sheath is removed (Fig. 10A.12b), allowing the stent to expand gently to full diameter. To ensure adequate lumen size to enable endoscopic examination, it may be necessary to inflate a 18 mm diameter balloon within the stent. Stent expansion may be speeded up by the injection of warm saline down the outer sheath via a 'butterfly' cannula. When the stent has expanded sufficiently, the introducer and guide wire are removed (Fig. 10A.12c). Following complete stent expansion patients should be able to receive a semisolid or normal diet.

10A.2.5   PROBLEMS POSTPROCEDURE

Stent insertion carries the risk of perforation and postprocedure the patients must be monitored carefully. A chest X-ray should be performed to ensure the oesophagus has not been perforated and the tube is in the correct position. Fluids may be commenced 4 hours after intubation if the patient has had no adverse events.

Prophylactic broad-spectrum antibiotics are sometimes given over a period of 24 hours commencing 1–2 hours prior to the procedure being performed.

Semisolid diet can be commenced on the next day and it is very important that dietary advice is given to the patient and relatives before discharge home.

Complications and precautions

Perforation
Perforation of the oesophagus may occur as a result of stent placement.

Blockage
Blockage of the tube or stent may be caused by overambitious eating by the patient. Insufficient chewing of food, especially products like meat or bread, may cause a food bolus to obstruct the tube. The patient will require an emergency gastroscopy to clear the bolus, which can be fragmented or removed by using biopsy forceps or a snare. Tubes may also become blocked as the tumour develops. In this situation it may be necessary to pass a smaller-sized stent through the original tube to allow the patient to swallow.

In patients with large tumours the stent may cause added pressure on the trachea, causing respiratory distress. The stent may have to be removed rapidly if this occurs to allow the patient to breathe. Removing the stent can be a very complex procedure, especially if there is tumour overgrowth. If tumour overgrowth occurs, the placement of a smaller stent above the first may benefit the patient. Some tubes deteriorate with time and may even begin to disintegrate. The stent may also migrate into the stomach but this normally causes no problems if left *in situ*.

In patients treated with metal stent insertion there is also a risk of tumour ingrowth through the stent wall, but in most cases the stent does not become completely occluded. Manufacturers are now coating stents to prevent tumour ingrowth, and this can be useful in the treatment of tracheo-oesophageal fistulae.

10A.2.6 DISCHARGE INSTRUCTIONS

Discharge instructions are very important when discharging patients with an oesophageal tube or metal stent. The patient and their relatives will then have something to refer to when they are coming to terms with coping with the tube. A contact telephone number is essential, not only for emergencies such as tube blockage, but also to answer any queries or alleviate worries that they may encounter.

Manufacturers of tubes publish their own leaflets for the patient. Other advice to be given includes:

1. A short explanation about the type of tube inserted.
2. Dietary advice, including the following points:
   - Any liquidized foods or fluids may be taken; solid foods may be eaten but it is advisable that they are cut into small pieces and must be chewed for at least twice as long as normal.
   - Foods that are difficult to chew because they are chunky, stringy or fibrous should be avoided as these can block the tube; avoid foods like citrus fruits, fruit skins, tough vegetables and cereals such as muesli. If taking medication ensure tablets are broken or crushed.
   - Always eat slowly, chewing adequately, as this reduces bulk. Dentures should always be worn when eating to aid in chewing.
   - Always sit upright when eating and use a high-backed chair.
   - Plenty of fluids should be taken during a meal and always have a fizzy drink after a meal as this will help to keep the tube clear.
   - To prevent acid coming up the oesophagus from the stomach causing heartburn, always sleep with at least three pillows or elevate the head of the bed.
   - If food begins to stick, do not continue eating; take a fizzy drink and walk about. If the problem does not resolve, contact the hospital as the tube has become blocked.

10A.3 COLONIC DILATATION

10A.3.1 INDICATIONS

Colonic dilatations (Plate 4) can be performed for benign colonic strictures, although most require surgery. They may be the result of surgical resection, with stricture formation occurring at the anastomosis site, or be due to conditions such as diverticular or Crohn's disease, ulcerative colitis, intestinal ischaemia or tuberculosis. Malignant strictures may be dilated as a palliative measure when the patient is too ill for surgical resection, and self-expanding metal stents may be inserted to keep the stricture open. Malignant inoperable strictures of the rectum and sigmoid colon are most commonly treated by dilatation.

10A.3.2 PROCEDURE

Contrast studies are performed to evaluate the stricture. The patient is prepared as for colonoscopy. Fluoroscopic screening is required during dilatation if it is wire guided. If Savary–Gilliard dilators are used (section 10A.1.6), a wire is passed down the biopsy channel and through the stricture under X-ray control until the correct position is achieved; the colonoscope is then removed leaving the guide wire in position. The dilator of choice is then inserted over the guide wire and the stricture is gently dilated. Wire-guided Savary-Gilliard dilators may be used for rectal and sigmoid strictures.

   Self-expanding metal stents can be inserted for inoperable malignant strictures as a palliative measure; however, this is a relatively new technique and its therapeutic value has yet to be assessed.

   Balloon dilatation of the colon may be performed using the same through-the-scope (TTS) technique as described for oesphageal balloon dilatation.

10A.3.3 SPECIFIC NURSING CARE

Nursing care is as for colonoscopy. If a self-expanding metal stent is placed, the patient will require an abdominal X-ray to ensure complete opening of the stent. At the time of stent placement a colonic balloon can be inflated to open the stent completely.

10A.3.4 COMPLICATIONS AND PRECAUTIONS

Recurrence of the stricture is a common complication following dilatation; repeat dilatations may be necessary to keep the stricture open. Insertion of a stent may prevent this in some cases.

Perforation of the bowel is a complication of colonoscopy, and with the added risk from dilatation the patient should be monitored closely postprocedure. This risk can be reduced if fluoroscopy is used when performing the dilatation.

10A.3.5   DISCHARGE INSTRUCTIONS

Patients will require close follow-up in the outpatient department for recurrence of stricture. They will need to see a dietitian for advice and education on diet, to ensure they do not become constipated and have daily bowel movements.

A contact telephone number is important, so patients can contact the unit in case they have further problems or require advice.

10A.4   FEEDING TUBE INSERTION (ENDOSCOPIC)

10A.4.1   INTRODUCTION

Endoscopically placed feeding tubes are designed for short-term feeding only in patients with a normal gastrointestinal tract.

They can also be used for gastric decompression. Nasogastric and nasojejunal tubes are normally placed using fluoroscopy or by the anaesthetist at operation, if required for postoperative drainage. It is only when this fails that they are placed endoscopically.

10A.4.2   INDICATIONS/CONTRAINDICATIONS

Short-term feeding or gastric decompression is the only indication for using this type of feeding tube. They should never be used for long-term feeding and if the patient requires feeding for longer than several weeks they should be assessed for percutaneous endoscopic gastrostomy (PEG) placement.

10A.4.3   PROCEDURE FOR NASOGASTRIC AND NASOJEJUNAL TUBE PLACEMENT

Through-the-channel method

A therapeutic large-channel 4.2 mm endoscope is preferred for this technique because its larger channel enables a large-bore tube to be passed. The tube is passed down the biopsy channel of the endoscope over a standard 0.035 inch (0.89 mm) diameter guide wire. The tube and guide wire are passed under direct vision through the pylorus. This can be checked by the use of fluoroscopy. Once the tube is correctly positioned the endoscope is removed carefully, whilst advancing the tube and guide wire through it. The guide wire is then removed and the tube rerouted through the nose. To do this the endoscopist passes a short piece of plastic tubing through the patient's nostril into the pharynx. The tubing is then caught with a pair of McGill forceps and guided out of the patient's mouth. The top of the nasogastric or nasojejunal tube is then passed through the tubing and the latter is withdrawn through the patient's nose until the tube lies directly in their pharynx. The small piece of plastic tubing is then removed and the nasogastric or nasojejunal tube is secured with tape at the patient's nose and to the side of the face for comfort.

Alongside-the-scope method

This allows placement of a tube that is bigger than the biopsy channel of the endoscope and can be used if a therapeutic endoscope is not available. For gastric decompression a larger bore tube is sometimes required. A short length of silk-type suture is attached to the tube of choice and is fastened to the end of the endoscope by passing a pair of biopsy forceps or a snare down the biopsy channel, grasping the suture material and pulling it back into the instrument channel.

The patient is then endoscoped in the usual way with the tube running alongside the endoscope. On reaching the pylorus, the tube can be positioned by using the biopsy forceps or snare. Positioning can be checked by fluoroscopy. The thread is then released and the endoscope removed. Care should be taken when withdrawing the endoscope not to dislodge the tube. If necessary, the tube can be made firmer by introducing a guide wire.

10A.4.4   SPECIFIC NURSING CARE

Tubes should always be flushed with water before and after feeding, to prevent blocking. They should be replaced about every 30 days (if required for that length of time). Tubes should have graduated markings to allow monitoring of tube migration. The tube should be removed straight away if migration occurs.

A guide wire should never be reinserted when the tube is in the patient.

If the tube is used for gastric drainage, never let the drainage bag become too full as it will be uncomfortable for the patient and the excess weight will pull on the tube.

10A.4.5   COMPLICATIONS AND PRECAUTIONS

Confused patients may not tolerate the tube very well and may pull it out. If left *in situ* too long the patient may develop gastro-oesophageal reflux disease. This is one of the main reasons why they are intended for short-term use only, and ideally should not be used in patients who have gastrointestinal problems to begin with.

The tube can irritate the patient's pharynx and cause them to develop a tickly cough.

10A.4.6   DISCHARGE INSTRUCTIONS

Patients are rarely discharged into the community with this type of feeding tube because they are intended for short-term use only and are usually removed before discharge.

10A.5   PERCUTANEOUS ENDOSCOPIC GASTROSTOMY AND PERCUTANEOUS ENDOSCOPIC JEJUNOSTOMY

10A.5.1   INTRODUCTION

Percutaneous endoscopic gastrostomy and percutaneous endoscopic jejunostomy are alternative measures used for long-term feeding in patients who are unable to take enough fluid or food to constitute a healthy balanced diet. It is a reasonably new technique and, because the feeding tube can be placed endoscopically, the ill, frail, patient does not have to undergo a surgical procedure. As the procedure is performed using sedation the patient does not require a general anaesthetic, thus reducing the risks further.

PEG and PEJ alter mortality by avoiding aspiration of food, reduce morbidity because of fewer intravenous lines, improve quality of life and speed rehabilitation by improving nutritional status. They are also well tolerated.

10A.5.2   INDICATIONS/CONTRAINDICATIONS

The choice of patients is as follows:

- Patients who have neurological disorders (e.g. cerebrovascular accidents) where the swallowing reflex has been impaired or failed to return following their stroke.
- Patients with neurological dysphagia, road traffic accident or other traumas.
- Patients with Huntington's chorea, multiple sclerosis and patients from younger disabled units.

- Patients undergoing major oropharyngeal and faciomaxillary surgery who will not be able to take anything orally following surgery.
- Patients who require radiotherapy or chemotherapy to maintain nutrition during their treatment.
- Children who have cystic fibrosis or require radiotherapy or chemotherapy.
- Unconscious patients are also considered. This type of patient may develop respiratory problems because of the risk of aspiration, and a minitracheostomy is sometimes necessary to prevent this occurring.

Contraindications include the following:

- Surgical options should be considered in patients who have ascites as endoscopic methods are more complex and hazardous in this group of patients.
- PEG and PEJ cannot be performed in patients who suffer from oesophageal strictures that are too tight to admit the endoscope.
- Patients who have previously undergone gastric surgery, as their anatomy becomes distorted, causing difficulty for the endoscopist.
- Obese patients cause particular problems because the thickness of the fat layer makes it difficult to place the trocar and cannula and illuminate the abdominal wall. However, these patients are sometimes considered.

10A.5.3   PROCEDURE TYPES

The PEG procedure set is shown in Fig. 10A.13.

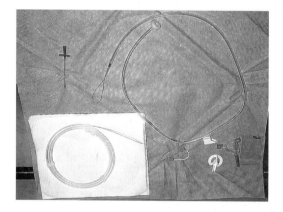

Fig. 10A.13 Percutaneous endoscopic gastrostomy (PEG) set (Merck), showing cannula, wire, tube and Y-connector (pull technique)

Pull

Two endoscopists are required to perform the procedure, one to insert the gastroscope and one to site the gastrostomy tube. The patient is gastroscoped in the usual way and a check made to ensure patency of the gastric outlet.

The patient is turned from the left lateral position so they are lying on their back. The stomach is inflated with air to improve vision and the room is darkened. The light at the tip of the endoscope is directed through the anterior abdominal wall (if a video endoscope is used it is particularly important to darken the room as illumination is decreased). Once transillumination is observed, the assistant indents the abdominal wall with their finger (Fig. 10A.14a), enabling the endoscopist to observe the indentation and check that the appropriate part of the body of the stomach has been chosen. The assistant then marks the area, which is then cleaned with skin preparation and draped with towels.

Local anaesthetic is infiltrated into the area where the tube is to be inserted. The assistant then makes a short cut of about 5 mm with a pointed scapel. A trocar and cannula are then inserted through the anterior abdominal wall and into the stomach, under endoscopic visualization. Once the trocar and cannula are in the correct position (verified by the endoscopist) the trocar is removed and a guide wire with loops at each end is inserted (Fig. 10A.14b). The endoscopist will observe passage of the guide wire into the stomach. A grasping forceps is then passed down the biopsy channel of the endoscope and the loop of the guide wire is grasped.

The endoscope and forceps carrying the guide wire are withdrawn carefully through the patient's mouth (Fig. 10A.14c), ensuring that the free end of the guide wire remains outside the abdominal wall. The guide wire is brought out at the patients mouth and is then attached to the gastrostomy tube by interlocking the wire loop on to the end of the tube through the placement wire loop (Fig. 10A.14d). The assistant then pulls the guide wire back through the cannula, pulling the gastrostomy tube down into the stomach. Once the tube reaches the skin the cannula is removed and the tube pulled through the previously made incision (Fig. 10A.14e). Most gastrostomy tubes have graduation marks on the tube to provide a guide as to how far the tube should be pulled through.

The endoscope is then reinserted to check that the button end of the tube is correctly positioned against the gastric wall. Once this is verified the assistant can then trim the tube to disconnect the guide wire (the tube should never be trimmed before positioning is checked, as air will escape via the tube and the endoscopist will not be able to inflate the stomach). The assistant then places a fixation device or bumper bar to hold the tube against the skin, ensuring that this is not too tight as it

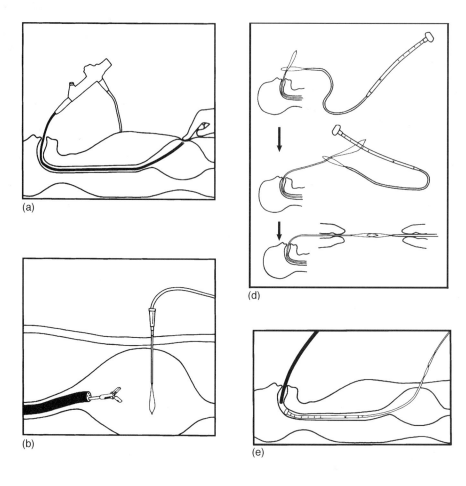

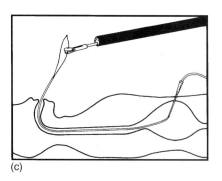

Fig. 10A.14 (a) The assistant indents the abdominal wall observed by the endoscopist who checks placement position. (b) Cannula with wire loop inserted through it into stomach. The loop is grasped by the endoscopist using biopsy forceps. (c) The wire loop is carefully withdrawn through the mouth. (d) Method of attaching tube to wire loop. (e) The wire loop is withdrawn, pulling the tube down the oesophagus, into the stomach and through the incision in the abdominal wall

may cause the patient some discomfort. A clamp is then placed on to the tube, and the 'Y' adaptor is attached. This allows the feed to be connected on to the tube; it also has a port for flushing the tube and to enable medication to be administered.

PEJ tubes can be inserted through gastrostomy tubes, supplied as an assembled kit to be used in conjuction with the PEG tube of choice.

The tube is placed under endoscopic guidance. The fixation device on the PEG tube is disconnected so that the PEG tube is at right angles to the abdominal wall. The jejunostomy tube is introduced via a special adaptor that attaches to the PEG tube (Fig. 10A.15). It also has an adjustable sleeve that connects, on completion, to the 'Y' adaptor.

The patient is endoscoped and the stomach inflated with air. The jejunostomy tube is inserted through the PEG by an assistant until it is visualized exiting the tube into the stomach. The tip of the jejunostomy tube is then grasped by inserting grasping forceps down the biopsy channel. The endoscopist then advances the forceps through the pylorus whilst the assistant feeds the other end through the PEG. Once the desired length has been inserted the stylet is removed and the tube secured by the adjust-a-sleeve to the 'Y' adaptor. Placement may be confirmed by fluoroscopy. The fixation device is reconnected and positioning of the PEG button confirmed before removing the endoscope.

Fig. 10A.15 Jejunal extension (Merck) showing attachment to Y-connecter and special tip, which allows it to be grasped by the forceps

Push

This technique involves pushing the gastrostomy tube through the abdominal wall rather than pulling it down from the mouth (Cotton and Williams, 1990).

The patient is endoscoped, the stomach distended and the abdominal wall illuminated as with the pull technique. Local anaesthetic is infiltrated into the skin and subcutaneous tissue. It is necessary to infiltrate the tissues thoroughly as a wider and deeper skin incision is required for this technique. A large-bore needle is then inserted through this incision into the stomach under endoscopic vision, and a guide wire is passed through the lumen of the needle. The needle is withdrawn and a cannula which has an outer peel-away catheter is passed over the guide wire and into the stomach. Placing the trocar takes pressure and rotation, which is why a larger skin incision is required. Once the catheter is observed entering the stomach, the trocar is withdrawn and the gastrostomy tube is inserted through the catheter. The peel-away catheter is then gently removed and the feeding tube left in position. The endoscope is removed once the correct position is achieved and the tube fixed to the abdominal wall.

The main advantage of this method is that the patient needs only one endoscopy and the feeding tube is not contaminated by passage through the mouth, although difficulty may arise when placing the trocar and cannula through the abdominal wall. PEJ tubes can also be placed through this type of gastrostomy tube.

10A.5.4 SPECIFIC NURSING CARE

Explanation to the patients and their relatives about the procedure and postprocedure care is essential. Informed consent is very important because of the risks and long-term implications, and consent may have to be obtained from relatives if patients themselves are too ill to consent. Ensure that adequate information is provided; preprocedure visiting is important to discuss any queries with the patient and relatives.

The patient should not be given anything orally or via the tube for at least 4 hours postprocedure.

10A.5.5 COMPLICATIONS AND PRECAUTIONS

Infection

Local skin sepsis around the tube placement site can be reduced by giving prophylactic antibiotics and by ensuring a safe aseptic technique when placing the tube. Even so infection rates of 20–30% have been reported and many centres use prophylactic antibiotics routinely.

Pain

For abdominal pain, check that the tube fixation device is not too tight against the abdominal wall. Prolonged tightness may cause ischaemic necrosis of the gastric mucosa.

Pneumonia

Aspiration pneumonia can be prevented by the insertion of a mini-tracheostomy prior to the procedure if the patient is at risk from aspiration.

Diarrhoea

Diarrhoea may be a problem when feeding is commenced. This can be due to hyperosmolar solutions being infused through the gastrostomy too quickly.

Fistula

A rare complication of tube placement is gastrocolic fistula, in which the patient presents with severe diarrhoea after feeding is commenced.

The fistula is usually caused initially by transcolonic puncture or nipping of the colonic wall between the stomach and the abdominal wall, resulting in fistula formation. This complication may not present until the tube is changed when it is positioned in the colonic lumen; once the gastrostomy tube is removed the fistula will heal without any further treatment.

Tube blockage

Tube blockage is common but can be prevented by flushing the tube after feeds and administration of medication with water or soda water.

Granulation tissue

Granulation tissue may occur at the stoma site. Silver nitrate applied to the granuloma will reduce the granulation tissue. If applying silver nitrate, be sure to protect the normal tissue with petroleum jelly to prevent burning. Skin excoriation is also common and can be prevented by the use of barrier creams.

PEG tube falling out

Gastrostomy tubes can be left *in situ* for 2 years or more without requiring changing because the high-grade polyurethane used in their manufacture is compatible with human tissue. If the tube falls out it will need replacing straight away to keep the stoma open. It can be replaced by insertion of another PEG or by a replacement tube with a balloon system. This gastrostomy does not require endoscopy for placement and can be inserted by the nurse or by patients themselves if taught correctly. A skin-level gastrostomy feeding kit or button can also be placed in a developed stoma. These are ideal for patients as they give a better cosmetic appearance and are flush with the skin; there is no excess tube. Buttons are used commonly in children with cystic fibrosis as they are more acceptable.

10A.5.6   ADVICE FOR WARD NURSES

Information on postprocedure care should be sent back to the ward with the patient, to advise the ward nurses on immediate care.

1. Give bolus feed postprocedure and if no problems then commence continuous feed as prearranged with the dietitian. If there are any problems contact the medical team.
2. The patient will need an intravenous infusion postprocedure until feeding is commenced via gastrostomy tube, especially if the patient is aged, frail and in poor health. This is to prevent dehydration.

3. If the tube falls out a Foley catheter or a replacement tube with a balloon system should be inserted.
4. If there are any problems concerning the gastrostomy tube a contact telephone number should be available.

10A.5.7   DISCHARGE INSTRUCTIONS

Care in the community is very important for patients with feeding tubes. Manufacturers of tubes and buttons supply excellent leaflets explaining how to care for their tubes. However, patients should always be educated before leaving the hospital and be observed caring for their tubes. The tube should be flushed after feeding and medication. If it becomes blocked it is advised that patients first attempt to unblock the tube with water, using a small-diameter syringe, as this will exert more pressure than a large-diameter syringe. If water does not remove the blockage then soda water or fizzy fluid such as lemonade may be tried as they contain carbon dioxide, which will help to unblock it. Pineapple juice is helpful as this contains an enzyme that helps to dissolve any blockage. If this fails they must telephone the contact number they are supplied with on discharge, as the tube may have to be changed.

Care of the stoma site is essential to prevent local sepsis. It is important that the stoma site is cleaned and dried daily and the tube rotated as this will prevent the build-up of scar tissue. Once the stoma site is formed, after about 2-3 weeks, patients will be allowed to bathe, shower and go swimming. Until that time they should not immerse the site in water.

If the 'Y' connector becomes damaged they should contact the nurse or doctor to get a replacement. If the tube falls out the nurse or doctor should be contacted straight away so a replacement tube can be inserted to keep the stoma open. If the patient puts on weight then the fixation device may have to be loosened as it will become tight.

Oral hygiene is important as the patient may be taking everything via their tube and they will get a build-up of plaque. Frequent mouth washes will prevent this, but ensure the patient knows not to swallow the mouthwash. On discharge many endoscopy units care for their patients in the community, and clinics have been set up for patients to see a nurse specialist and dietitian for follow-up care.

10A.5.8   PERCUTANEOUS FEEDING BUTTONS

Once a PEG tube has been in place for approximately 6–8 weeks (sometimes earlier in children), and the fibrous tract around the tube is well established, it is possible to remove the PEG and replace it with a percutaneous feeding button (Fig. 10A.16).

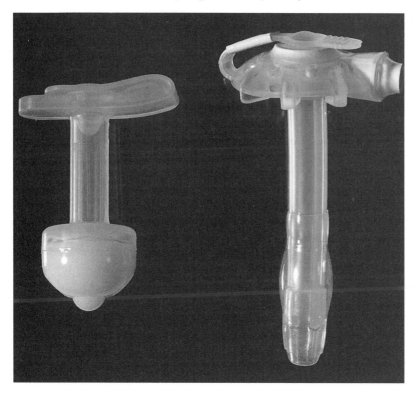

Fig. 10A.16 Percutaneous buttons: Bard (left) and Mic-Key (right)

Percutaneous feeding buttons are short tubes that lie flush with the skin surface and which carry out the same function as a PEG. Because of their small size, they are cosmetically very acceptable and can easily be worn under normal clothing. They are of particular use in children and other groups of patients liable to dislodge the relatively long PEG tube, and in adolescent patients such as those with cystic fibrosis where sexuality and body image are important factors.

The button is inserted down the established fibrous tract by distortion of the tip using a metal trocar, or by passing the insertion tube down the tract and then inflating a retaining balloon.

The buttons are available in several sizes, and it is important that the correct tract length is chosen (tract length plus 1 cm). **Note:** Obese patients will require a longer tube than normal as their apron of fat will drop downwards when standing, tending to pull the tube out. Extreme obesity may contraindicate the use of this type of feeding device.

Manufacturers provide various types of measuring devices that vary in their accuracy. The best type is that similar to a balloon catheter where the catheter is inserted through the tract into the stomach (it may be possible to aspirate gastric juice for testing), the balloon is then inflated, the catheter withdrawn until resistance is felt and the tract then measured. There have been reports of death following incorrect button placement, so it is best to check endoscopically that both the measuring device and the retaining device of the button chosen are in the correct position in the stomach when inserted.

Feeding buttons are generally very well tolerated and may remain in position for 2 or more years before they require replacement. The balloon types are easier to replace (the patient may be able to do this), but also tend to fall out more easily. Choice of which type to use is the preference of the endoscopist.

10A.6   FOREIGN BODY REMOVAL

It is often necessary to attempt endoscopic removal of foreign bodies accidentally, or in some cases deliberately, introduced into the gastro-intestinal tract. Of these, 80 to 90% pass through unhindered, usually within a 48-hour period, with the rest (10–20%) requiring endoscopic removal or very occasionally surgery (1%).

Foreign body ingestion most commonly occurs in the 6-month to 4-year age group when toys, crayons, coins and ballpoint pen caps are the most common objects ingested; in adults, bones and food boluses are the most common causes. Prisoners and psychiatric patients may deliberately introduce foreign bodies into the upper gastrointestinal tract, whilst in the lower gastrointestinal tract foreign bodies are mainly found in adult males between 24 and 65 as a result of either homo-sexual activity or criminal assault. Iatrogenic origins are uncommon but documented, and include retained instruments (mainly dental) as well as parts of biopsy forceps, small-bowel biopsy capsules and other parts of medical equipment.

The potential danger of ingested foreign bodies is from:

1. Physical obstruction.
2. Chemical poisoning.

Physical obstruction most commonly occurs in the oesophagus at either the cricopharyngeal or the cardiac (lower oesophageal) sphinc-ters. Normally, if an object can pass into the stomach it will pass unaided through the bowel unless its shape or size causes it to lodge in either the pylorus, duodenal loop or ileocaecal valve. (As a general guide, an object that will pass through the cricopharyngeal sphincter will also pass through the anal sphincter.)

Surgical removal should not be attempted unless the object can be seen radiologically or symptomatically not to have moved for a number of days. The only exception to this is in the case of objects containing lead or mercury (e.g. alkaline batteries) or sharp objects likely to cause haemorrhage or perforation, in which case urgent intervention is required.

10A.6.1 METHODS OF REMOVAL

A description of the foreign body is very helpful in deciding the method of removal. It is important to be aware that symptoms suggestive of perforation, peritonitis, haemorrhage or septicaemia may be a direct result of foreign body ingestion.

Upper gastrointestinal foreign bodies

The method chosen depends on the size, location and composition of the foreign body. Points to note are:

- Objects above or in the cricopharyngeal sphincter can often be removed using a laryngoscope and a pair of McGill forceps.
- Food boluses can be broken up by using either the endoscope tip or a variety of instruments such as biopsy or grasping forceps. A solid bolus may be removed using a Dormier basket.
- Long narrow objects such wires or paper clips can be removed using a polypectomy snare or grasping forceps.
- Coins and round objects like stones and batteries can often be removed using a Dormier basket or snare.
- Other smooth-shaped objects can often be grasped with rat-toothed or alligator forceps.
- Rubber-toothed forceps or magnetic devices are useful in the removal of sharp metallic objects such as nails, screws and needles.
- Objects with small central openings such as washers can be successfully removed using forceps or any similar instrument that will pass through the opening if closed, but not if open.

An overtube should always be used if sharp or pointed objects are to be removed as this will protect the oesophageal mucosa and prevent possible airway obstruction as it is removed. The use of an overtube should be considered in all cases of foreign body removal to minimize trauma, particularly if multiple passings of the endoscope are required of if intubation is difficult.

Procedure

The patient is placed in the left lateral position as for a diagnostic upper gastrointestinal examination. Patients can often be agitated and disturbed and may require premedication prior to attending the endoscopy unit. Foreign bodies lodged at the cricopharyngeal sphincter or in the upper oesophagus often cause excessive salivation, hindering vision, and it may be necessary to dry up secretions using atropine or other antisecretory agents.

Vital signs should be monitored during endoscopy, and the patient should be closely observed for signs of perforation, severe pain or respiratory distress.

Excess secretions should be removed regularly from the mouth and oropharynx to keep the airway clear.

Use of an overtube

An overtube (Fig. 10A.17) should be used in all cases where sharp or pointed objects are to be removed, in cases where repeated intubation is required (e.g. multiple objects or where food boluses or bezoar need breaking up) and if intubation is difficult and needs repeating.

The overtube should be at least 2 mm diameter larger than the endoscope and should be well lubricated inside and out with lubricating gel. It is loaded on to the endoscope, the patient is intubated and the overtube slid into place leaving the proximal end outside the mouth. There is a small risk of perforation with this procedure, but this is less than the risk from leaving the foreign body *in situ*. The object is grasped and pulled back into the overtube before removal, thus protecting the oesophageal mucosa and airway as it is removed.

Where a foreign body is larger than the overtube, a latex hood may be attached to the distal end of the endoscope. This lies at the side of the endoscope during insertion, but is pulled back over the foreign body as it is removed. A condom may be used for this purpose or may be used to 'trawl' the object into it prior to removal.

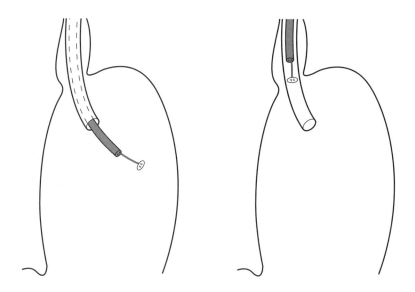

Fig. 10A.17 Use of an overtube to remove a foreign body (button) from the stomach

Postprocedure care

Vital signs (blood pressure, pulse, respirations) should be recorded regularly until patient has fully recovered, and the patient should be observed carefully for signs of haemorrhage, abdominal or chest pain, abdominal distension or surgical (subcutaneous) emphysema.

Lower gastrointestinal foreign bodies

Foreign bodies introduced via the rectum or passed down from the upper gastrointestinal tract can be removed endoscopically using a colonoscope and instruments similar to those used to remove an object from the upper gastrointestinal tract. Foreign bodies in the sigmoid colon may be similarly removed, using a flexible sigmoidoscope or rigid sigmoidoscope and a pair of grasping forceps. Rectal foreign bodies may be removed using a proctoscope. The removal of foreign bodies from the lungs is considered in Chapter 15.

A general anaesthetic may be required in order to produce adequate anal sphincter relaxation if large foreign bodies require removal and surgical intervention may be required.

10A.6.2 SPECIAL PROBLEMS

Alkaline batteries

These are readily available to and easily swallowed by children and when acted on by gastric secretions, may break down releasing a strong alkali that attacks the mucosa, causing caustic burns and tissue necrosis leading to perforation and potentially fatal complications such as tracheo-oesophageal or oesophagoaortic fistulae.

Narcotic drugs

Cocaine, heroin and other narcotic drugs may be swallowed, sealed in condoms, often in an attempt to conceal possession. If these burst, it is extremely dangerous, and potentially fatal (1–3 g of cocaine is an average lethal dose). Endoscopic removal is likely to cause the condom to burst and is therefore not indicated, and surgical removal is the treatment of choice in this situation.

Bezoar

Bezoar are collections of food and foreign matter that have undergone digestive changes in the gastrointestinal tract. Symptoms include epigastric fullness, pain, and periodic nausea and vomiting, with gastric outlet and intestinal obstruction as common complications.

There are two types:

1. Trichobezoar, made from matted hair.
2. Phytobezoar, formed from plant material.

The latter can usually be broken up endoscopically using biopsy forceps or a snare so that the residue passes naturally or can be dissolved using a combination of liquid diet and a substance such as cellulase or acetylcysteine. Surgical intervention is occasionally required.

Trichobezoar are often large, difficult to break up and cannot be dissolved. Surgical removal is indicated.

REFERENCES

Baillie, J. (1992) *Gastrointestinal Endoscopy: Basic Principles and Practice*, vol. 1. Butterworth Heinemann, Oxford, pp. 27–51.

Bardman, D. (1977) *Perspectives in Duodenal Ulcer*, Smith, Kline & French, pp. 48–51.

Bennett, J.R. (1981) *Therapeutic Endoscopy and Radiology of the Gut*, vol. 1, Chapman & Hall, London.

Bennett, J.R. (1991) *Management Guidelines for Gastro-oesophageal Reflux Disease*, vol. 1, Astra Pharmaceuticals, Kings Langley, UK.

Cotton, P.B. and Williams, C.B. (1990) *Practical Gastrointestinal Endoscopy*, 3rd edn, Blackwell Scientific, Oxford.

D'Silva, J. (1994) Treatment advances in reflux disease. *Nursing Standard*, 8(44), 25–9.

Hawkins, E.E.C. (1985) *Lecture Notes on Gastroenterology*, vol. 1, Blackwell Scientific, Oxford, pp. 149–51.

Ravenscroft, X. and Swan, C. (1984) *Gastro-intestinal Endoscopy and Related Procedures*, vol. 1, Chapman & Hall, London, pp. 81–5.

Wojciech, C. (1995) in *Stents. State of the Art and Future Developments* (ed. D. Liermann), Polyscience, pp. 218–21.

Haemostasis and tumour ablation 10B

Mike Shephard

10B.1 INTRODUCTION

Many of the techniques used endoscopically to control haemorrhage or to ablate tumours (Table 10B.1) are similar, and for this reason are described together here.

10B.1.1 HAEMOSTASIS

Gastrointestinal haemorrhage has an annual incidence of between 50 and 100 cases per 100 000 population in the UK. It has an associated mortality rate of between 6 and 10%: some studies have put this figure at more than 10% in the elderly patient with other coexisting medical conditions. Possible causes are listed in Table 10B.2.

With the exception of the emergency situations detailed in the list below, which may require immediate intervention, if an upper gastrointestinal source is suspected then endoscopy should be carried out within 24 hours of the bleed as the chance of finding the cause of bleeding is much higher in this period. It should be noted that 70–80% of upper gastrointestinal bleeds are self-limiting.

If a lower gastrointestinal source is suspected then endoscopy should not be performed until the gut has been cleansed.

Gastrointestinal haemorrhage situations requiring emergency endoscopy include:

- When a patient has known or suspected varices.
- Where there is evidence of continued and severe active bleeding which is life threatening.
- When the patient has had an aortic graft.

Practical Endoscopy Edited by M. Shephard and J. Mason. Published in 1997 by Chapman & Hall, London. ISBN 0 412 54000 2

Table 10B.1   Endoscopic therapies available for haemostasis and tumour ablation

Haemostasis	Tumour ablation
Monopolar diathermy (rare)	Monopolar diathermy
Bipolar diathermy	— polypectomy
— haemostatic probe	— piecemeal removal
Heater probe	Bipolar diathermy
	— tumour probe
Laser	
— photocoagulation	Laser
	— photovaporization
Injection therapy	
— adrenaline (ephedrine)	Injection therapy
— sclerosants	— Sclerosants
— alcohol	— Alcohol
— fibrin	
Endoscopic band ligation	
Oesophagogastric tamponade	
Endo-clip	
Endo-suture	

Table 10B.2   Causes of gastrointestinal haemorrhage

	Upper gastrointestinal	Lower gastrointestinal
Conditions amenable to endoscopic therapy	Oesophageal ulcers Gastric ulcers Duodenal ulcers Neoplasms Oesophageal and gastric varices Angiodysplasia Telangiectasia Polyps (rare) Mallory–Weiss tear (if actively bleeding)	Polyps (benign or malignant) Neoplasms (non-polypoid) Angiodysplasia Telangiectasia Haemorrhoids (occasionally)
Conditions not usually treated endoscopically	Erosive oesophagitis Gastritis/duodenitis Mallory–Weiss tear	Diverticular disease Inflammatory bowel disease Haemorrhoids

● To check that the cause of severe rectal bleeding is due to a colonic lesion (i.e. to exclude an upper GI cause).

Preparation is similar to that for a routine upper or lower gastro-intestinal investigation but care should be taken in the patient with a significant bleed because:

1. A patient with a reduced haemoglobin level is more susceptible to the respiratory depressant effects of the sedative used. In the severely respiratory compromised patient it may be better to attempt endoscopy without sedation.
2. A patient who is already hypotensive from severe blood loss will be further compromised by the use of sedatives and/or narcotic agents because of their known blood pressure-lowering effects.

Resuscitation

1. **IV access**
   Central Line (internal jugular probably best)
   –lower risk of pneumothorax
   –pressure can be applied if coagulation problems arise.

   PERIPHERAL VENOUS ACCESS
   Venflon – 16 G (Grey)
   One or both arms.
2. **FLUID REPLACEMENT**
   Colloid or packed cells
   Avoid saline and other Na-containing products as they may precipitate ascites (HAEMACEL is high in sodium).

   REMEMBER ... too much fluid will raise portal vein pressure and may precipitate further bleeding.
3. Maintain **CENTRAL VENOUS PRESSURE** at 0 to 5 cm H_2O (measure from sternal angle).
4. Patients with serious liver disease may have **COAGULATION** problems.
   Correct using: **FFP** (fresh frozen plasma); vitamin K (intramuscularly); ?platelet infusions?
5. **BEWARE!** Patients with impaired liver function who receive multiple blood transfusions are at risk of **CITRATE TOXICITY**. This causes **CARDIAC DYSRHYTHMIAS** because citrate chelates calcium. For this reason calcium gluconate may be given periodically.
6. Monitor **FLUID OUTPUT** – urinary catheter.
   A nasogastric tube helps keep stomach empty and is a useful means of assessing bleeding. This does not affect bleeding varices.

---

3. Medication such as hyoscine or glucagon may be required to reduce peristalsis when investigating or treating gastrointestinal haemorrhage, but it should be noted that the administration of the former (or any other anticholinergic drugs) to an already tachycardic patient could have serious consequences for the patient as one effect of this group of drugs is to increase the heart rate.

It is not usual to take biopsy specimens from acutely bleeding lesions, both because it may worsen the situation, and also because the patient's clotting status may not be known at that time. Once the acute phase is over, the patient may be re-endoscoped and specimens taken.

The young patient with a single episode of haematemesis following excessive alcohol intake is not a suitable candidate for endoscopic investigation unless there are other indications such as a previous history of gastrointestinal bleeding or further haematemesis which make further investigation necessary.

10B.1.2   TUMOUR ABLATION

The palliative ablation of endoscopically assessable gastrointestinal tumours is an important part of the endoscopy workload. What is generally a simple although often time-consuming procedure can produce a vast improvement in the quality of life of a patient who has a short life expectancy. There are two main indications for the use of ablation procedures:

1. Palliative treatment of inoperable gastrointestinal tumours.
2. Treatment of tumour overgrowth following stent insertion.

10B.2   METHODS OF HAEMOSTASIS AND TUMOUR ABLATION

10B.2.1   MONOPOLAR DIATHERMY (ELECTROSURGERY)

Haemostasis

The closed tip of hot biopsy forceps can be used to coagulate bleeding areas in the gastrointestinal tract. However, this method is not currently popular and is seldom used. If attempted, the forceps need regularly removing from the endoscope and the tip cleaning, otherwise coagulated blood on the tip prevents good electrical contact.

Tumour ablation

Polypoid lesions, whether in the upper or lower gastrointestinal tract, can be treated using the snare method described in Chapter 12.

Larger lesions can be debulked in parts using a snare, but care must be taken to ensure the tumour is not 'cheese-wired' rather than diathermically cut as this may cause severe haemorrhage. In these cases, the bleeding from a tumour can sometimes be stopped by using hot biopsy forceps as described above.

The method of action of monopolar diathermy, together with its safe use and complications, is described in Chapter 18A.

10B.2.2   BIPOLAR DIATHERMY

Haemostasis

Haemostasis can be achieved using a specially designed haemostatic probe that incorporates a high-pressure water-jet system for clot removal. The top of the probe (Fig. 10B.1) consists of a series of either longitudinal or circumferential electrodes that act as the active and return electrodes. Heat that is sufficient to coagulate tissue is therefore supplied to the contact area very precisely. Bipolar haemostatic probes are available in 5, 7 and 10 French sizes. The 5-French probe can be used via a bronchoscope to arrest bronchial haemorrhage. The 7-French probe is the most commonly used, whilst the 10-French probe can be used only with a large-channelled endoscope.

Advantages of bipolar haemostatic probe

There are a number of advantages to bipolar diathermy:

- It is clinically as effective as monopolar diathermy.
- It needs no metal or adhesive patient electrode (compared with monopolar diathermy).
- Equipment is compact, portable, easy to use and requires minimal special safety equipment or precautions (compared with laser).
- Can be used with any upper or lower gastrointestinal endoscope with minimum 2.8 mm diameter channel (a twin-channelled scope is preferred for simultaneous suction). A 2 mm probe is available for bronchoscopic use.
- Heat is transmitted from the tip and sides of the probe for good tissue contact.
- The probe can be used to apply direct pressure to the bleeding point.
- It is inexpensive.

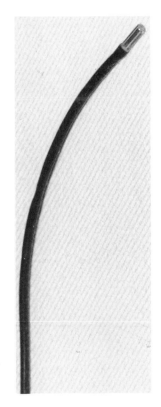

Fig. 10B.1 Bipolar haemostatic probe

Contraindications to bipolar diathermy

The main contraindications are:

- Massive haemorrhage obscuring view of bleeding site, and where surgery is indicated.
- Clinical evidence of perforation.
- Unco-operative, violent patients.

Equipment

Most bipolar units have settings to control the level of current delivered to the tip (usually on a scale of 1–10) and a variety of time settings varying from 1 second to infinity (i.e. continuous) (Fig. 10B.2). There is also a two-pedal foot control to activate the current to the probe, and control the water jet.

The water bottle (for the jet) should be filled with sterile water and the probe primed using the foot pedal.

To test the equipment is working:

1. Set the current control to 10, and the time to infinity.
2. Place a small drop of water on the slide or similar flat surface, and place the tip of the probe on it.
3. Depress the foot pedal. After a short while, the water should start to bubble.

The use of a silicone lubricant to the probe will make passage through the endoscope easier.

Procedure

Once the bleeding site is identified, the probe is passed down the endoscope, and is applied to tissue within 2–3 mm of the bleeding

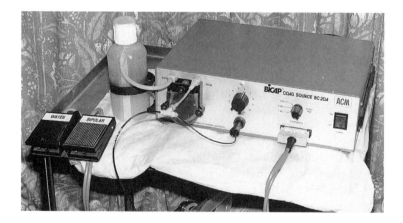

Fig. 10B.2   Bipolar diathermy equipment

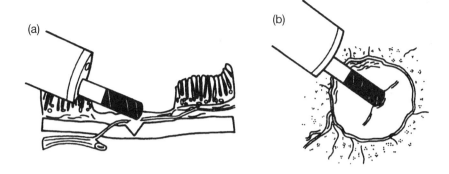

Fig. 10B.3   (a and b) Bipolar coagulation

vessel (Fig. 10B.3). The water jet can be used to remove excess clot and mucus. Pressure is used when applying the probe, and the probe is activated using 1- or 2-second bursts. The method therefore uses a combination of pressure and heat to achieve haemostasis. The procedure is continued circumferentially around the vessel until haemostasis is achieved. The probe will require removing periodically to clean the tip so as to ensure continued good electrical contact.

Tumour ablation

Bipolar tumour probes (Fig. 10B.4) shaped similarly to Eder–Puestow oesophageal dilators are available in various diameters for the ablation of tumours. It is also possible to have probes designed to provide heat either circumferentially or to a 45 ° or 90 ° arc. Each probe consists of:

1. A distal flexible tip.
2. An olive-shaped electrode.
3. A flexible shaft with 1 cm markings.
4. An electrical connection for the bipolar unit.

Procedure
Endoscopic evaluation of extent and position of the tumour helps decide whether a circumferential or directional probe is required. Radiographic studies (barium swallow or enema) may be required to judge the length of an endoscopically impassable tumour.

    Steps for ablation are as follows:

1. A guide wire is passed distal to the tumour, as for any dilatation procedure (section 10A). If the tumour obscures the lumen then fluoroscopy may be required to achieve this.

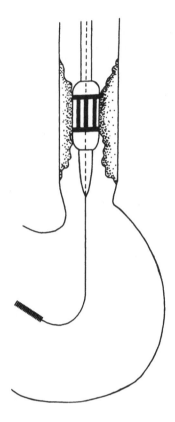

Fig. 10B.4   Bipolar tumour probe

2. If required, the tumour can be dilated using conventional dilators (balloon or Savary) to just under the approximate diameter of the tumour probe to be used. It is important not to overdilate the tumour as good contact is required between the tumour and the probe.
3. The selected tumour probe is then passed over the guide wire so that the olive is distal to the tumour.
4. The probe is slowly withdrawn through the tumour whilst heat is applied continuously. A white area of burn should be clearly seen. This can be repeated with progressively larger probes until the desired result is obtained.

   Sometimes burnt tissue adheres to the probe and is pulled off, leaving raw haemorrhagic areas. Some endoscopists will pass a small diameter endoscope alongside the probe so that the process can be observed.

Postprocedure care
The patient should be kept 'nil by mouth' for at least 4 hours, after which clear fluids may be commenced (some units do this overnight and perform a barium swallow to check patency prior to allowing clear fluids).

Complications of bipolar diathermy include:

- Perforation.
- Haemorrhage (immediate or delayed).
- Deep ulceration.

The patient should be observed for these signs of complications. A low-grade fever and retrosternal chest pain are not uncommon, and it is usual for the patient to experience initial dysphagia owing to tissue oedema following the procedure.

Many units repeat endoscopy after 48–72 hours to assess whether a further treatment is required, with monthly follow-up thereafter.

Note: Bipolar units are available with either 30 W or 50 W power; 30 W are usually sufficient to coagulate a bleeding vessel, but are insufficient for tumour ablation where the 50 W version is required. The 50 W version is suitable for both procedures.

10B.2.3   LASER THERAPY

Depending on the power supplied, laser treatment can either photo-coagulate or photovaporize tissue. Photocoagulation produces a white area with surrounding oedema and is useful for treating areas that are not actively bleeding such as ulcers with visible vessels and angiodysplasia. Photovaporization destroys tissue, with charring of surrounding areas and smoke production.

Indications/contraindications

Indications for photocoagulation and photovaporization are listed in Table 10B.3. Contraindications include the following:

1. Severely deranged coagulation mechanism.
2. Very large blood vessels.
3. Lesions that are inaccessible or where there is a very poor view.
4. Unco-operative, violent patients.

Equipment

The types of laser and the safety requirements needed in their use are considered in Chapter 18. The majority of lasers used in gastrointestinal

Table 10B.3 Indications for laser therapy

Photocoagulation	Photovaporization
Haemorrhagic conditions of gastrointestinal tract, especially: oesophageal, gastric or duodenal ulceration	Neoplasms
	Benign oesophageal webs
Angiodysplasia and telangiectasia	Anastomotic strictures
Mallory–Weiss tears	Polyp obliteration
Neoplasms	Neoplasia/erosions in flexible hysteroscopy
Haemorrhoids	Biliary obstruction: intra- or extrahepatic due to stricture or stones in common bile duct
Control of haemorrhage during bronchoscopy	

endoscopy are of the Nd:YAG variety (95%) with argon lasers accounting for the remainder (Table 10B.4).

The most common method of laser energy transmission is through a flexible quartz waveguide. This is usually protected by a plastic catheter passed through the endoscope. There is a space between the plastic sheath and the fibre that allows a cooling agent such as air, carbon dioxide or helium to be passed around it. Because of this, a major

Table 10B.4 Indications for laser therapy

Nd:YAG laser	Argon laser
Accounts for 95% of all lasers used in gastrointestinal endoscopy	Accounts for about 5% of all lasers used endoscopically
Tissue penetration approx. 4 mm	Tissue penetration approx. 1 mm
Penetrates blood clots	Absorbed by haemoglobin so cannot penetrate clots
Invisible to human eye Requires additional (visible) aiming beam	Visible to human eye
More likely to inflict eye damage Higher risk of perforation	Less likely to inflict eye damage Unlikely to cause perforation

complaint by patients can be abdominal distension, which may require medication or further intervention to settle. To help alleviate this, and also to remove potentially harmful smoke/fumes, it is recommended that an endoscope with two working channels is used so that in-sufflated gas and laser-produced smoke/vapour can be removed more easily.

Technique

Two methods may be employed:

1. Non-touch technique, using a conventional quartz waveguide, where the laser is 'fired' at the tissue from a distance.
2. Touch method, with tip in contact with tissue. This requires the use of a special sapphire tip that attaches to the end of a conventional waveguide. This has the effect of concentrating the energy to the tip of the waveguide so that a lower power setting can be used. Because the tip can actually be placed in contact with the tissue, it is also a more precise method.

Flexible endoscopes can be damaged by incorrect use of lasers and most equipment suppliers exclude laser-induced damage from any warranty or service contract. Damage can be minimized by:

1. Ensuring the laser tip is well outside the endoscope before it is activated. The operator should never activate the laser unless the tip can be seen.
2. Using endoscopes with white porcelain or stainless steel tips specifically designed for endoscopic laser use. These will reflect the beam, unlike the conventional black tip, which absorbs the energy, thus causing damage.
3. Ensuring sufficient distance is maintained between the endoscope and the target area.

The target area needs to reach a temperature of 60 °C or over to coagulate tissue (e.g. protein), and 100 °C to vaporize tissue.

To coagulate a bleeding point using a conventional waveguide, the laser is applied circumferentially around the area required at a distance of 1–2 cm; 60–90 W of energy in half-second bursts is usually sufficient. It may be necessary to perform a gastric lavage prior to laser therapy to remove excess clotting, and frequent irrigation of the bleeding site is often required using a 20 ml syringe through the working channel of the endoscope. A pair of graspers, biopsy forceps or a snare can be used to help break up large adherent clots. Occasionally, laser therapy can cause uncontrollable haemorrhage requiring immediate resuscitation.

Tumour ablation requires a higher level of energy, usually 80–100 W in 2-second bursts (longer bursts are possible but may cause excessive damage). The tumour will usually need dilating prior to laser therapy. Treatment should be delivered commencing at the distal end of the tumour. The laser is applied in increasingly larger concentric circles. Concentric rectal tumours should have only a 270 ° arc treated to minimize the risk of stenosis. Treating the distal portion first prevents oedema produced by the treatment obliterating the view.

Procedure

The patient is prepared as for a diagnostic endoscopy. Before the procedure commences, the following should be checked.

1. All staff and patient are wearing protective goggles or glasses.
2. The protective lens cover is in place on the ocular head of the endoscope (unless video endoscope). This allows the endoscopist to use the laser without the use of protective goggles or glasses.
3. All personnel should wear special 'laser' masks that prevent inhalation of smoke and tissue aerosol. The use of a smoke evacuator is beneficial in this situation.
4. The laser and cooling system should be checked for any malfunction.
5. All safety systems (illuminated signs, door locks, etc.) are working correctly.

A fuller explanation of the safe use of lasers is to be found in Chapter 18.

A minimum of two endoscopy assistants are required, the first acting as a 'technician' looking after the laser and associated equipment, and the second reassuring and monitoring the patient.

The 'technician'
When not in immediate use, the laser should be set on 'standby' to prevent accidental firing. It is the responsibility of the endoscopy assistant in charge of the laser to switch between standby and 'fire', and to alter the power setting and duration under the direction of the endoscopist.

The tip of the waveguide requires frequent cleaning if the 'touch' method is used as tissue will adhere to surface. This should be cleaned using hydrogen peroxide solution and a soft toothbrush. If a single-channel endoscope is used, this is also a good opportunity to remove excess smoke and vapour. It is often necessary to debride the treatment area of necrotic tissue periodically using conventional biopsy forceps.

After use, all equipment should be cleaned in line with manufacturers' instructions.

Patient reassurance and monitoring

The endoscopic use of laser can be very time consuming, and some treatments can last for an hour or longer. It can also be painful. The patient will require reassurance and encouragement during the procedure, and may require further sedation or analgesia to maintain co-operation and comfort. There should be monitoring of vital signs (pulse, blood pressure, respiration and oxygen saturation) and the abdomen should be watched for excessive distension due to gas insufflation. This can cause a vasovagal reaction that is hard to detect in the sedated patient without adequate monitoring facilities.

Postprocedure

The patient should be kept 'nil by mouth' for 4 hours, but should be checked for signs of complications (e.g. perforation, haemorrhage) before clear fluids are given. If an oesophageal lesion is treated, dysphagia may initially be worse owing to oedema. It may be necessary to pass a nasogastric tube to help relieve abdominal distension, and it is not unusual for the patient to exhibit signs of mild fever for up to 48 hours following laser therapy.

Angiodysplasia

Vascular abnormalities such as angiodysplasia can be obliterated endoscopically using both the argon and the Nd:YAG laser. These lesions are found throughout the digestive tract, but gastric or duodenal lesions are responsible for most bleeds from this cause. Application of a laser to these abnormalities usually causes initial bleeding, which is stopped with further laser application. With colonic lesions, the risk of perforation is higher on the right side because the intestinal wall is thinner in this area than in other areas of intestine.

10B.2.4   HEATER PROBES

These work in a similar way to the bipolar haemostatic probe but they are unable to ablate tumours. The basic design consists of a 2.4 or 3.2 mm probe with a Teflon-coated hollow aluminium tip (Fig.10B.5). (An endoscope with a large working channel is required for the 3.2 mm probe.) A heater coil is located inside the hollow tip, which, because of its excellent thermal conductivity, uniformly distributes heat to the surrounding tissues, causing it to coagulate. A high-powered water jet is incorporated into the probe to allow blood, clots and other debris to be

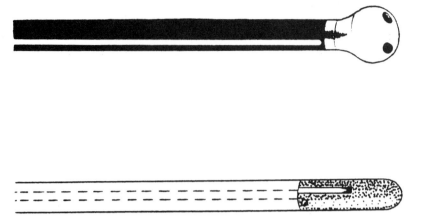

Fig. 10B.5   The heater probe

washed away. The Teflon tip discourages tissue adhesion, and requires less cleaning during the procedure.

The patient preparation, procedure and postprocedural care are similar to that for a bipolar haemostatic probe except that the probe tip is applied directly to the bleeding site (not around it) with several brief applications of up to 30 joules being required to cause haemostasis.

Note: As the tip of the probe reaches temperatures in excess of 60 °C, it must be allowed to cool before it is withdrawn through the endoscope to prevent damage to the working channel.

10B.2.5   ENDOCLIP LIGATION

This technique allows a metal clip (Fig. 10B.6) to be placed endoscopically over a bleeding vessel to achieve haemostasis. Experience suggests this is often not successful and that its main use is to mark accurately a bleeding vessel so that surgical intervention can effect haemostasis.

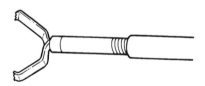

Fig. 10B.6   The Endoclip

10B.2.6   ENDOSCOPIC SUTURING

Prototypes of an 'endoscopic sewing machine' have been developed recently (P. Swain, Royal London Hospital, personal communication). The device allows a series of sutures to be placed endoscopically, and theoretically a bleeding vessel could be occluded using this method. The equipment and the procedure are still in their infancy, but have potential for the future.

10B.2.7   INJECTION THERAPY

Endoscopic injection therapy is the most commonly used procedure for producing haemostasis and can also be used for tumour ablation. A bleeding lesion may be injected with (Table 10B.5):

1. *Adrenaline 1:10 000 (ephedrine)*; this causes local vasoconstriction. (Accidental intravenous injection may cause a transient tachycardia.) Recent research has suggested that the injection of a combination of adrenaline and thrombin is an even more effective method for producing haemostasis.
2. *Dehydrated alcohol (ethanol)*; injected around the bleeding site, this causes tissue destruction by drawing water from the tissue and by fixing it; the ulcer produced eventually heals with fibrosis.
3. *Sclerosants*; sclerosants as used for the treatment of oesophageal varices (section 10C) are effective in causing haemostasis if injected around a bleeding vessel. The sclerosant causes vasoconstriction and

Table 10B.5   Chemical agents used in endoscopic injection therapy

Chemical agent	Haemostasis	Tumour ablation
Adrenaline 1:10 000 (ephedrine)	X	
Sclerosants:		
Sodium tetradecyl-sulphate (STD)	X	X
Sodium morrhuate	X	X
Polidocanol	X	X
Ethanolamine oleate	X	X
Dehydrated alcohol (ethanol 95%)	X	X
Fibrin	X	

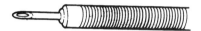

Fig. 10B.7   Sclerotherapy needle

tissue necrosis with ulceration and subsequent fibrous tissue formation.

4. *Fibrin*; this is the only method that augments the body's natural reaction to haemorrhage and causes no tissue damage. This is discussed in more detail below.

Because of their tissue destruction properties, sclerosants and absolute alcohol can also be used to ablate tumours. The chosen treatment is injected directly into the area of tumour requiring debulking.

Procedure

The procedure is similar to that described above. A two-channel endoscope is best as this allows simultaneous suction.

The injector (Fig. 10B.7) consists of a flexible inner sheath with a Luer lock or slip connection proximally, which allows a syringe to be attached and a needle at distal end. An outer sheath is added for increased rigidity; this also allows the needle to be retracted inside whilst not in use. These items are usually disposable.

Fibrin injection

With the exception of fibrin injection, all other methods of haemostasis involve the destruction (by chemicals or heat) of already damaged tissue. Fibrin injection (Beriplast P) provides haemostasis without tissue necrosis by submucosal injection of a fibrin sealant.

Initially, the sealant was applied direct to a bleeding area in an attempt to stop haemorrhage, but this proved ineffective. The sealant is now delivered direct to the bleeding site by a special dual-channelled needle designed specifically for the purpose.

The fibrin sealant is supplied as two separate dry powders, both of which have to be activated by mixing with a solution. For ease the vials are colour coded blue and red:

Vial 1 plus solution = fibrinogen (blue)
Vial 2 plus solution = thrombin (red)

fibrinogen + thrombin = fibrin clot

It is important that the two do not mix until actually in the submucosa (hence the use of a dual-channelled needle); a complex procedure is required to deliver the sealant to the area required.

Equipment required includes:

- Two 2 or 3 ml Luer lock syringes (for two components).
- One 5 or 10 ml syringe filled with molar saline (1 mol/l) (to prime the probe).
- One double lumen probe.
- Two 2 or 3 ml Luer lock syringes filled with saline for each fibrin clot to be introduced.
- Permanent red and blue markers to mark syringes.

Method

1. Prepare fibrinogen (blue) and thrombin (red) solutions as on the manufacturer's instructions, and place them in appropriately labelled Luer lock syringes.
2. Prepare a duo-probe as follows:
   (a) Check the needle will push out of sheath.
   (b) Fill both lumens with molar saline so that no air remains.
   (c) Retract the needle and lock in position.
   (d) Attach the blue-coded syringe to the blue-coded probe attachment.
   (e) Attach the red-coded syringe to the red-coded probe attachment.

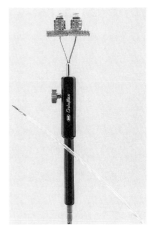

Fig. 10B.8 (a) The duo-probe

The probe is now ready for use.

Note: It is recommended that a probe such as the Endoflex duo-probe (Fig. 10B.8) Neumuhl type B is used as the different viscosities of the thrombin and fibrinogen solutions are matched by different lumen sizes. (Manufacturer: Endoflex GmbH, D-46562 Voerde, Germany.)

Procedure

1. The patient is prepared as for an upper gastrointestinal endoscopy.
2. The endoscope is passed and the bleeding lesion found.
3. The probe is inserted through the endoscope and the needle pushed out.
4. The endoscopist then inserts the needle at an angle deep into the submucosa under direct endoscopic vision.
5. The needle is retracted about 2 mm to create a small space in the submucosa for the solutions.
6. On the endoscopist's verbal instruction, the assistant simultaneously injects both solutions by pushing down on the plungers with the heel of the hand (the saline is now in the tissue and the Beriplast P in the probe).
7. The two empty colour-coded syringes are removed and replaced with two 2 or 3 ml syringes containing molar saline.

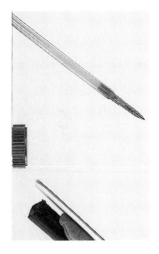

Fig. 10B.8 (b) Tip showing the two separate needles (reproduced with permission of Endoflex GmbH)

8. Inject 1.5 ml of molar saline down both channels of the duo-probe (the Beriplast P is now in the tissue).
9. Withdraw the endoscope and needle slightly.

This procedure may be repeated as many times as is required to achieve haemostasis.

Results

A large clinical trial of 955 patients with gastrointestinal bleeding (Friedrichs, 1994) showed a very low rate of rebleeding following therapy, with associated low mortality and need for emergency (surgical) intervention. The majority of patients (716) required only one injection of Beriplast endoscopy, with 239 requiring a second course and 72 requiring a third session. Nine patients required seven sessions in total. The treatment was particularly successful in the elderly patient with multiorgan disease who would have been at risk from other forms of intervention.

The treatment appears to be an effective alternative endoscopic method of haemostasis, but is dependent on:

- Accurate visualization of the bleeding source and placement of clots.
- Close endoscopic follow-up (at least daily in the beginning), so it places increased demands on the endoscopy service.
- A skilled team who are familiar with the procedure.

REFERENCES

Fredrichs, O. (1994) Submucosal fibrin glueing. Early elective therapy of bleeding peptic ulcers. *Endoskopie Heute*, 7(1), 16–22.

Oesophageal varices 10C

Jean Harvey

10C.1 INTRODUCTION

Effective management of a patient who presents with bleeding oeso-phageal varices depends upon the utilization of skills and expertise of both the medical and nursing teams. Bleeding from oesophageal varices is an extremely fearful and distressing experience for the patient, whose fears and anxieties may be amplified by the urgency of the situation and should be acknowledged by those responsible for their care.

The patient's condition will be critical if bleeding is severe and will therefore require meticulous management and constant observation. Potential problems that may occur as a result of bleeding from oeso-phageal varices include:

- *Hypervolaemi* related to blood loss.
  - Monitor blood pressure.
  - Arterial catheter will directly monitor blood pressure.
  - Central venous pressure will monitor fluid loss.
  - Assess urine output.
- *Risk of bleeding*
  - Advise the patient to avoid straining.
  - Observe for retching or vomiting.
  - Maintain a stool chart.
- *Impaired gas exchange* related to aspiration pneumonia
  - Check blood gases.

The management of bleeding oesophageal varices continues to be a subject of debate. Despite the increase in therapeutic options, morbidity and mortality remain high.

The range of endoscopic options available for the treatment of bleeding oesophageal varices includes endoscopic sclerotherapy,

Practical Endoscopy Edited by M. Shephard and J. Mason. Published in 1997 by Chapman & Hall, London. ISBN 0 412 54000 2

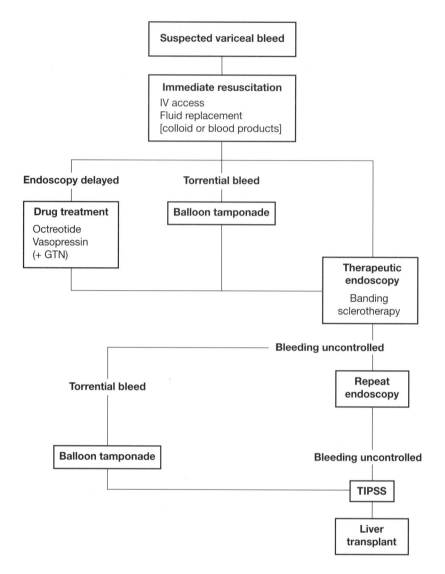

Fig. 10C.1   Flowchart: treatment of suspected oesophageal varices

variceal banding and balloon tamponade (Fig. 10C.1, Table 10C.1). Other options include surgical and drug intervention.

This chapter will focus on the various medical and surgical options available in the management of the patient with bleeding oesophageal varices, with particular emphasis on the various endoscopic methods available and the use of balloon tamponade.

Table 10C.1 Tubes available for oesophagogastric tamponade

Tube type	Oesophageal aspirate	Oesophageal balloon	Gastric aspirate	Gastric balloon	Comments
Sengstaken–Blakemore		X	X	X	Oesophageal aspiration by passing a separate tube (Salem pump or similar) orally or nasally above the oesophageal balloon
Linton	X		X	X	Absence of oesophageal balloon prevents pressure necrosis Manometer used to measure balloon inflation pressure
Minnesota	X	X	X	X	Large 18 Fr adult tube allows gastric lavage and aspiration, and administration of medication via gastric aspiration port

10C.2 AETIOLOGY

Oesophageal varices are tortuous veins that occur in the submucosa of the oesophagus and the upper part of the stomach. They are secondary to portal hypertension, which is commonly the result of:

- Cirrhosis of the liver owing to, for example, alcoholism, viral hepatitis or biliary cirrhosis.
- Obstruction of the portal venous system, for example owing to portal vein thrombosis.

As a result of portal hypertension, the flow of blood from the portal vein through the liver may meet with resistance owing to disease and cirrhotic changes in the liver. Pressure rises within the portal venous system, resulting in portal hypertension. Due to obstruction of the flow of blood through the portal system there is a 'back-pressure' down the system, resulting in engorged dilated veins.

In order for the body to cope with this problem, collateral circulatory channels develop between the portal vein and the systemic circulatory system to bypass the liver. These 'bypass' veins are most commonly found around the lower oesophagus and the stomach. These are known as oesophageal and gastric varices.

The 'bypass' veins are performing a useful function, but as they become engorged and tortuous the walls are weakened, predisposing them to rupture. The tension in the variceal wall, which is related to the radius of the varix as well as intravariceal pressure, is believed to be critical in the pathogenesis of rupture.

10C.3   INDICATIONS OF BLEEDING FROM OESOPHAGEAL VARICES

Variceal bleeding may occur in up to 30% of patients with chronic liver disease. The risk of bleeding depends on several risk factors (e.g. the degree of liver disease, the size of the oesophageal varices and endoscopic red signs on varices).

Mortality from bleeding is related to the severity of liver disease. There is a correlation between the severity of liver impairment, the extent of the varices, the frequency and severity of bleeding and the mortality from bleeding.

Some patients have varices for many years and never bleed from them. Non-bleeding varices are asymptomatic and may go undiagnosed. Bleeding from varices may be a slow ooze indicated by vomiting coffee-ground vomit and the passing of melaena. Alternatively, bleeding from varices can be very severe and sudden with the vomiting of large quantities of blood and passing of melaena. The perforation and bleeding may be caused by mechanical trauma from the strain of coughing, vomiting or defecation, rough food passing over a varix or ulceration of the oesophageal mucosa and venous wall by gastric acid secretion.

As reflux oesophagitis is thought to trigger variceal bleeding, patients with known varices may be given medication to control gastric acidity.

Note: Any degree of bleeding in a patient with known portal hypertension must be taken seriously and medical advice sought urgently as a small bleed may lead to a severe, possibly fatal, bleed.

Throughput in the endoscopy department is usually rapid and patient stay short.

If you are aware that you will be receiving a patient with bleeding oesophageal varices, it will be helpful to find out as much as you can about them before they arrive.

Points to note are:

- Make sure you know how much blood is available for the patient.
- Ensure the patient has a wide-bore cannula *in situ*.

- Have available full blood count and clotting screen results.
- Have available and checked:
  - resuscitation equipment
  - suction
  - oxygen
  - ligation or banding kit
  - Sengstaken–Blakemore tube
  - sclerotherapy equipment.
- Ensure the endoscopy nursing and medical teams have an updated broad clinical knowledge in the management of a patient with bleeding oesophageal varices.

10C.4 ENDOSCOPIC EVALUATION

Endoscopy is of high diagnostic value in a patient with oesophageal varices. It allows assessment of the oesophageal varices, can estimate the risk of bleeding and can provide first-line treatment for bleeding oesophageal varices.

10C.4.1 ENDOSCOPIC APPEARANCE OF OESOPHAGEAL VARICES

Endoscopically, oesophageal varices appear as irregular, serpiginous, bluish structures running longitudinally in the submucosa of the oeso-phageal wall. They are usually most prominent distally (Plate 5). They can appear as blue, white, red or of normal oesophageal colour. Neither white or blue coloration correlates with the risk of bleeding. Red colour signs do, however, correlate with the risks of bleeding, e.g.:

- A cherry red spot on the varices less than 2 mm in diameter.
- A haematocystic spot – a larger red spot on the varices.
- A diffuse redness of an area of the varices.

Any red colour sign increases the risk of bleeding significantly (Plate 6).

The location of varices is also predictive of the risk of bleeding. Varices extending proximally are indicative of a high portal pressure, thus increasing the risk of bleeding.

10C.5 ENDOSCOPIC OESOPHAGEAL SCLEROTHERAPY

By using a flexible retractable needle, a sclerosing agent can be injected endoscopically into the portal circulation to create a variceal thrombo-sis and control bleeding. The sclerosing agent is injected directly into each varix. Each injection consists of 1–2 ml of sclerosant. This therapeutic form of injection of varices is quite effective but can be difficult to perform during active bleeding. Sclerotherapy controls bleeding in approximately 85–90% of cases (Silverstein and Tytgat, 1987).

Types of sclerosants include:

- Sodium tetradecylsulphate (STD) 1–3%.
- Sodium morrhuate 5%.
- Polidocanol.
- Ethanolamine oleate.

Note: STD 3% solution carries a higher risk of causing perforation than either of the other sclerosants or 1–1.5% strength STD.

10C.5.1 PREPROCEDURE PREPARATION

The required amount of sclerosing agent is drawn up prior to the procedure.

The syringes are sealed with a blind-end hub and immersed in warm water. This makes the substance easier to inject. The outer sheath of the sclerotherapy needle should be checked for any damage.

Remember that the sclerosing agent is an irritant so ensure that all personnel involved in the procedure, including the patient, are wearing safety goggles or a visor.

10C.5.2 PROCEDURE

The patient is prepared for sclerotherapy as for a routine gastroscopy. The endoscopy nurse will explain the procedure to the patient and at this stage it is advisable to inform the patient that he or she may experience some retrosternal discomfort following the sclerotherapy procedure.

Vital signs are recorded and act as a baseline to observe for a deterioration during the procedure and also postprocedure. Oxygen is administered and saturation of oxygen monitored by pulse oximetry.

A small amount of sclerosing agent is then injected in the lumen of the varices needle in order to expel any air. The patient is positioned in the left lateral position and sedation is given. The endoscopy nurse positioned at the head of the patient will closely monitor vital signs and ensure that the airway is kept clear by pharyngeal suction as required. If active bleeding occurs it is important to observe the amount of blood lost and inform the endoscopist.

The second endoscopy nurse will assist the endoscopist during the procedure. When the endoscopist has located the varix to be injected, the endoscopy nurse passes the loaded needle to the endoscopist. A full syringe containing the sclerosing agent is attached securely to the needle lumen. A gauze swab is wrapped around the connection between the swab and the needle to absorb any leak of sclerosant.

The sclerotherapy needle is passed down the biopsy channel of the endoscope. When the varix is located the nurse will be asked to advance the needle out and inject the sclerosing agent. During injection the endoscopy nurse must inform the endoscopist how much sclerosant is being injected. The amount of sclerosing agent used during the procedure is documented in the patient's notes.

Following the procedure the needle, if reusable, must be cleaned in accordance with cleaning and disinfection guidelines. If single-use only, then it is disposed of in the sharps container.

10C.5.3   POST-THERAPY PATIENT CARE

The patient is reassured that the procedure is complete and is advised to inform the nursing staff should pain or discomfort occur. Absolute rest is encouraged and the head of the bed elevated unless contraindicated by shock. This position may reduce the flow of blood into the portal system. The patient is observed for further bleeding and for signs of oesophageal perforation. Hourly pulse and 4-hourly temperature are recorded. Signs of oesophageal perforation will be indicated by an elevated temperature and tachycardia. The patient may complain of chest pain, abdominal pain, pleuritic pain or pain extending to the shoulders. On physical examination there may be obvious signs of subcutaneous emphysema. The medical team must be informed if the patient presents with any of these symptoms. A chest and abdominal X-ray will be requested.

If the patient remains pain free with no tachycardia or pyrexia, fluids and soft diet will be introduced in accordance with the endoscopist's instructions.

10C.6   BALLOON TAMPONADE

The purpose of balloon tamponade is to exert pressure on the oesophageal wall to arrest bleeding from oesophageal or gastric varices and prevent accumulation of blood in the gastrointestinal tract, which could precipitate hepatic coma. The use of balloon tamponade is indicated only if bleeding cannot be controlled by therapeutic or drug intervention and endoscopy has confirmed that bleeding is from oesophageal or gastric varices.

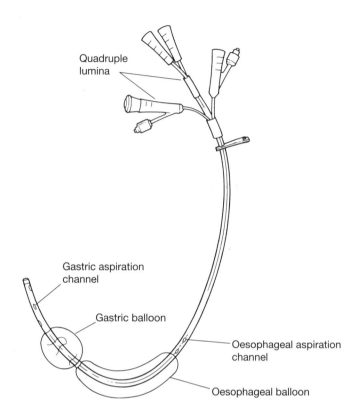

Quadruple lumina

Gastric aspiration channel

Gastric balloon

Oesophageal aspiration channel

Oesophageal balloon

Fig. 10C.2 The quadruple lumen Sengstaken–Blakemore (Minnesota) tube

The type of balloons available for balloon tamponade do vary so it is therefore vital to ensure that the manufacturer's instructions are checked before use. The tube most commonly used for balloon tamponade is the Sengstaken–Blakemore tube. Sengstaken and Blakemore (1950) described the use of a triple-lumen oesophagogastric tube that compressed both fundal and oesophageal varices with a provision of a third channel for gastric aspiration. Edlich *et al.* (1968) of the University of Minnesota developed a quadruple-lumen oesophagogastric tube. The additional fourth channel allows aspiration of the oesophageal contents above the oesophageal balloon. The quadruple lumen Sengstaken–Blakemore tube is sometimes referred to as the Minnesota tube. It has two inflatable balloons and four channels (Fig. 10C.2).

10C.6.1   PREPARATION FOR INSERTION OF THE SENGSTAKEN–BLAKEMORE TUBE

It cannot be overemphasized that insertion of the Sengstaken–Blakemore tube should be performed only by experienced medical personnel supported by a nursing team with broad clinical knowledge of the total management of a patient requiring balloon tamponade.

Equipment should be checked and prepared prior to the procedure. A checklist for this procedure includes:

- Senstaken–Blakemore tube.
- Artery forceps × four pairs.
- Lubricant.
- Gauze swabs
- 30 ml syringe.
- Suction equipment.
- Drainage bag.
- Disposable gloves.
- Adhesive tape.
- Sphygmomanometer.
- Oxygen.
- Crash trolley.

The availability of a dedicated 'bleeder' trolley or a 'bleeder' box will ensure that the equipment required for this type of emergency is readily available for immediate use, therefore saving precious time. It is important to remember that the patient's condition may be critical so therefore it may be useful to obtain as much relevant information as possible.

10C.6.2   CHECKING THE TUBE PRIOR TO USE

The nurse must ensure that the proximal end of each lumen is identified and clearly labelled to prevent possible error in inflation or deflation of tubes after insertion. It is essential to prepare the tube before insertion – this is to partly check for leaks and to establish a baseline with which measurements will be compared once the tube has been inserted.

The gastric balloon is deflated and then inflated with the required amount of air. This ensures that the gastric balloon is large enough to keep it in the stomach. Balloon pressure is measured using a sphygmomanometer and then recorded. Then the gastric balloon is completely deflated.

The oesophageal balloon is deflated and then inflated with the required amount of air, measured and recorded. It is then completely deflated.

The required amount of air for balloon inflation may vary in accordance with the type of tube that is being used. Therefore, it is important to check the manufacturer's instructions before use.

Storing the Sengstaken–Blakemore tube in the fridge allows for easier intubation.

10C.6.3 MANAGEMENT DURING PROCEDURE

The patient is placed in the left lateral position. It is necessary to ensure that suction is at hand. The Sengstaken–Blakemore tube is well lubricated and inserted via the mouth. The tube is advanced until 50 cm has been inserted. The tube is then placed securely in position by the endoscopy assistant.

The gastric balloon is inflated with the required amount of air. Insertion of air into the balloon must be a gradual process. During inflation the patient is observed for signs of pain and discomfort. If pain occurs this may indicate that the balloon is in the oesophagus. Therefore, it is important to stop inserting air, deflate the balloon, reposition and reinflate the balloon.

When the required amount of air has been inserted into the gastric balloon the balloon pressure is measured and recorded. The pressure should correlate with the preinsertion pressure. If not this may indicate wrong positioning or that the tube is leaking.

The tube is then pulled gently upwards until resistance is felt. At this stage the inflated gastric balloon fits snugly into the fundus of the stomach (Fig. 10C.3). A slight tension is applied to maintain correct positioning of the tube.

The oesophageal balloon is inflated slowly until the predetermined volume of air has been inserted. If pain occurs then it is important to stop inserting air. The pressure in the oesophageal balloon should be 25–45 mmHg. The pressure in the balloon is checked and the air reduced until the patient is comfortable.

The level of the tube at the incisors is checked and recorded.

Aspiration of oesophageal contents is a common complication of balloon tamponade therefore frequent aspiration may have to be undertaken to minimize retention of regurgitated secretions.

10C.6.4 POSTPROCEDURE MANAGEMENT

Following intubation of the Sengstaken–Blakemore tube, patients will require constant observation in a designated area where they can be closely monitored at all times by a qualified nurse. Qualified nursing and medical staff should be aware of how to remove the Sengstaken–

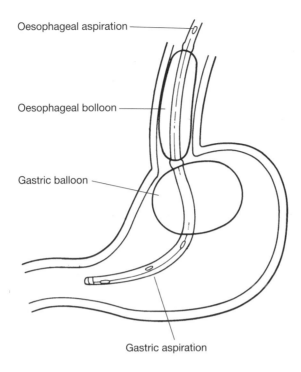

Oesophageal aspiration

Oesophageal bolloon

Gastric balloon

Gastric aspiration

Fig. 10C.3 Tube *in situ*; gastric and oesophageal balloons inflated

Blakemore tube should a patient show signs of respiratory distress. The tube can be removed immediately by cutting across the entire tube with scissors. A chest X-ray may be performed to check correct positioning of the tube and to check for complications or aspiration of oesophago-gastric contents.

Continual low-pressure suction is applied to the oesophageal aspiration channel and a drainage bag is connected to the gastric aspiration channel. The gastric aspiration channel can also be used to administer medications (e.g. lactulose).

Balloon pressures are checked every 30 minutes and recorded. To avoid oesophageal ulceration and tissue necrosis the oesophageal balloon is deflated for 5 minutes every hour.

It is important to note that, depending on the type of tube used, it may be necessary to clamp the oesophageal and gastric lumen to prevent leakage of air from the balloons.

The level of the tube at the incisors is checked regularly to ensure the tube has not become displaced. It may also be necessary to irrigate the gastric tube with 30 ml normal saline every 1–2 hours to prevent occlusion of the tube.

10C.6.5   COMPLICATIONS

The most common complication of balloon tamponade is aspiration of oesophageal and gastric contents (Garden and Carter, 1992). The use of the four-lumen Sengstaken–Blakemore tube will minimize the risk of aspiration and respiratory complications.

Asphyxia may occur if the oesophageal balloon is allowed to migrate upwards into the pharynx. If the patient shows signs of respiratory distress, then this must be relieved immediately either by reinserting the tube or if this is not possible, by removing the tube completely using the method described previously. A perforated oesophagus can occur if the gastric balloon is inflated while in the oesophagus or if the tube is pulled out while the balloons are both inflated. Oesophageal ulceration and tissue necrosis can occur if the oesophageal balloon is not deflated every hour.

10C.6.6   REMOVAL OF THE SENGSTAKEN–BLAKEMORE TUBE

The Sengstaken–Blakemore tube should not remain inserted for more than 24 hours as prolonged pressure from the balloon within the oesophagus may result in tissue necrosis. However, some clinicians will leave the tube *in situ* for a further 24 hours with the oesophageal balloon completely deflated. Therefore, if the patient rebleeds the oesophageal balloon can be inflated and balloon tamponade applied quickly.

Removal of the tube should be decided by the medical team and meet with a definite plan of further treatment. To remove the tube, disconnect it from the suction source and clamp both the stomach and oesophageal aspiration lumen to prevent aspiration of oesophagogastric contents within the tube. Completely deflate the oesophageal balloon, following it by deflation of the gastric balloon. Instruct the patient to inhale and exhale slowly. During exhalation withdraw the tube with one continuous gentle motion.

The patient should remain nil by mouth following removal of the tube for 6–8 hours. Provided that patient observations are satisfactory, fluids and soft diet may then be introduced according to the instructions from the medical team.

10C.7   ENDOSCOPIC LIGATION OF VARICES

A recent advancement in the endoscopic management of variceal bleeding is the use of the endoscopic variceal ligation technique. This therapeutic management of bleeding varices controls bleeding in at least 90% of cases. It has been proved to be equally as effective as sclerotherapy but has fewer side-effects. Some studies have revealed a reduction in rebleeding following banding of oesophageal varices.

There are several banding devices currently in use and the equipment used is gradually becoming more efficient and user friendly. Banding ligation of varices is performed by attaching a device to the forward viewing end of the endoscope (Fig.10C.4a). A prestressed rubber band is already positioned at the distal end of the device, which is held in place by a tripwire. The device comprises an inner and outer cylinder attached to a wire that runs through the biopsy channel of the endoscope (Fig.10C.4b).

Once the device is positioned close to the variceal cord, endoscopic suction is applied to suck the varix into the device, the tripwire is pulled and the band is released over the entrapped varix. The varix will eventually slough off leaving a small ulcer.

10C.8   MEDICAL TREATMENT

The beta-blocker propranolol is widely used for the long-term medical treatment of portal hypertension. Propanolol has been shown in most controlled studies to reduce the risk of rebleeding in portal hypertension, although some trials have shown no benefit (Garden and Carter, 1992). The aim is to reduce the portal venous pressure and prevent bleeding from oesophageal or gastric varices. By controlling portal venous pressure this may prevent the development of portal hypertension and varices.

10C.8.1   VASOPRESSIN

Vasopressin has been used for over 40 years and controls bleeding in only 75% of cases (Fogel *et al.*, 1982).

It reduces portal vein flow by splanchnic vasoconstriction. This reduces portal venous pressure and may stop active bleeding from varices by allowing haemostasis and clotting. However, vasopressin is now not widely used owing to its side-effects. These include:

- Cardiac ischaemia.
- Hyponatraemia.

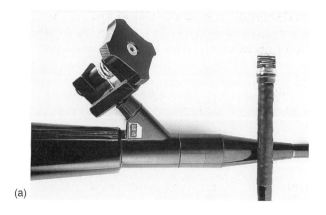

(a)

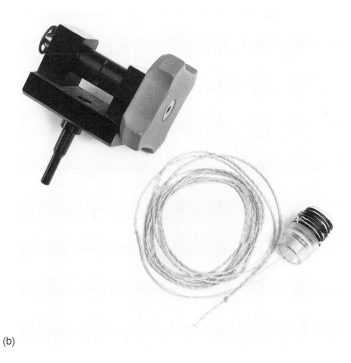

(b)

Fig. 10C.4 (a) Variceal band ligation. The 'six-shooter' multibander (W. Cook). (b) Composition of multibanding device

- Abdominal cramping.
- Bowel infarction.
- Involuntary bowel evacuation.

Vascular side-effects are reduced if a nitroglycerin infusion is administered concurrently. Vasopressin is contraindicated in patients with coronary artery disease.

Dose

Bolus of 20 units of vasopressin diluted in 100–200 ml of dextrose 5% in water to be administered over 10–20 minutes.

10C.8.2   OCTREOTIDE

This is a synthetic analogue of somatostatin that reduces portal venous pressure without the cardiovascular side-effects of vasopressin. It has been shown to be at least as effective as vasopressin in arresting variceal bleeding.

Dose

50 m bolus IV followed by 50 µg/h infusion.

Both somatostatin and octreotide are considered the drugs of choice for the treatment of bleeding oesophageal varices, mainly because of the ease of administration and reduction of side-effects.

10C.9   SURGICAL TREATMENT

Surgical shunting procedures aim to reduce portal pressure and control bleeding oesophageal varices by diverting the blood from the portal venous system to the inferior vena cava. Surgical portasystemic shunting can also be carried out, but this has a very high mortality rate so is not often used.

10C.9.1   TRANSJUGULAR INTRAHEPATIC PORTASYSTEMIC STENT SHUNTS (TIPSS)

This method has been developed more recently. The aim is to reduce portal venous pressure and stop variceal bleeding. In it, a catheter is passed intravenously via the internal jugular vein, and a stent is inserted between the systemic and portal venous systems. Encephalopathy may occur as a result but can be treated conservatively.

10C.9.2   OESOPHAGEAL TRANSECTION

Transection of the oesophagus using a staple gun with or without devascularization of the superficial veins of the oesophagus was once the treatment of choice for the endoscopic treatment-resistant active variceal bleed. However, the mortality rate in an emergency situation is over 28% and oesophageal stricture and gastropathy due to worsening portal hypertension are common complications. TIPSS is considered to be superior to oesophageal transection, mainly because the clinical condition of many patients is too poor for major surgery.

10C.9.3 LIVER TRANSPLANTATION

More recently, liver transplantation has been considered for patients presenting with oesophageal varices due to cirrhosis of the liver. Many centres will not consider transplantation in patients with cirrhosis due to alcohol abuse unless they can be shown to have abstained from alcohol for at least 3 months.

Liver transplantation is now a well-established surgical technique, and over 70% of patients treated in this way survive for 5 years or more.

REFERENCES

Edlich, R.F., Lande, A.J., Goodale, R.L. and Wangensteen, O.H. (1968) Prevention of aspiration pneumonia by continuous oesophageal aspiration during oesophageal tamponade and gastric cooling. *Surgery*, **64**, 405–8.

Fogel, M.R., Knauer, M., Ljudevit, L. *et al.* (1982) Continuous intravenous vasopressin in active upper gastrointestinal bleeding – a placebo trial. *Ann Intern Med*, **96**, 565–9.

Garden, O.J. and Carter, D.C. (1992) Balloon tamponade and vasoactive drugs in the control of acute variceal haemorrhage, in *Clinical Gastroenterology in Portal Hypertension* 6(3) (ed. R. Shields), Baillière Tindall, London, pp. 451–9.

Sengstaken, R.W. and Blakemore, A.H. (1950) Balloon tamponade for the control of haemorrhage from oesophageal varices. *Ann Surg*, **131**, 781–9.

Silverstein, F.E. and Tytgat, G.N.J. (1987) *Slide Atlas of Gastrointestinal Endoscopy*, Gower Medical, London.

BIBLIOGRAPHY

Brewer, T.G. (1993) Treatment of acute gastroesophageal variceal haemorrhage. *Medical Clinics of North America. Gastrointestinal Emergencies*, 77(5), 993–1007.

Brunner, L.S. and Suddarth, D (1990) *Lippincott Manual of Medical and Surgical Nursing*, Harper and Row, London, 518–22.

Thompson, J.M., McFarland, G.K., Hirsch, J.E. *et al.* (1989) *Mosby's Manual of Clinical Nursing*, C V Mosby, New York.

Watson, J.E. and Royle, J.A. (1988) Nursing disorders of the liver, biliary tract and exocrine pancreas, in *Watson's Medical–Surgical Nursing and Related Physiology* (ed. J.E. Watson), 602–5.

Williams, S.G.J. and Westaby, D. (1995) Recent advances in the endoscopic management of variceal bleeding. *Gut*, **36**(5), 647–58.

Endoscopic retrograde cholangio-pancreatography

11

Hazel French

11.1 INTRODUCTION

Endoscopic retrograde cholangio-pancreatography (ERCP) is a combined endoscopic and radiological technique used to visualize the biliary and pancreatic ducts. Initially this was a purely diagnostic procedure, but as techniques have advanced more therapeutic procedures have become possible and nowadays in the modern endoscopy unit up to 80% of ERCP work will be therapeutic. ERCP is probably the most complicated part of the endoscopy assistant's work and something which can be initially very daunting. However, once mastered it becomes a challenging and fulfilling part of their work, and one which involves close co-operation with the endoscopist, anticipating equipment needs and, where appropriate, suggesting possible solutions to problems encountered. It is therefore essential that the endoscopy assistant is fully conversant both with the procedure and with the equipment involved. As with other endoscopic procedures, each endoscopist tends to develop his or her own individual approach to ERCP so that although the procedures described in this chapter may vary from those performed in a particular unit, the principles will be very much the same.

11.2 ANATOMY

The liver is the largest internal organ of the body, weighing approximately 1.36 kg (3 lb) and is situated in the right upper quadrant of the abdomen tucked against the inferior surface of the diaphragm (Fig.

Practical Endoscopy Edited by M. Shephard and J. Mason. Published in 1997 by Chapman & Hall, London. ISBN 0 412 54000 2

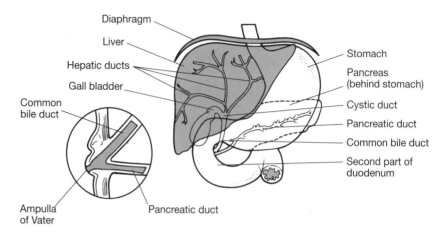

Fig. 11.1   Anatomy of liver and pancreas

11.1). The right and left hepatic ducts transport bile from the liver and unite to form a single common hepatic duct. The cystic duct originates from the gall bladder and joins the common hepatic duct to form the common bile duct (CBD). The CBD empties into the duodenum at the ampulla of Vater, and it is joined by the pancreatic duct between 1 and 10 mm from its orifice. Very rarely the CBD and pancreatic ducts remain separate with individual orifices in the duodenum. The ampulla is surrounded by a ring of circular muscle called the sphincter of Oddi, which regulates the flow of bile and pancreatic enzymes into the duodenum. The 'nipple-like' structure formed where the CBD enters the duodenum is referred to as the papilla.

The gall bladder is a sack-like structure that lies on the under surface of the liver and is approximately 8 cm long and 4 cm wide, although it can become much larger if filled with gall stones. Its function is to store bile after it is secreted by the liver.

The pancreas consists of a 'head', 'body' and 'tail', and has both an endocrine and exocrine function. It lies transversely across the abdomen with the head situated in the duodenal loop and the tail located close to the spleen. There is an accessory papilla situated approximately 2 cm above and slightly to the right of the main papilla (when viewed endoscopically). This drains the pancreas via Santorini's duct.

11.3   RELATED PHYSIOLOGY AND PATHOLOGY

The purpose of the biliary system is to concentrate and store bile for use in the digestive process. Under normal conditions the ampulla of Vater remains slightly open, allowing a small quantity of bile to leak naturally into the duodenum. (For this reason it is usually easy to cannulate.) When food enters the duodenum a hormone is released that causes the gall bladder to contract and push its store of bile into the intestine. Bile is a greenish yellow fluid secreted continuously by the liver; initially it contains up to 97% water. Whilst being stored in the gall bladder, up to 90% of this water is removed resulting in a concentrated solution made up of bile salts, cholesterol, lecithin, fatty acids, electrolytes, conjugated proteins and other organic substances. It plays an important part in fat digestion and the absorption of fat-soluble vitamins and minerals, and it also acts as the excretion pathway for substances such as cholesterol, bilirubin and certain hormones. If the flow of bile through the CBD is obstructed for any reason then the bile constituents are forced into the bloodstream where its pigments are deposited in the skin and mucous membranes, causing a yellow discoloration known as jaundice. This situation may also occur in haemolytic anaemia where there is excessive destruction of red blood cells or in patients with gross liver dysfunction. Symptoms of disease usually first present during middle age. Between the ages of 20 and 50 years the incidence is six times higher in women than in men, but once over the age of 50 the incidence becomes roughly equal.

11.3.1 BILIARY STONES

The presence of stones in the CBD is the most common cause of disease in the biliary system. There are two types of biliary stones:

1. Cholesterol stones, which include both pure cholesterol and other constituents of bile and are associated with a very high concentration of cholesterol in the bile produced by the liver. These account for three-quarters of all biliary stones and are more likely to occur in females during pregnancy and in those taking oral contraceptives or on hormone replacement therapy. They are dark coloured and generally soft.
2. Pigment stones, which account for the other quarter of biliary stones and are made up of bilirubin and inorganic calcium salts. These stones are black or brown in colour and can be extremely hard. They are more common in people with alcoholism or alcoholic cirrhosis, and those requiring parenteral nutrition.

Not all stones cause symptoms and, even when they do, the intensity, extent and nature vary considerably. Symptoms usually consist of a steady pain that occurs 3 to 6 hours after a heavy meal, frequently during the night, and often radiates to other parts of the abdomen, middle of the back or the tip of the right shoulder. The patient may also be nauseated and vomit. In severe cases the patients exhibit symptoms of fever (shivering, temperature, malaise) and acute pancreatitis. Less severe cases often present with symptoms of upper abdominal discomfort, dyspepsia and belching.

11.4 PREPARATION FOR ERCP

11.4.1 PREPARING THE ROOM

ERCP is made a lot easier if the room used is set up logically and methodically. Room size is important as cramped conditions can cause problems in some of the more complex procedures. As the patient lies on their left side during the investigation, it is usually best to set up the room with the patient in the reverse position to that used for conventional radiography (i.e. with their head where the feet would normally be) (Fig. 11.2). It is important that the endoscopist, radiologist (if

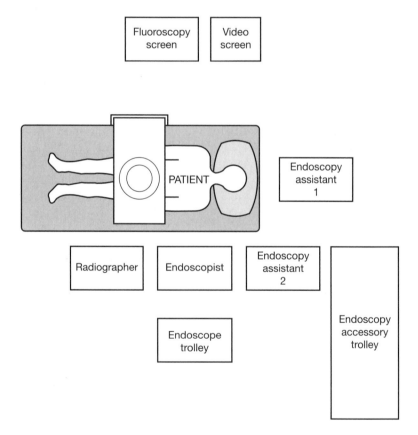

Fig. 11.2 Room layout for ERCP

present) and endoscopy assistant are able to see the fluoroscopy and endoscopy monitor screens, and experience will show the best positions for these. In addition to the screens, the following will always be required:

- Endoscopy trolley together with light-source, suction and diathermy equipment.
- Accessory trolley(s) containing adequate stock of all ERCP equipment and accessories.
- Oxygen and suction equipment for the patient.
- Resuscitation equipment, which should be readily available either in or close to the procedure room.
- Pulse oximetry, together with non-invasive blood pressure monitoring if available. Monitors should be placed in such a position that the endoscopy assistant caring for the patient can easily see them without having to turn or strain.
- ERCP patients can be severely ill and/or may be unable to move themselves, so appropriate lifting and handling aids should be readily available.

Disinfection

Disinfection is of paramount importance for ERCP procedures because of the possibility of serious infection from organisms such as *Pseudomonas*, which may be present either in the endoscope or in the accessories used. Endoscopes should be cleaned meticulously, paying particular attention to the 'bridge' area. The raiser bridge channel may have to be disinfected manually as many automatic disinfectors are unable to pump fluid through such a small-diameter channel. Instruments should be particularly clean because infection of the biliary or pancreatic systems can have serious consequences. The use of automated systems that sterilize rather than disinfect the endoscope are worth consideration for ERCP, as is the use of sterile high-quality filtered water for rinsing all reusable equipment. ERCP accessories should be either single-use presterilized items or reusable items that can be adequately cleaned and resterilized according to manufacturers' instructions.

11.4.2   DUODENOSCOPES

Duodenoscopes differ from the conventional upper gastrointestinal endoscope in that they have:

1. Side viewing with a wide-angle lens system, to allow vision of the duodenal wall.

2. An additional elevator (bridge) mechanism, which allows fine manipulation of instruments. The elevator mechanism is situated at the distal end of the instrumentation channel and enables the instruments used to be finely controlled when used in conjunction with the angulation controls. The channel containing the elevator control wires can also be flushed to allow adequate decontamination.

3. A longer insertion tube to aid intubation of the duodenum and also to provide a more comfortable working position.

11.4.3 PATIENT PREPARATION

The general preparation is the same as for upper gastrointestinal endoscopy. Many units admit the patient to hospital the day before the investigation, although this is becoming less common. In addition, the following are required:

1. Patient should be kept nil by mouth for at least 4–6 hours prior to the ERCP (usually overnight), although this may need to be longer if there is any reason to suspect gastric outlet obstruction.

2. Informed written consent should be obtained from all patients as with other endoscopic procedures, but this may need to be broadened to include any possible therapeutic interventions anticipated.

3. Haematological investigation of blood-clotting mechanism should be performed to check this is within normal limits. Some centres will carry out diagnostic ERCP without this, but it is considered good practice to perform this for all ERCP patients. A sample should also be taken for blood cross-matching in case an emergency transfusion is required.

4. An intravenous cannula should be inserted in patient's **right** hand to allow easy intravenous access (the patient will be lying on their left arm).

5. Many centres routinely give prophylactic antibiotic cover for all the ERCP patients.

11.5 DIAGNOSTIC ERCP

11.5.1 INDICATIONS/CONTRAINDICATIONS

Indications for ERCP include:

● Evaluation of acute recurrent chronic pancreatitis.
● Investigation of symptoms suggestive of malignancy, particularly if abdominal ultrasound or computerized tomography (CT) scans are normal or equivocal.

- Unexplained abdominal pain of suspected biliary origin.
- Confirmation of sclerosing cholangitis.
- Investigation of jaundiced patients suspected of having a biliary obstruction.
- Investigation of patients with deranged liver function on haemalogical investigation.
- Investigation of patients to detect CBD stones prior to laparoscopic cholecystectomy.
- Manometry of the sphincter of Oddi and CBD.
- Confirming patency of biliary tree following biliary surgery or liver transplantation.

Note: In many countries, especially the USA, biliary manometry is performed routinely as part of diagnostic ERCP. A fuller description of this procedure is to be found in section 11.6.7.

The need for ERCP in children is rare and is limited to investigation of recurring pancreatitis of unknown origin, obstructive jaundice where causes such as sclerosing cholangitis or congenital stricture of the CBD are suspected, and as part of the preparation of patients for pancreatic surgery where knowledge of the anatomy of the biliary and pancreatic ducts is required.

Contraindications to diagnostic ERCP are rare, but it should be avoided in patients with a history of recent myocardial infarction, and performed with caution in those with a severely deranged blood-clotting mechanism or in the acute phase of pancreatitis. ERCP should be avoided wherever possible during pregnancy and caution should be observed in patients with a known allergy to contrast media.

11.5.2 PREPARATION FOR DIAGNOSTIC ERCP

1. *Endoscopy trolley*; a duodenoscope usually with a 2.8 or 3.2 mm diameter biopsy channel is adequate for diagnostic ERCP as it will easily take a size 5 French (Fr) cannula. Check optics, air/water, suction and elevator (bridge) mechanism prior to use.
2. *Medication*;
   (a) sedative (e.g. midazolam or diazepam);
   (b) analgaesia (e.g. pethidine or nalbuphine);
   (c) anticholinergic (e.g. hyoscine);
   (d) glucagon or glycerine trinitrate spray.
   Specific reversal agents for benzodiazepines (flumazenil) and narcotic analgesics (naloxone) should also be available.
3. *Accessory trolley*.
4. *Radiation protective wear*.

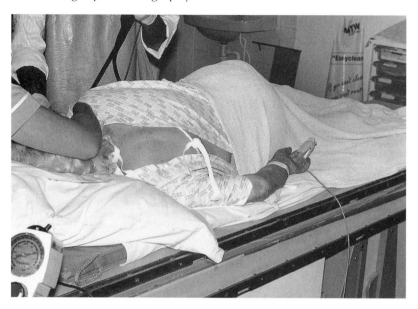

Fig. 11.3   Patient position for ERCP. Note left arm placed behind back

11.5.3   PATIENT POSITION DURING ERCP

The patient is prepared as for a diagnostic upper gastrointestinal endoscopy, with the exception that they are required to lie with their left arm behind their back (Fig. 11.3). The patient should remain on their side whilst the duodenoscope is passed through the pylorus and into the second part of the duodenum. Once in the duodenum, cannulation is easier if the patient is lying on their stomach. Assisting the patient to change to this position is faciliated by having their left arm behind their back.

(**Note:** Some patients find this uncomfortable, and may find it easier if a pillow or foam wedge is used to help support them.)

Should the duodenoscope 'fall back' into the stomach then it is sometimes necessary to temporarily move the patient back on to their side whilst the pylorus is again negotiated.

11.5.4   PROCEDURE

The catheter should be primed with the chosen contrast (Fig. 11.4). The three-way tap allows filling of the 10 ml syringe without letting any air into the catheter. Diagnosis may be difficult if air has been introduced by the operator as air bubbles can be mistaken for stones.

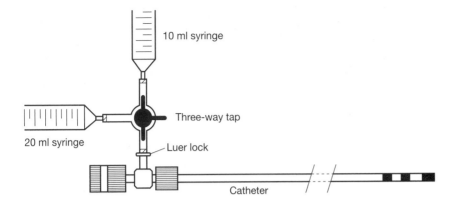

Fig. 11.4   Standard catheter primed with contrast

The endoscopist will pass the endoscope into the duodenum and find the ampulla (papilla) (Fig. 11.5). This can usually be easily identified from its colour, shape and position at the top of the vertical fold, although sometimes the papilla is small or flattened and may be hidden by a fold of tissue or in a diverticulum.

The previously prepared cannula is passed through the endoscope and the endoscopist will then cannulate the ampulla (Fig. 11.6). This may not be straightforward and can be very difficult. Either the bile duct or the pancreatic duct or both may be cannulated.

Care must be taken when the assistant is injecting contrast into the pancreatic system as overfilling of the pancreatic duct can cause pancreatitis. It is important to inject slowly watching the X-ray screen and stop injecting if you are injecting into the pancreatic duct. No more than 3–5 ml of contrast should be injected into the duct, and often less than this is required for adequate visualization (Fig. 11.7).

TIPS FOR ERCP

Excess bubbling in the duodenum can seriously impair vision. Either:

1. Give patient a silicone-based drink about 30 minutes before the procedure as a matter of routine.

or

2. Mix 1 ml of a silicone-based liquid (Infacol or similar) with water in a 20 ml syringe (it needs shaking well) and introduce into the duodenum via either the ERCP catheter or the instrumentation channel of the endoscope.

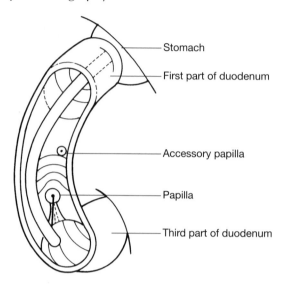

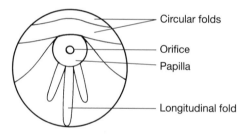

Fig. 11.5 Landmarks during ERCP (adapted from Cotton and Williams, 1990)

If injecting contrast is difficult, stop injecting and consult the endo-scopist; it may indicate a submucosal injection (Fig. 11.8). Submuscosal injection occurs mainly with a short taper-tipped or metal-tipped cannula (section 11.5.5) as these are more likely to traumatize tissue, but it may also occur with a friable ampullary tumour.

Cannulation is sometimes difficult and different solutions can be tried:

1. Changing the type of catheter, to a long taper for biliary cannulation or a short tapered catheter for pancreatic duct cannulation.

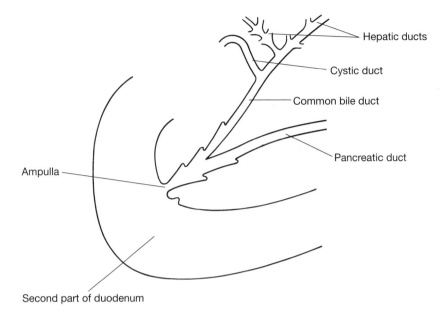

Fig. 11.6   Relationship of bile and pancreatic ducts

2. For a floppy ampulla try a metal ball tip.
3. A sphincterotome can be used to angle the tip into the bile duct using the bowing wire. It is easier to use a sphincterotome with a dedicated wire channel so that all of the contrast is injected into the duct rather than some refluxing into the duodenum.
4. A taper-tip cannula can also help to cut down reflux of contrast into the duodenum if the ridge of the catheter (a millimeter from the tip) is pushed upwards against the ampulla.
5. Occasionally sphincterotomy is performed using a needle knife to cut an access into the bile duct but this can be dangerous and is usually done only if diagnosis is essential.
6. A guide wire pushed through the catheter can sometimes help (flush out the contrast with sterile saline first before putting the guide wire into the catheter otherwise the guide wire will 'stick' in the catheter). The catheter is then advanced up the guide wire and the procedure repeated, until deep cannulation is obtained. A side-arm adapter should be attached to the catheter to allow contrast to be injected with a guide wire *in situ*. This enables the endoscopist to check the position of the catheter during placement.

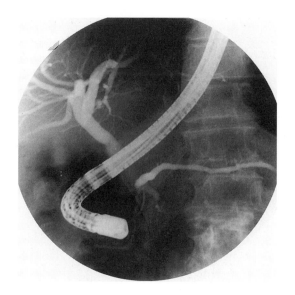

Fig. 11.7   X-ray of bile duct and pancreatic duct

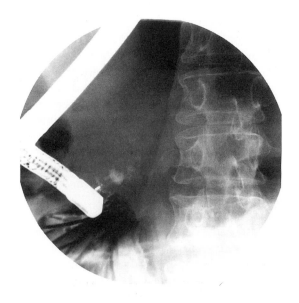

Fig. 11.8   X-ray: submucosal injection of contrast

11.5.5   ERCP CATHETERS

The majority of ERCP catheters are of 5 Fr diameter although some are 6 Fr tapering to 5 Fr at the distal tip. Most incorporate a steel 'stiffening' wire at the proximal end to aid instrumentation, together with a side arm for injection of contrast medium. A radio-opaque tip is provided to allow easy visualization as well as graduated markings (usually in 2 mm increments) for easy assessment of cannulation depth. Nowadays virtually all catheters accept guide wires, the standard size being 0.89 mm (0.035") but some of the finer tipped catheters will only accept 0.53 mm (0.021") or 0.63 mm (0.025") wires. There are five basic types (Fig. 11.9):

1. *Standard catheter*; this may be square ended or have a slight taper. It is the first-line choice for cannulation, and accepts a 0.89 mm diameter guide wire.
2. *Short taper tip*; this is useful in difficult cannulations, particularly of the pancreatic duct. It is often used as an alternative to the standard ERCP catheter, and accepts a 0.89 mm guide wire.
3. *Long taper tip*; this usually accepts only 0.53 or 0.63 mm diameter guide wire. It is useful in difficult cannulations where the CBD is

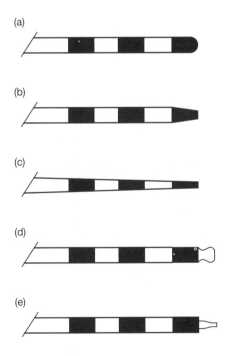

Fig. 11.9   ERCP catheters: (a) standard; (b) short taper tip; (c) long taper tip, (d) metal 'ball' tip; (e) conical metal tip

required. If this is used, it is best to exchange it for a stiffer 0.89 mm guide wire if therapeutic work is contemplated.

4. *Metal 'ball' tip*; this is useful if a 'floppy' papilla is encountered. It usually accepts 0.89 mm guide wires. The tips are very easy to see, but are more traumatic to tissue (see submucosal injection above).

5. *Conical metal tip*; this is especially useful if the papilla is very tight or if a minor papilla is to be cannulated. It will usually take only 0.53 or 0.63 mm guide wires. The tip can be particularly traumatic to tissue.

There are many variations available, including a peel-away variety for guide wire work, and precurved ones that allegedly provide easier cannulation. In the end, personal preference is usually the deciding factor.

11.5.6 BABY CHOLEDOCHOSCOPES

Some units have baby choledochoscopes that can pass into the biliary duct. These are expensive and easily damaged and for these reasons are not widely used. The baby choledochoscopes can be inserted into the biliary tree, allowing the endoscopist to examine the ducts and take biopsies under direct vision.

11.5.7 DIAGNOSTIC OR THERAPEUTIC ERCPs IN PATIENTS FOLLOWING BILLROTH II GASTRECTOMIES

ERCP can be difficult in patients who have had a Billroth II gastrectomy. This is because it can be difficult to identify endoscopically

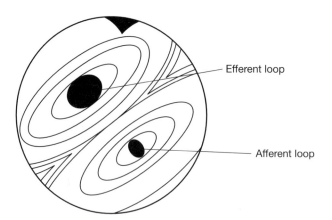

Fig. 11.10 Billroth II gastrectomy: loop orientation – as seen endoscopically

the afferent and efferent loops of bowel in the stomach: The efferent loop is usually more obvious (Fig. 11.10).

The correct orifice is usually found in the '2–5 o'clock' sector. Once in the loop, the usual landmarks are not visible until the papilla is recognized. If the wrong loop is identified it may be helpful to mark it by taking a few biopsies at the entrance or by injecting dye submucosally. Cannulation is often very difficult as everything is upside down. This unit has found either a paediatric duodenoscope or a gastroscope more useful with this group of patients. Either a new catheter with no curve on it or a Billroth II papillotome is useful cannulation in these circumstances (Fig. 11.11).

Cannulation is often very difficult in this group of patients and a combined radiologic and endoscopic approach is sometimes necessary to achieve cannulation. This approach is described later in the chapter.

11.6 THERAPEUTIC ERCP

11.6.1 INDICATIONS

Indications for therapeutic ERCP include:

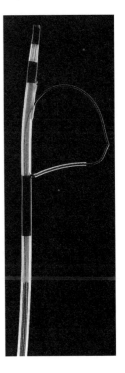

Fig. 11.11 Billroth II papillotome (W. Cook)

- Dilated common bile duct or intrahepatic ducts found on ultrasound (with or without duct stones present).
- Patients who present with an obstructive jaundice.
- Problems thought to be of biliary origin following laparoscopic cholecystectomy (i.e. ?retained stone or incorrect technique).

11.6.2 SPHINCTEROTOMY

Endoscopic sphincterotomy uses electrosurgery (diathermy) to cut through the sphincter of Oddi, which surrounds the ampulla, using a sphincterotome (papillotome). This allows drainage of the bile duct and clearance of any stones or debris present in the bile duct. Stone size, shape and quantity can vary greatly (Fig. 11.12).

As a guide the diathermy should be set on blend level 4 for a braided wire sphincterotome and blend level 3.5 for single-wire sphincterotomes, although this will vary with equipment used. Different sphincterotomes are used for different situations. For routine sphincterotomy use a 6 Fr catheter with a 30 mm length cutting blade that takes a 0.89 mm (0.035") guide wire. A protective (insulated) guide wire should always be used if it is to be left in place while diathermy is being

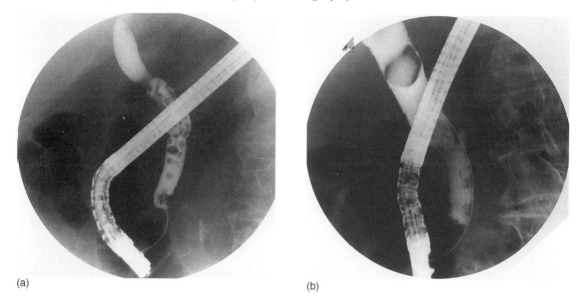

(a)

(b)

Fig. 11.12 (a) X-ray: multiple small stones in common bile duct. (b) X-ray: single large stone in a dilated common bile duct

used. Uninsulated guide wires must be removed completely before diathermy is used.

Sphincterotomes (papillotomes)

Sphincterotomes are available in many forms: however, there are four basic types (Fig. 11.13):

1. *Standard*; this accepts a 0.89 mm guide wire. It has a short (2 mm approx.) tip, and a 30 or 35 mm cutting blade, either single filament or braided.
2. *Long nosed*; this is generally the same as above, but the tip is longer (3 or 4 mm), making it more likely to stay engaged once cannulation is achieved. It can be harder to manoeuvre, however.
3. *Precut*; the cutting blade originates at the tip of this cannula, allowing a cut to be made with a very shallow cannulation.
4. *Needle knife (precut knife)*; this is used where no cannulation is possible. It is probably the most dangerous of endoscopic therapeutic interventions.

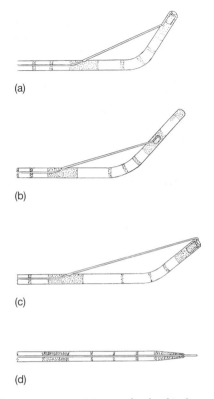

(a)

(b)

(c)

(d)

Fig. 11.13 Sphincterotomes: (a) standard; (b) long nosed; (c) precut; (d) needle knife

Procedure

The endoscopist cannulates the duct with the sphincterotome and inserts it until the desired length of blade is inside the bile duct. It is important to ensure that the sphincterotome is not in the pancreatic duct before electrocautery is performed and this can be confirmed radiologically either by its position on the screen or by injection of more contrast medium.

When instructed the endoscopy assistant should bow the sphincterotome slowly, watching the wire on the video screen. The endoscopist will control the cutting by intermittent use of the foot pedal. It may be necessary to slacken and tighten the wire several times, before a satisfactory cut is made (Plate 7).

Plate 8 shows the correct placement of the sphincterotome in the ampulla, and the correct amount of wire in and out of the duct.

If the sphincterotome does not work check that the wire is fully in view. If not it may be 'shorting' on to the scope. It may be necessary to increase the diathermy setting by half a point or reduce the length of wire in contact with the mucosa to initiate cutting. (If there is still a problem, check the diathermy (Chapter 18).)

11.6.3 IMPACTED STONES

Stone impaction usually causes the papilla to bulge into the duodenum and forces the orifice downwards. It is not always possible to inject contrast past an impacted stone.

Cannulation may be achieved with a bowed sphincterotome by 'hooking' the tip into the orifice. Often a needle knife can be used to incise the face of the papilla over the stone. The needle knife's bare wire is inserted in the papilla orifice. Pressure is then applied at the '12 o'clock' position and diathermy commenced. Sometimes the needle knife can be used to make a direct drill incision above the papilla into a dilated bile duct or into the face of a swollen papilla.

Precutting is more dangerous than standard sphincterotomy and should be reserved for use by the expert in patients with a strong indication for sphincterotomy and when all other standard techniques have been exhausted.

Note: Endoscopic sphincterotomy is one of the most risky of the therapeutic procedures currently performed by endoscopists. The usual quoted morbidity and mortality rates are approximately 10% and 1% respectively (Cotton and Williams, 1990).

Stone extraction

Most stones (at least those less than 1 cm in diameter) will pass spontaneously in the days or weeks following sphincterotomy (Fig. 11.14). Therefore many endoscopists leave small stones in the ducts to pass naturally and recheck by repeat ERCP after 6 weeks.

Stone extraction devices
Two types of extraction devices are available:

1. *Dormier baskets* (Fig. 11.15); the majority are four-, six-, or eight-wire rectangular or spiral shaped baskets, with a 3.5 to 6 cm length and 1.5 to 3 cm diameter. Wire-guided baskets are available, and some have long filiform tips to aid cannulation.
2. *Stone extraction balloons* (Fig. 11.16); the catheter is usually a 5 or 7 Fr diameter with a 8.5 to 18 mm diameter balloon. Generally, the larger the catheter size, the larger is the balloon. Wire-guided balloons are available.

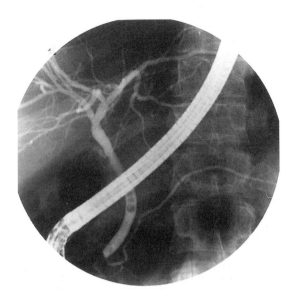

Fig. 11.14   These stones passed spontaneously following adequate sphinc-terotomy. The duct was clear at 6 weeks follow-up ERCP

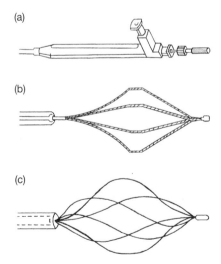

Fig. 11.15   Stone retrieval baskets: (a) handle with Luer port for con-trast medium; (b) four-wire rectangular basket; (c) six-wire helical [spiral] basket

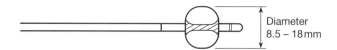

Fig. 11.16   Stone extraction balloon

Procedure

Stones can be removed using balloon-tipped catheters or baskets (either four-, six- or eight-wire baskets, according to the personal choice of the endoscopist).

Balloon catheters and baskets should always be checked before use and primed with contrast if possible. The deflated balloon is advanced into the common bile duct and positioned beyond the stone or stones using fluoroscopic guidance (Fig. 11.17a). The balloon is then inflated. By watching the screen the endoscopy assistant can inflate the balloon to a size sufficient to almost match the diameter of the duct without jamming it in position (Fig. 11.17b).

The inflated balloon is then retracted slowly, drawing the stone down the duct and through the papilla (Fig. 11.18). (It is best not to try to pull too many stones out in one go, as this may cause damage to the duct.) The procedure is repeated until the duct is clear.

In cases of impacted stones, multiple stones or extremely tortuous ductal anatomy, over-the-wire balloon catheter placement is indicated (Fig. 11.19). The wire can be advanced first and positioned above the stone. The balloon catheter can then be tracked over the guide wire into position. Once initial cannulation has been obtained and a guide wire inserted, all other accessories can be passed over the guide wire until the procedure is complete.

It is reasonable to attempt removal of stones with a balloon catheter, but if this fails, an ERCP stone-removing basket can be tried. The basket is passed into the common bile duct beyond the stone. The basket is then opened fully, taking care not to push any stones into the hepatic ducts. It is then pulled downwards to engage the stone. It may be necessary to move the basket up and down the duct to encourage the stone to engage. The basket is then closed around the stone smoothly and firmly (Fig. 11.20). The endoscopist will then extract the stone under fluoroscopic guidance.

Mechanical lithotripter

If a stone is found in the bile duct that is too large to extract using the above methods then a mechanical lithotripter can be used to fragment the stone prior to extraction. A large-channel duodenoscope is best for this procedure. A sphincterotomy is first performed. The catheter

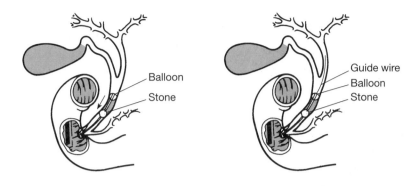

(a)

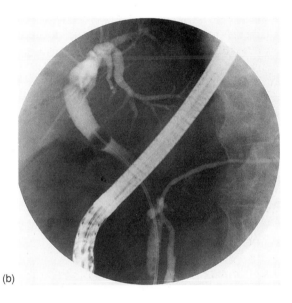

(b)

Fig. 11.17 Balloon stone extraction (reproduced with permission of Boston Scientific Corporation). (b) X-ray: inflated balloon catheter in common bile duct

containing the basket is then introduced into the bile duct and the stone is trapped in the basket. The metal sheath is then passed over the plastic catheter, and the torque handle attached. The basket is slowly closed using the mechanical torque, which crushes the stone against the metal sheath. If the stone is very hard, the basket may break instead.

If it is not possible to crush the stone then nasobiliary drainage or biliary stenting should be considered to allow adequate drainage of the biliary system.

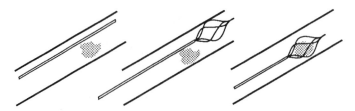

Fig. 11.18 Stone extraction using a helical basket (reproduced with permission of Boston Scientific Corporation)

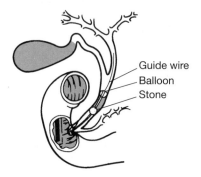

Guide wire
Balloon
Stone

Fig. 11.19 Balloon stone extraction using over-the-wire technique (reproduced with permission of Boston Scientific Corporation)

Stone and basket impaction

Impaction of a basket can normally be avoided by ensuring the sphincterotomy is large enough for the stone to pass through. However, if the stone becomes impacted at the ampulla it is important to establish biliary drainage in order to avoid a potentially fatal cholangitis. If a stone cannot be pulled out of the duct and the basket is caught, then the following may be attempted:

1. Try pushing the basket back into the duct. Once in the duct it may be possible to open the basket and try to release the stone. The sphincterotomy can then be widened and the stone removed or a biliary stent can be inserted.
2. Remove the basket handle using wire clippers and wrap the end of the basket around a pencil and turn to either crush the stone or break the basket.

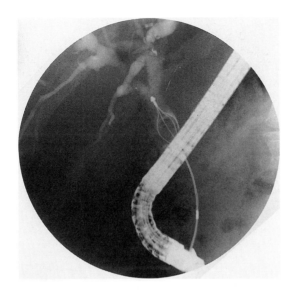

Fig. 11.20 X-ray: stone engaged in basket

Alternatively, use a Soehendra lithotripter. A flexible spiral metal sleeve is passed over the cut wires of the basket. The sleeve and the wires are then firmly reeled in on a winding mechanism. The stone is either crushed or the basket breaks.

3. Pass a guide wire alongside the basket and the stone, then pass a nasobiliary drain. This will stabilize the situation and give time to consider the options.

4. Cut the basket, remove the scope, reintubate and increase the size of the sphincterotomy.

   If all fails the patient will need to undergo urgent surgery to provide biliary drainage and to remove the basket.

11.6.4 BILIARY STENTING

Biliary stenting is performed for:

- Biliary strictures.
- Bile leaks following surgery.
- Large stones.

Biliary strictures

Biliary strictures prevent normal bile flow and produce a variety of complications (Fig. 11.21).

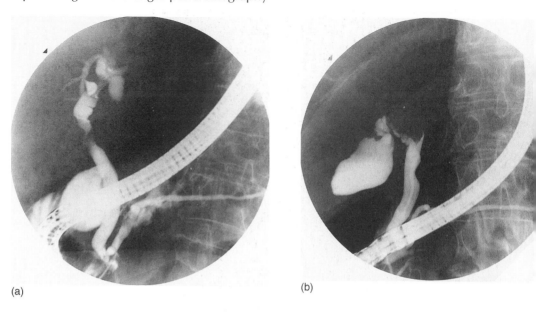

(a)   (b)

Fig. 11.21   (a) X-ray: high irregular biliary stricture. (b) X-ray: complete obstruction of biliary system just above cystic duct

The goal of treatment is twofold:

1. To relieve the obstruction by dilating the lumen.
2. To maintain an unobstructed passage.

This is achieved either by stenting or by biliary dilatation.

Biliary pancreatic stents

Stents are available in a variety of shapes, lengths and diameters (Fig. 11.22), and which one is used is often the personal choice of the endoscopist.

Lengths are usually 5, 7 or 12 cm although there is wide variety, and it is possible to obtain 15 or 18 cm stents commercially or to make your own.

Diameter varies depending on use, and the diameter of the instrument channel of the duodenoscope used.

5 Fr stents are almost exclusively for pancreatic use.

7 Fr stents may be inserted into the biliary or pancreatic duct through a diagnostic duodenoscope with a 2.8 or 3.2 mm working channel.

10 or 12 Fr stents can be inserted only with a 3.8 mm (10 Fr) or 4.2 mm (up to 12 Fr) working channel.

Expanding metal stents such as the Strecker stent require a large-channelled 3.8 or 4.2 mm duodenoscope.

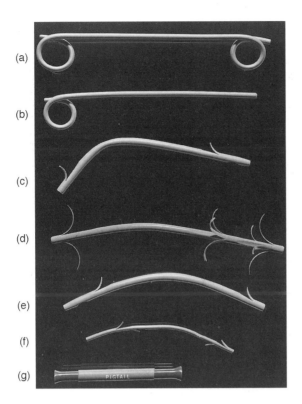

Fig. 11.22   Biliary stents: (a) double pigtail; (b) single pigtail; (c) Cotton–Huibregtse; (d) Tannenbaum; (e) Lueng–Cotton; (f) pancreatic; (g) introducer tube

Techniques of stent placement

It is usual to use a large-channel 4.2 mm duodenoscope as this allows inserts of 10 or 12 Fr stents. However, a 7 Fr stent may be inserted using a 2.8 or 3.2 mm diameter channel endoscope, although these are more prone to blockage.

A diagnostic ERCP is first performed to identify the stricture. There are two requirements for the successful stenting of biliary strictures:

1. It must be possible to pass a guide wire through and beyond the stricture.
2. There must be an indication of the stricture length.

If it is possible to pass the ERCP cannula through the stricture then the guide wire can easily be passed through and beyond the stricture into the hepatic tree. If this is not possible then an attempt must be made at passing a guide wire through the stricture from below.

Guide wires with hydrophilic coating are often best in this situation, with or without a torque-controlled tip. It is sometimes necessary to use initially a very fine guide wire and then exchange it for a larger stiffer one prior to stent insertion. The tip of the guide wire should ideally be placed in a major intrahepatic duct to prevent the wire flicking out during stent insertion.

TIPS FOR ERCP

When carrying out equipment exchanges over a guide wire, always wipe the wire dry with gauze and then apply silicone oil to lubricate it. This makes introduction of the new instrument a lot smoother!

Guide wires

Endoscopic guide wires are generally 260 to 480 cm in length; the 400 to 480 cm lengths are most often used in ERCP. The most commonly used diameter is 0.89 mm but 0.63 and 0.53 mm diameters are also available (section 11.5.5). All have soft atraumatic flexible tips and are of four basic types:

1. *Teflon coated*; this is used for routine procedures.
2. *Insulated*; this is used with a sphincterotome. The insulation allows the guide wire to remain *in situ* whilst a sphincterotomy is performed. (Teflon-coated guide wires must be removed.) An example is 'Protector' wire (W. Cook).
3. *Hydrophilic*; this is supplied in a protective sheath that requires priming with molar (1 mol/l) saline prior to use. The wet surface of the guide wire attracts the liquid, which makes it extremely slippery. It is used to negotiate tight strictures. Some have curved 'J'-shaped tips and will allow torque to be applied.

   Note: These wires quickly lose their slippery surface so need to be 'exchanged' for a stiffer wire suitable for therapeutic procedures if this is contemplated. Examples are 'Tracer' wire (W. Cook) and 'Terumo' wire (Kimal).
4. *Exchange (therapeutic) wires*; these are usually stiffer to ease stent insertion and are often insulated and torqueable. They 'kink' less easily and are ideal for exchanging with the hydrophylic type above. An example is 'Zebra' wire (Boston Scientific).

Passing a guide wire though tortuous strictures can be difficult and frustrating. The secret of success is to attempt only one bend at a time. The wire is pushed through the first bend. The endoscopist then

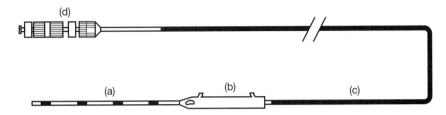

Fig. 11.23 'Oasis' single-action stent introducer system (W. Cook): (a) guiding catheter; (b) stent; (c) pusher; (d) Luer lock fitting

advances the catheter along the guide wire, and the wire is then advanced around the next bend. This process is repeated until the stricture has been successfully trasversed.

There are two different methods of stent introduction:

1. *Single-action stent introducers* (Fig. 11.23); the correct size stent is mounted on to the guiding catheter and the insertion set is threaded on to the guide wire. As the insertion set is pushed into the scope by the endoscopist, the nurse assistant pulls slightly on the guide wire to prevent looping in the duodenum, stopping when the stent reaches the endoscope. Care must be taken at this point whilst the endoscopist manoeuvres the stent into the biopsy port. The assistant continues to apply gentle backwards pressure on the guide wire, whilst the endoscopist advances the stent, again to prevent the guide wire looping in the duodenum. The guide wire should not move position in the hepatic duct. Fluoroscopic checks frequently during the placement will confirm that the guide wire has not moved. The guiding catheter enters the bile duct first and is passed well above the stricture. At this point the assistant releases the pusher, by undoing the Luer lock fitting at the injection port. The stent is then pushed into place by the endoscopist (Fig. 11.24). The assistant pulls backwards on the guiding catheter slightly to assist the smooth passage of the stent. The stent position can be checked by injecting more contrast medium down the guiding catheter, although this necessitates the removal of the guide wire.

   (**Note:** If the guide wire is removed for injecting contrast medium, then it is best to replace the wire at least part way down the guiding catheter before this is removed. This adds stiffness to the catheter and helps it to be removed.) When the stent is correctly placed, the endoscopy assistant will remove the guiding catheter whilst the endoscopist maintains the position of the pusher to keep the stent in place.

2. *Traditional method of stent introduction* (Fig. 11.25); this set is useful when placement may be difficult, especially when the guide

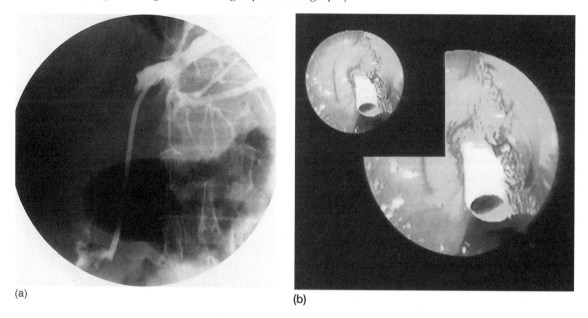

(a)   (b)

Fig. 11.24 (a) X-ray: stent *in situ*. Distal tip is in the hepatic duct, proximal end in the duodenum. Contrast can be seen draining into the duodenum. (b) Proximal end of stent placed in the duodenum. Bile draining from the stent

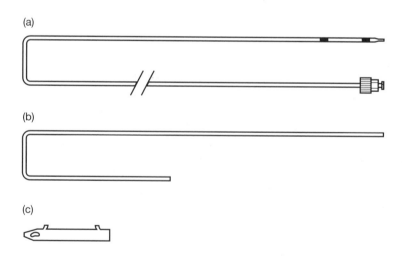

Fig. 11.25 Conventional stent introducer set: (a) guiding catheter with detachable Luer connector; (b) pusher; (c) stent

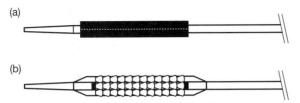

Fig. 11.26 Strecker biliary stent: (a) unexpanded stent mounted on delivery system; (b) balloon inflation secures stent position (reproduced with permission of Boston Scientific Corporation)

wire has been difficult to pass or the stricture is very tight. The placement is similar to above; the only difference is that the guiding catheter is fully introduced into the biliary system before the stent is mounted on to the guiding catheter with the pusher mounted behind. The stent is then pushed into place as above. The advantage of this system is that the guiding catheter can be manipulated more easily before the stent is placed on the catheter. (Also if the wire should dislodge from the bile duct, the guiding catheter can be used to reintroduce the guide wire.)

Occasionally it may also be necessary to dilate the duct before inserting a stent. There are many different dilators, from balloons to graduated dilators. These are passed by a guide wire in the same way a stent is introduced. Some endoscopists perform a sphincterotomy prior to insertion of a stent or biliary dilatation.

Metal expanding stents

Strecker biliary stents (Fig. 11.26) can also be used, especially where there are very tight malignant strictures. The stent is supplied preloaded on to a balloon dilatation catheter. This is then introduced over a guide wire that has been placed well above the stricture. When the stent is accurately placed the balloon is inflated to expand the stent. The balloon is then deflated. This may need to be repeated several times to expand the stent fully. The balloon and guide wire are then removed using an anticlockwise movement, leaving the stent expanded and in place. This stent has high radio-opacity and provides excellent visibility. It is indicated for difficult malignant strictures. Metal expanding stents are more expensive than other types of stents.

Hilar lesions

Hilar strictures not involving the bifurcation can be managed with a stent placed in the same fashion as above. Strictures involving the bifurcation are more difficult to manage and carry a greater risk of

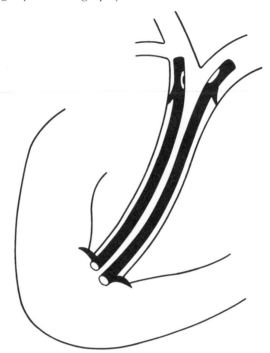

Fig. 11.27   Hilar lesions. Two stents placed side by side

complications. Often adequate palliative measures can be achieved by placement of just one stent into one of the major hepatic ducts. Alternatively, two stents can be placed side by side, one into the left hepatic duct and one into the right duct (Fig. 11.27).

Most stenting procedures are straightforward. Antibiotics are continued overnight. The patient is discharged the next day if there are no complications. They can eat a normal diet on discharge.

Stent changes and stent removal

There are two possibilities for changing and removing stents:

1. *If the stent is still well situated in the duodenum*; pass a standard catheter into the tip of the stent, and inject contrast to check the biliary tree. It may be necessary to replace it with a longer stent. Flush out the contrast from the catheter with a saline flush. Then insert a guide wire into the catheter, placing the wire high into the hepatic ducts. The catheter is then removed, leaving the guide wire in the hepatic ducts. Periodic fluoroscopic screening can check the position of the wire.

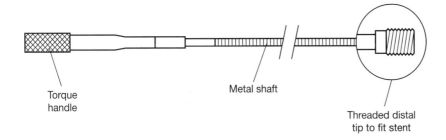

Fig. 11.28   The Soehendra stent retriever (W. Cook)

A Soehendra stent retriever (Fig. 11.28) is then passed down the guide wire and screwed into the end of the stent. This is achieved by the endoscopist assistant turning the handle clockwise. When the stent remover has engaged the stent, it is pulled back bringing the stent with it.

The endoscopy assistant pushes the guide wire inwards as the stent remover is pulled out so that it remains *in situ* within the hepatic duct. The normal stenting procedure can then be followed if the stent has to be replaced.

2. *If the stent is in a poor position*; where the above method cannot be used, it may be removed by use of a snare, Dormier basket or grasping forceps, the snare being either pulled out through the biopsy channel of the endoscope or by the endoscope being removed completely from the patient. The complete stenting process will then have to be repeated if the stent is to be replaced.

11.6.5   COMBINED PROCEDURES

This involves use of a percutaneously placed guide wire to gain access to the bile duct, when endoscopic access has failed and therapeutic treatment is required. It is most commonly used for stent placement, but can also be used to perform a sphincterotomy.

The radiologist performs a standard percutaneous drainage of the bile duct, and leaves a catheter *in situ*, with the catheter tip situated in the duodenum, and the side holes of the catheter draining the biliary ducts. This catheter can be left in for a few days to decompress the biliary system.

The radiologist then passes a 480 cm long guide wire into the drain. (For sphincterotomy use an insulated wire.) The endoscopist finds the catheter situated in the duodenum and catches the wire as it emerges from the catheter using standard biopsy or grasping forceps. It may be necessary for the radiologist to pull the catheter back slightly for the wire to be grasped.

The guide wire is drawn slowly and smoothly up through the duodenoscope (a 3.8 or 4.2 mm channel endoscope is ideal). When the wire is out of the endoscope it is pulled so that the radiologist has just a small amount left at the skin (about 15 cm).

The combined stent set is then threaded into the guide wire with the chosen stent mounted near the pusher. The endoscopist pushes the system down the endoscope until the distal end reaches the skin surface. This is grasped by the radiologist who pulls on both ends. It is important not to form loops in the duodenum throughout this procedure. Gentle traction is applied at the opposite ends by the endoscopy assistant and the radiologist respectively. The stent is then passed down the catheter with all three staff working together to achieve satisfactory placement. Great care must be taken as the radiologist pulls on the puller. Without due care and attention it is possible to pull the stent into the liver so it is important at this stage that observation of the ampulla is maintained at all times so that the stent can be placed accurately into the bile duct.

On completion the combined introducing set is pulled out by the nurse assistant. Sometimes a percutaneous drain is left in place overnight to check biliary drainage the following day.

11.6.6 NASOBILIARY DRAINAGE

Nasobiliary drains are long polyethylene tubes of 5 or 7 Fr gauge. There are several differently designed drains. All seem to be effective and the choice is decided by the personal preference of the endoscopist. They are placed in the biliary tree either over a guide wire or inserted as a catheter (the drains with a distal pigtail have to be placed over a guide wire).

When the nasobiliary catheter is situated in the bile duct the endoscopist removes the endoscope whilst pushing the catheter inwards. It is important to leave a large loop of the nasobiliary drain in the duodenum. This keeps the nasobiliary drain in place. The tube is then rerouted through the nose following the manufacturer's instruction.

The position of the drain can be checked by injecting contrast and screening the patient. It can be left in place for several weeks if necessary. It can be infused with saline to flush out biliary debris or infused with solvents to dissolve stones.

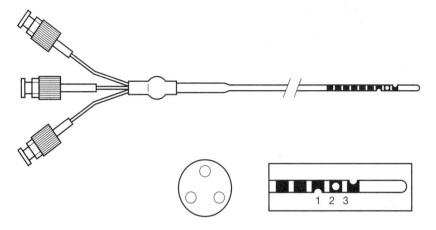

Fig. 11.29   Biliary manometry catheter: (1) proximal port, (2) middle port, (3) distal port

11.6.7   MANOMETRY

Some patients present with classic gall stone pain but on investigation no gall stones are found. This can also be caused by insufficient emptying of the gall bladder. Manometry is performed during ERCP using a manometry catheter (Fig. 11.29). This measures the pressure of the sphincter of Oddi. The pressure should not exceed 5 kPa (40 mmHg). Sphincterotomy can be performed after the measurement has been taken if it is necessary.

11.6.8   COMPLICATIONS OF ERCP

The main complications of therapeutic ERCP are:

- Perforation.
- Bleeding.
- Pancreatitis.
- Infection.

   Perforation is more likely to occur with small CBDs, sphincterotomy off-centre (beyond the '2 o'clock' position) and bile ducts situated in the diverticulum. If perforation is recognized whilst there are still stones in the duct, surgery is indicated (unless the patient is at severe risk). When there are no stones present, many patients have been treated successfully by conservative means using a biliary stent or nasobiliary drainage catheter placed on low-pressure suction.

Bleeding that does not obscure the endoscopic view will either stop naturally or can be injected with adrenaline (ephedrine) (1 in 10 000) into the raw sphincterotomy, using a standard sclerotherapy needle. Surgery may be necessary, especially if bleeding is sufficient to obscure the view within 1–2 min. This type of bleeding is unlikely to stop spontaneously.

It is impossible to eliminate the risk of pancreatitis after sphincterotomy. It can be reduced by minimizing the number of pancreatic duct injections and the amount of coagulation in the region of the pancreatic duct or orifice. Some of the worst cases of pancreatitis have resulted from the use of contaminated equipment (particularly with *Pseudomonas*).

It is unusual for cholangitis to occur if drainage is instituted either by removal of stones or by placement of a biliary stent.

Most complications are obvious within 24 hours. Late complications (up to 10 years) have been described in about 10% of patients, including stenosis of the orifice, new stone formation and recurrent attacks of cholangitis despite apparent adequate drainage.

11.6.9 POSTPROCEDURE CARE

1. Observations to be taken include temperature, pulse, respirations and blood pressure:
   1/4-hourly for 2 hours
   1/2-hourly for 2 hours
   1-hourly for 2 hours
   4-hourly until the next day
   to recognize signs of complications from:
   (a) drugs given;
   (b) bleeding;
   (c) CBD obstruction;
   (d) sepsis;
   (e) perforation.
2. Report any pain or vomiting to the doctor.
3. Recheck blood the following day before discharge.
4. The patient oral intake over night should be clear fluids only.
5. Normal diet can be resumed the following day if all observations are satisfactory.

> ### TIPS FOR THERAPEUTIC ERCP
>
> 1. The training of all endoscopy staff and full understanding of equipment used is essential.
> 2. Ensure all staff fully understand what is required (including radiography staff).
> 3. Keep everything as sterile as possible.
> 4. Plan enough time for each patient.
> 5. Work together as a team; wire exchanges take co-operation between the endoscopy assistant and the endoscopist.
> 6. Make sure the patient has adequate drainage of the bile duct at the end of the procedure.

REFERENCES

Boston Scientific Corporation (1993) *Products for Endoscopy*, Boston Scientific, Watertown, USA.

Cotton, P. and Williams, C.B. (1990) *Practical Gastrointestinal Endoscopy*, Blackwell Scientific, Oxford.

BIBLIOGRAPHY

Ravenscroft, M. and Swan, C. (1983) *Gastrointestinal Endoscopy and Related Procedures*, Chapman & Hall, London.

Society of Gastroenterology Nurses and Associates (1993) *Gastroenterology Nursing – a Core Curriculum*, Mosby, St Louis, USA.

Lower gastrointestinal endoscopy 12

Diagnostic procedures 12A

Jean Wicks

12A.1 INTRODUCTION

The lower gastrointestinal tract was first inspected by rigid instruments. Hippocrates is recorded as having inspected the rectum with a candle, whilst in 1795 Bozzini used a rigid sigmoidoscope. Rigid sigmoidoscopes and proctoscopes still play a very important role in the examination of the rectal and distal colonic mucosa.

The development of flexible fibreoptic instruments and, more recently, electronic endoscopes with a couple device chip (CDC2) camera at the tip, has resulted in superior resolution and colour quality, and has revolutionized colonoscopy. Endosonography, or transintestinal ultrasonography, can be used to give detailed imaging of intestinal wall structures and rectal carcinoma. This is considered more fully in Chapter 13.

Colonoscopy was first introduced in the 1970s and for the first time allowed accurate visualization of the colonic mucosa and lesions. Biopsies may be taken and regular follow-up of adenomatous polyps and the prevention of cancer is a real possibility. Improvements in technique have allowed the bowel to be examined with speed and safety and with reasonable comfort for the patient.

Examination of the colon is easier if the anatomy is clearly understood, the patient has had an effective bowel preparation, if well-maintained instruments are used, and if properly trained endoscopy assistants are available.

Practical Endoscopy Edited by M. Shephard and J. Mason. Published in 1997 by Chapman & Hall, London. ISBN 0 412 54000 2

12A.2   ANATOMY AND PHYSIOLOGY

The large intestine runs from the ileocaecal valve to the anus. From the ileocaecal valve it is divided into the caecum, ascending colon, transverse colon, descending colon, sigmoid colon, rectum and anus (Fig. 12A.1).

The layers of the colon comprise the mucosa, submucosa and serosa. The longitudinal muscular layers are gathered together into three broad bands called 'taeniae'; they pucker the colon into its characteristic folds.

The main function of the colon is to transport waste material from the alimentary system out of the body. Absorption of fluid from waste

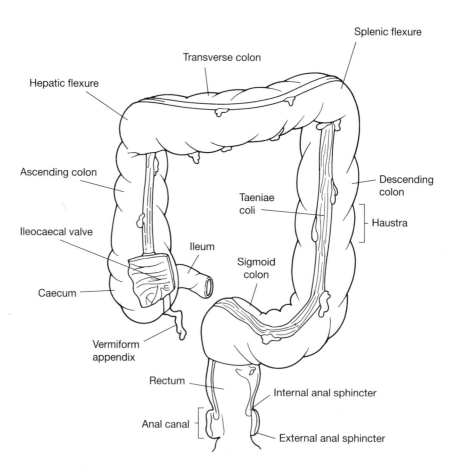

Fig. 12A.1   Anatomy of large intestine (adapted from original by David Brown, *Anatomy and Physiology,* Mosby Publications)

material conserves the body's water and makes the consistency of the faeces suitable for evacuation, and therefore able to be propelled along the colon by peristalsis. This process of passage along the colon with reabsorption of water takes place under the influence of the autonomic nervous system; when the faeces reach the rectum a desire to defaecate is prompted by a feeling of distension in the rectal area. Control of the reflex actions required to defaecate can be voluntarily halted so that the desire to pass faeces abates. Chronic constipation can occur if long-term inhibition of the process of defaecation happens.

12A.3 COLONOSCOPY

12A.3.1   INDICATIONS

The large bowel is examined to investigate bleeding from the bowel, diarrhoea, lower abdominal pain, polyps and abnormal barium studies (Table 12A.1).

The following procedures may be undertaken using a colonoscope:

- *Diagnostic*:
  – biopsy
  – brush cytology.
- *Therapeutic*:
  – diathermy for angiodysplasia
  – stricture dilatation
  – injection therapy for acute bleed and for tumour ablation
  – laser for tumour ablation
  – bipolar diathermy for tumour ablation.

12A.3.2   BOWEL PREPARATION

Colonoscopy can be an unpleasant procedure so it is important to avoid the need for re-examination if possible. Repeat examination is also expensive. Successful colonoscopy depends on good bowel preparation.

Bowel preparation prior to endoscopic examination may include:

1. *Colonic lavage*; machine cleansing the colon by a regulated flow of warm water. This is not easily tolerated by the patient and time consuming for nursing staff. Side-effects include nausea and vaso-vagal attacks.
2. *Whole-bowel washout*; includes 2–3 days with clear fluids only, and rectal washout with warm water. The disadvantage is excessive fluid retention in the colon.

Table 12A.1   Differential diagnosis

Disease	Symptoms
Angiodysplasia	Rectal bleeding
Carcinoma	Rectal bleeding Change in bowel habit Abdominal pain
Crohn's disease	Abdominal pain Diarrhoea Rectal bleeding Weight loss
Diverticular disease	Pain in left iliac fossa Abdominal distension Change in bowel habit Occasional rectal bleeding Local tenderness
Irritable bowel syndrome	Long-standing abdominal pain Altered bowel habit
Ischaemic colitis	Abdominal pain Bloody diarrhoea
Polyps	Rectal bleeding Abdominal pain Increased mucus in stools
Ulcerative colitis	Rectal bleeding Diarrhoea Abdominal pain Weight loss

Side-effects include vomiting, electrolyte imbalance and vasovagal attacks.

3. *Iso-osmotic bowel preparation*; polyethylene glycol-balanced electrolyte solution avoids water absorption and the risk of dehydration. The action is to flush out bowel contents. The whole preparation should take 4–6 hours. Advantages are that colonoscopy can be performed at short notice as there is no dietary restriction required. Disadvantages include the fluid in colon; the preparation is unpalatable and patients are often unable to drink adequate volumes of it. Contraindications are gastrointestinal obstruction/perforation, gastric retention, acute intestinal or gastric ulceration and toxic colitis or megacolon.

Side-effects include nausea, vomiting and abdominal fullness.

4. *Purgative*; Sodium picosulphate is a stimulant laxative with an osmotic bowel-cleansing action. Large amounts of clear fluid need to be drunk throughout the day that the preparation is taken. Dietary restriction is important (Fig. 12A.2). Advantages are that it is cheap and efficient. Disadvantages are that occasionally a sodium phosphate enema may be required if the patient's bowel is not considered satisfactorily prepared.

    Side-effects include dehydration and griping.

Occasionally patients will have to be admitted to hospital prior to colonoscopy for preparation of the bowel or if other coexisting medical conditions (e.g. diabetes or anticoagulant therapy) make this necessary.

    There are many important aspects to consider when administering a bowel preparation:

1. The patient's age and condition.
2. Patient compliance.
3. Preparation as an outpatient resulting in a shorter hospital stay and a reduction in nursing time.
4. Extent of the disease.
5. Tolerance of the preparation.
6. Safety of the preparation.
7. The need to avoid any risk of dehydration.
8. Purgation, its accompanied discomfort and unpredictability.
9. The embarrassment of undergoing rectal washouts and enemas. (The patient must have easy access to toilet facilities.)
10. Dietary restriction (e.g. in diabetics).

It is important to stop oral iron 1 week prior to examination because this tends to cause constipation and may prevent an adequate bowel preparation from being achieved.

12A.3.3 PROCEDURE

The patient may be an inpatient or an outpatient, depending on their condition and the method of bowel preparation.

    On arrival at the department the patient is assessed (Chapter 6) and the nurse ensures that he or she understands about the procedure. Informed written consent is obtained by the referring clinician.

    If a bowel preparation has been taken by the patient the nurse should ensure that it is considered satisfactory to proceed to colonoscopy. The patient is dressed in a hospital gown and positioned comfortably in the left lateral position on the trolley. Ideally the knees should be drawn up

PICOLAX BOWEL PREPARATION

It is important that you should carry out the following instructions as the success of your examination depends on your bowel being as clear as possible.

We ask you to co-operate by:

1. Taking no iron tablets for 1 week before your examination.
2. Be prepared for frequent bowel movements starting 2–3 hours after the first dose of the Picolax. Ideally stay at home and be near a toilet.
3. For 2 days before your examination take a light diet.

SUGGESTED LIGHT DIET

BREAKFAST   8–9 am
One–two boiled eggs and one piece of white bread
LUNCH   12–2 pm
Chicken or fish with white rice

NO VEGETABLES, POTATOES OR FRUIT

TEA   4–6 pm
As for lunch

4. **On the day before the examination:**
   Throughout the day and evening drink at least 1 pint (half a litre) of clear fluid every hour (e.g. water, fizzy or squash drinks, tea, coffee without milk, Oxo, Bovril or clear soup). **PLEASE FILL IN THE FLUID CHART ON THE NEXT PAGE.**

   8 am – Before breakfast dissolve powder contained in one of the packets into half a cup of cold water. The solution will become hot. Wait for 5 minutes to cool. Fill the cup with cold water and drink all of it.

   4 pm – Repeat the above instructions using the contents of the second packet.

   NO FOOD TO BE TAKEN AFTER THE SECOND POWDER. BOILED SWEETS MAY BE SUCKED.

5. On the day of the examination you may drink but have nothing at all to eat.

FLUID CHART

PLEASE TICK BOX (   ) DRINK ONE PINT (HALF LITRE) HOURLY

9 am		4 pm	
10 am		5 pm	
11 am		6 pm	
12 md		7 pm	
1 pm		8 pm	
2 pm		9 pm	
3 pm		10 pm	

Fig. 12A.2   Instructions for Picolax bowel preparation

Table 12A.2   Drugs for colonoscopy

Intravenous sedation	Diazemuls or midazolam titrated to patient's age and condition
Intravenous analgesia	Pethidine if necessary
Intravenous benzodiazapine reversal drug	Anexate
Intravenous hyposcine (Buscopan)	May be given as a smooth muscle relaxant

Extreme care should be taken when mixing benzodiazapines with opioids.

level with the hips. An incontinence sheet is placed under the buttocks. It is necessary to remember that it is important to preserve the patient's dignity at all times.

An intravenous cannulae should be *in situ*. Oxygen therapy at 2 litres per minute is administered either by mask or nasal catheter, and a pulse oximeter sensor placed in position and the levels documented.

Drugs for colonoscopy are listed in Table 12A.2.

Equipment for colonoscopy or flexisigmoidoscopy is as follows:

- Colonoscope or flexisigmoidoscope and accessories.
- Video processor or light-source.
- Diathermy equipment.
- Snare and hot biopsy forceps.
- Suction machine.
- Sputum trap to collect small polyps via suction channel.
- Trolley 1 – gauze swabs
     lubricating jelly
     disposable gloves
     drugs for sedation
     benzodiazapine reversal drug.
- Trolley 2 – histology specimen containers
     slides for cytology
     cytology brushes
     biopsy forceps
     request forms for histopathology
     histology record book.
- Resuscitation equipment.

When the patient is fully relaxed and after digital examination of the rectum, the colonoscope is inserted into the anus. Adequate lubrication of the endoscope by the assistant ensures smooth insertion and reduces

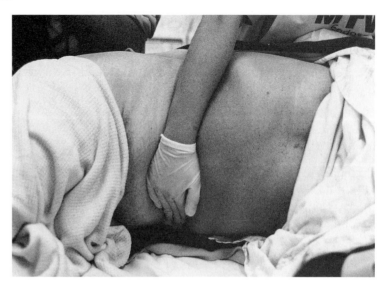

Fig. 12A.3   Straightening a sigmoid loop: pressure is applied with the flat of the hand downwards and towards the left iliac crest

patient discomfort. The assistant maintains the position of the endoscope when the endoscopist is manipulating the controls in order to prevent it from slipping back.

During the examination the colon is inflated with air to facilitate the passage of the endoscope. An excess of air can cause patient distress, and can precipitate a vasovagal attack.

Patients with a stoma will have the colonoscope inserted into the colostomy or ileostomy.

During the examination a trained nurse will monitor and reassure the patient. During the course of the examination the patient may be turned from the left lateral to a prone or supine position to help facilitate the examination.

Abnormal areas of mucosa should be biopsied or brush cytology obtained. Polypectomy may also be performed and electrosurgery applied for angiodysplasia. This is considered in more detail in section 12B and Chapter 18.

During the examination external pressure may be applied to aid the passage of the endoscope. If a sigmoid loop is formed it may be straightened by the endoscopist and held in position by an assistant applying pressure with the flat of the hand downwards and towards the left iliac crest (Fig. 12A.3). If a loop is formed in the transverse colon the colon can be 'splinted' by the assistant's hand pushing upwards just above the umbilicus (Fig. 12A.4). If the endoscopist is experiencing

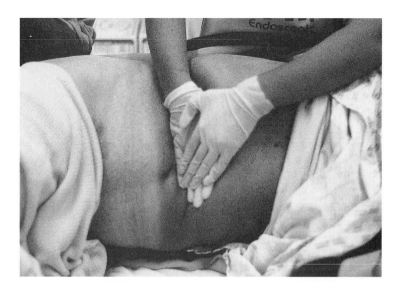

Fig. 12A.4 'Splinting' the transverse colon: pressure is applied upwards towards the rib cage, with the hand placed just above the umbilicus.

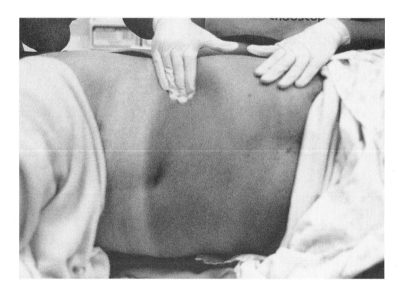

Fig. 12A.5 Negotiating the hepatic flexure: light pressure with the finger tips may help the tip of the scope around the hepatic flexure

difficulty in manoeuvring around the hepatic flexure then light pressure from the assistant's hand on this area may help (Fig. 12A.5). It should be noted that these manoeuvres can cause the patient distress, so caution is advised.

After the procedure the patient is made clean and comfortable and transferred to the recovery area.

12A.3.4 SPECIFIC NURSING CARE

Bed rest is maintained until the effects of the sedation have subsided. Vital signs are monitored and pulse oximetry and oxygen therapy may be continued if necessary until the patient is fully recovered.

The patient should be checked for abdominal distension to see whether flatus is passed. The intravenous site should be checked and the cannulae removed only when the patient is fully recovered. (This may take 2–3 hours depending on the patient's age and condition and the medication used.) If polypectomy has been performed it is important to retrieve the polyp for histological examination, and if it has not been retrieved during the examination, the patient should be placed on a bed pan, and any material passed examined and 'sieved' to retrieve the polyp.

Patients may eat and drink (not alcohol) once fully recovered and the endoscopy assistant is happy that there are no complications.

12A.3.5 COMPLICATIONS

Complications after the procedure may include reaction to sedation, perforation of colon, haemorrhage, and colic due to air in the colon. The patient should be encouraged to pass flatus.

Hypotension or respiratory arrest may also occur during the procedure as a result of a combination of benzodiazapines and opioids or the patient being given too much sedation for their age or condition.

Perforation of the colon may be caused if there is excessive use of force by an inexperienced operator or resulting from the tip of the instrument or a loop forming during the examination. Bleeding from a snare polypectomy may be copious and perforation may be caused by the diathermy snare during polypectomy.

A rarer complication is leakage of current, which may cause burns to the patient, endoscopist or nurse, so care should be taken not to touch extraneous metal such as trolley sides.

12A.3.6 DISCHARGE INFORMATION

When the patient is fully recovered he or she is allowed to get up, transferred to the second-stage recovery and given a drink and something to eat.

ENDOSCOPY DEPARTMENT

Today you have had an endoscopic examination of your bowels. You are unlikely to have any serious side-effects.

1. If you have any abdominal discomfort, this is most likely due to the air put in by the doctor during the examination and this effect will not last long.

2. If you pass small traces of blood from the back passage this could be because you had 'biopsies' taken during the examination. SHOULD THIS PERSIST OR INCREASE PLEASE CONTACT US. IF WE ARE NOT AVAILABLE YOU SHOULD CONTACT YOUR DOCTOR.

Please do not hesitate to get in touch if you are worried about these or any other problems related to the examination.

REMEMBER THE WARNING GIVEN TO YOU ON YOUR APPOINTMENT LETTER REGARDING THE SEDATIVE INJECTION.

Please go and see your general practitioner in 10 days, by which time a report regarding your examination will have been received.

Fig. 12A.6 Discharge instructions following colonoscopy or flexible sigmoidoscopy

With a relative or escort present, the results of the examination are then given to the patient. The reason for having a second person present is that the sedation can cause amnesia in some patients and they may forget important details.

A standard written discharge sheet is finally given to all patients, warning about the after-effects of the sedation and other important information (Fig. 12A.6).

12A.4 FLEXIBLE SIGMOIDOSCOPY

Flexible sigmoidoscopy is a limited endoscopic examination of the large bowel, usually to the descending colon, which is often performed in the outpatient department. The large bowel is examined to investigate bleeding from the bowel, diarrhoea, lower abdominal pain, polyps and abnormal barium studies (Table 12A.1).

The following procedures may be undertaken using a flexible sigmoidoscope:

● *Diagnostic*:
  – biopsy
  – brush cytology.

- *Therapeutic*:
  – diathermy for angiodyplasia
  – polypectomy.

12A.4.1   BOWEL PREPARATION

Oral iron should be discontinued 1 week prior to examination (section 12A.3.2).

Depending on the preparation prescribed by the clinician, bowel preparation may be as follows:

1. Bowel washout (as described in section 12A.3.2).
2. Sodium phosphate enemas – one or two depending the patient's age or condition.
   Note: If the patient is suffering from an exacerbation of inflammatory bowel disease, extreme care should be taken when preparing the bowel. It is usually considered to be safer to examine the bowel without any previous preparation.

   Disadvantages are vaso-vagal attacks, and abdominal pain.
3. Sodium picosulphate – Picolax (section 12A.3.2 and Fig. 12A.2).

12A.4.2   PROCEDURE

The patient may be an inpatient or an outpatient. On arrival at the department the nurse assesses the patient and ensures that he or she understands about the procedure and that informed consent is obtained by the referring clinician.

If bowel preparation has been taken by the patient the nurse should ensure that it is considered satisfactory to proceed to flexible sigmoidoscopy. If preparation is to be given in the department the nurse should consider the important aspects of bowel preparation discussed earlier.

The patient is given a hospital gown to wear and positioned comfortably in the left lateral position with an incontinence sheet under the buttocks. To preserve the patient's dignity, he or she should be covered with a blanket at all times. It is also important for the nurse to reassure the patient throughout the examination and inform the endoscopist of any distress the patient may suffer.

Flexible sigmoidoscopy is usually carried out without sedation. However, if sedation is used, the same procedure as for colonoscopy should be used (section 12A.3.3).

The endoscopist should perform a digital examination of the rectum prior to inserting a well-lubricated flexible sigmoidoscope. Adequate lubrication of the endoscope by the assistant ensures smooth insertion and reduces patient discomfort. The assistant maintains the position of the endoscope when the endoscopist is manipulating the controls to prevent it from slipping back. The colon is inflated with air to facilitate the passage of the endoscope.

After the examination the patient is made clean and comfortable and taken to the recovery area to rest for a while before getting up. Some patients may want to get up immediately. The abdomen should be checked for distension and whether flatus has been passed.

12A.4.3   COMPLICATIONS

Complications include the following:

- Perforation of the colon.
- Haemorrhage if polypectomy performed.
- Colic due to excessive air in the colon.

12A.4.4   DISCHARGE INFORMATION

(see section 12A.3.6).

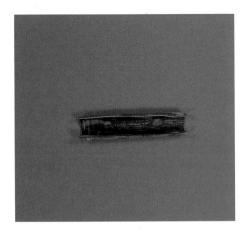

Plate 1 Inside of a suction/biopsy channel; this endoscope had regularly undergone a recognized decontamination programme

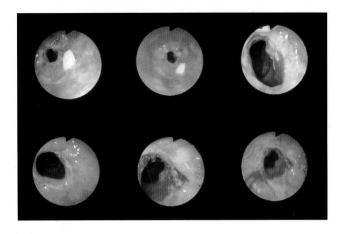

Plate 2 A benign oesophageal stricture: before and after dilatation

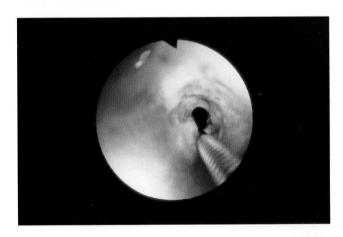

Plate 3 Guide wire passing through stricture

Plate 4 Colonic balloon dilatation

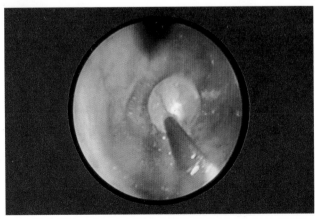

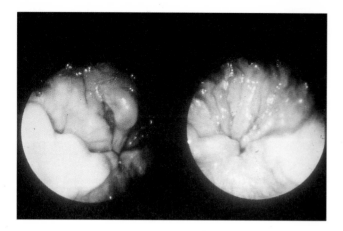

Plate 5 Endoscopic view of oesophageal varices showing blue discolouration (reproduced with permission, from Silverstein and Tytgat (1987) *Slide Atlas of Gastrointestinal Endoscopy*, Gower Medical, London)

Plate 6 Varices showing positive red signs [streaks and spots] with a haematocystic spot at distal end of lower varix indicating possible recent bleeding (reproduced with permission, from Silverstein and Tytgat (1987) *Slide Atlas of Gastrointestinal Endoscopy*, Gower Medical, London)

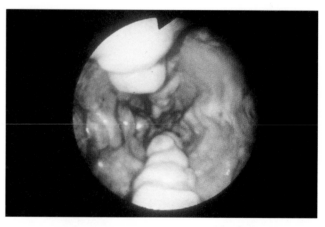

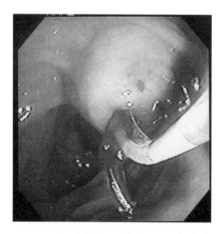

Plate 7 Cutting wire placement

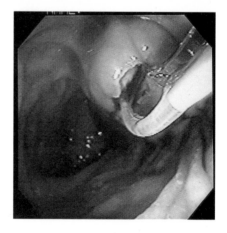

Plate 8 Spincterotomy

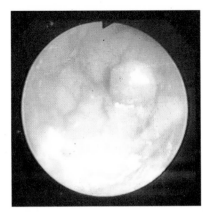

Plate 9 Polyp

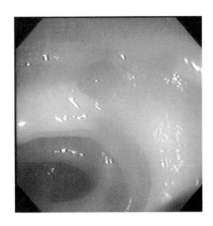

Plate 10 Polyp

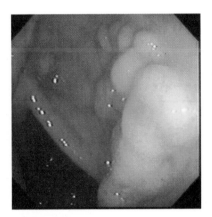

Plate 11 Polyp

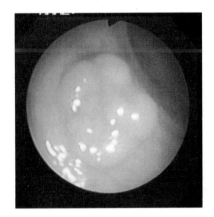

Plate 12 Polyp

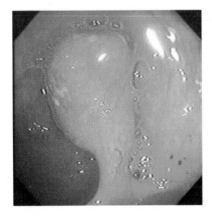

Plate 13 Pedunculated polyp

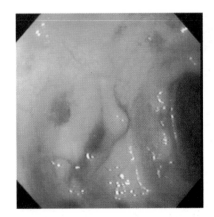

Plate 14 Raised 'islands' of mucus in a polyp

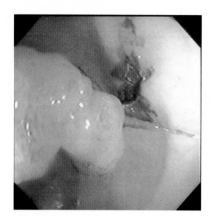

Plate 15   Adenocarcinoma

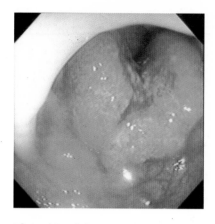

Plate 16   Adenocarcinoma

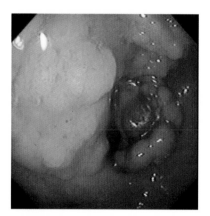

Plate 17   Tubular adenoma

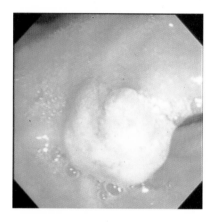

Plate 18   Large sessile polyp

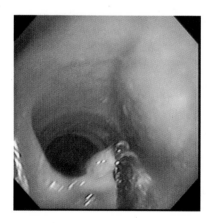

Plate 19   Hot biopsy polypectomy: polyp held by the forceps

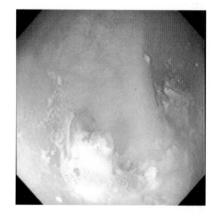

Plate 20   Hot biopsy polypectomy: coagulated base of polyp

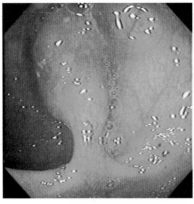 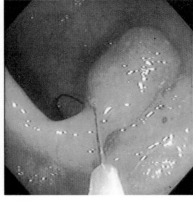 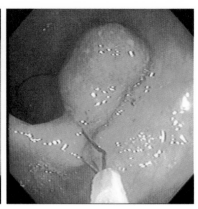

Plate 21 **Plate 22** **Plate 23**

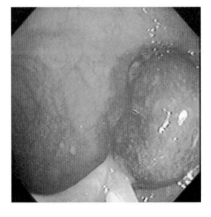

Plate 24

Plates 21, 22, 23 and 24: Snare polypectomy: snare manipulation and closure over the polyp

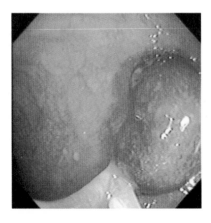 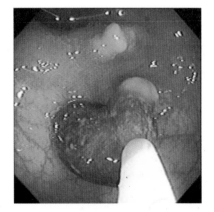

Plates 25 and 26 Snare polypectomy: pulling the polyp away from the surrounding walls

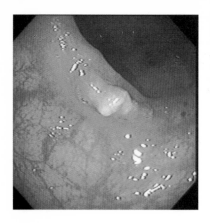

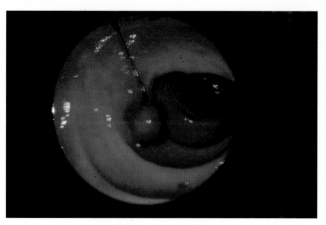

Plate 27 Snare polypectomy: site of removal

Plate 28 Ligating device placed over a polyp

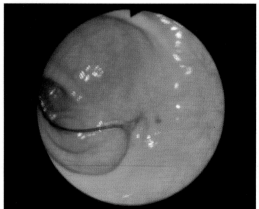

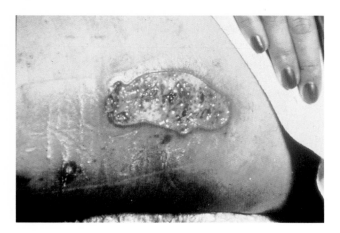

Plate 29 Polyp excised, with ligating loop preventing bleeding

Plate 30 Cutting tissue using an electrosurgical pencil

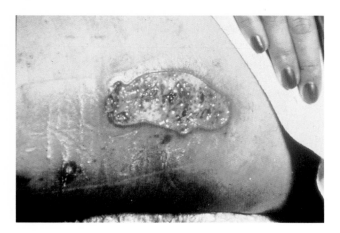

Plate 31 An accidental burn to a patient under the site of the return electrode

Therapeutic procedures: polypectomy 12B

Mark Hughes and Graeme Duthie

12B.1 INTRODUCTION

Polyps are amongst the commonest lesions to be found within the gastrointestinal tract, especially the large intestine. It is not the intention of this chapter to undertake a detailed study of the nature of polyps, which can be easily found in other texts. It is to describe how the different types of polyp are practically managed via the endoscope and, more importantly, how the care of the patient is managed. The principles and techniques described in this chapter, although mainly referring to the removal of polyps within the large intestine, also apply to the removal of polyps elsewhere within the gastrointestinal tract.

Central to this chapter is the care of the patient. Polyps and their removal, because of the common and routine nature of this procedure, can mean nothing more than that to the professional. However, all sorts of anxieties can occur to the patient, especially the fear of cancer, which for some can be very real. The nurse within the endoscopy unit fulfils a vital role in helping the patient to come to terms with these anxieties and highlights the importance of communication and information for patients who have had or are about to have a polypectomy.

12B.2 WHAT ARE POLYPS?

The term 'polyp' is used to describe a lesion that is raised above the level of the gastrointestinal mucosa. It is derived from the Latin 'polypus' which means 'many-footed like an octopus'.

Practical Endoscopy Edited by M. Shephard and J. Mason. Published in 1997 by Chapman & Hall, London. ISBN 0 412 54000 2

Polyps occur in a variety of shapes and sizes. However, there are just two basic shape types, of which the others are variations. Therefore these are described as either **sessile** or **pedunculated**. Pedunculated polyps are those that are attached to the intestinal mucosa by a 'stalk' somewhat resembling a 'lollipop'. The stalk can be short or long and can be thick or thin. Sessile polyps have no obvious stalk, instead spreading out along the mucosa, 'hugging' its surface. Plates 9 to 12 illustrate the variety of sessile polyp shapes; Plate 13 illustrates the classic pedunculated polyp.

There also exists a third polyp type, which actually is not a true polyp. This is the so-called **pseudopolyp**. This type of polyp is commonly found in inflammatory conditions of the bowel (e.g. ulcerative colitis). Here the mucosa of the intestinal tract is undermined by the inflammatory process and resulting scar tissue; this results in raised 'islands' of mucosa in the polyp, as seen in Plate 14.

This simple 'shape' distinction is valuable for the endoscopist because it provides a good guide to the method of polyp removal. But why remove the polyp at all? The single most important factor in the decision to remove polyps, especially those within the colon and rectum, is their potential to become malignant over time. The endoscopist needs to know the histology of the polyp and whether it is of the type at 'high risk' of developing into a cancer – the **adenomatous polyp**. The experienced endoscopist may well be able to differentiate by the naked eye certain types of polyp, but the only sure way of getting an identification is its removal and histology.

Polyps can either be **neoplastic** or **non-neoplastic**, that is to say either premalignant/malignant or benign. Table 12B.1 details this division and the common types of polyp found.

Table 12B.1   The nature of polyps

Neoplastic	
Adenoma	Tubular
	Tubularvillous
	Villous
Cancer	Adenocarcinoma
Non-neoplastic	
Metaplastic	Known also as hyperplasia
Hamartoma	Peutz–Jeghers polyps
	Juvenile polyps
Inflammatory	Crohn's disease
	Ulcerative colitis

Metaplastic polyps (also termed 'hyperplastic') are usually minute (2–5 mm), sessile and are the same colour as normal intestinal mucosa. They are often found in the elderly, although they can appear at all ages, and are frequently an incidental finding at endoscopy. They do not become dysplastic or cancerous as far as is known. Whether these polyps should be removed or not is up to the individual endoscopist and the unit policy.

Hamartomatous polyps are tumour-like malformations of mucosa in which the tissues of a particular part of the body are arranged haphazardly. An example of this would be the juvenile polyp.

Adenomata are the most important types of polyps. Not only do they invariably cause symptoms but they are widely believed to be the precursor of cancer, especially that of the colon and rectum.

Adenomata are classified according to their histological architecture. **Tubular** polyps are often pedunculated and range from 1 mm to 5 cm in size. The larger polyp tends to be darker in colour than the surrounding mucosa, owing to its vascularity and the haemorrhage within it, as a result of injury. **Villous** polyps are usually sessile and large, and can be described as having a 'cauliflower-like' surface. Again they are darker in colour and can occupy a large circumferential area. Large villous adenomata can completely obliterate the intestinal lumen, causing intestinal obstruction. There is a third classification of this type of polyp that exhibits the appearances of both the tubular and villous adenoma and represents an intermediate stage: the **tubularvillous** adenoma.

Adenomata are examined to see what type they fall into but also to see how well the cells resemble normal intestinal mucosa; that is, the degree of **dysplasia** is determined. Dysplasia is classed as mild, moderate or severe. Some pathologists consider severe dysplasia to be equivalent to carcinoma *in situ*.

Adenocarcinoma looks nothing like the intestinal mucosa. It can be flat, sessile, ulcerated or circumferential. Plates 15–17 show some of the appearances of adenocarcinoma. Plate 17 shows a tubular adenoma at the left and forefront of the picture. However, to its right there proved to be a cancer.

It can be seen that polyps occur in different shapes and sizes and are of different types. The decision to remove the polyp is based on a variety of reasons: its size, appearance, whether it is causing symptoms, etc. The important factor is the known risk of malignancy and it is this assessment of risk by the endoscopist that will determine polypectomy.

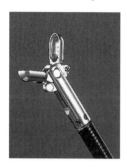

Fig. 12.B1   The tip of a pair of hot biopsy forceps

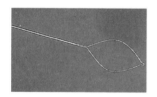

Fig. 12.B2   A snare

12B.3   EQUIPMENT USED FOR POLYPECTOMY

Polyps can be removed in one of two ways. The first is used for diminutive polyps, usually less than 5–8 mm, which in the majority of cases are sessile. In these cases, specially insulated biopsy forceps are used that are designed to carry a cautery current and deliver it to the grasping end of the forceps. Figure 12B.1 shows the working end of this forceps. Because they carry a current and therefore heat, this type of forceps is called '**hot biopsy forceps**' (Chapter 18). The removal of the polyp is therefore termed '**hot biopsy**', compared with the more common form of biopsy of gastrointestinal tissue, which is referred to as '**cold biopsy**'.

The second is the use of a wire **snare**. This technique is used in the majority of cases for pedunculated polyps, but it is also used for larger sessile polyps (Plate 18). The snare is composed of a long plastic sheath; through this sheath is a wire. At the operator end it is attached to an electrically insulated plastic handle that advances and retracts the wire in the sheath. At the working end the wire is shaped into a loop. Using the handle, the loop can be retracted into the plastic sheath so protecting the patient and the endoscope from injury and damage until it is ready for use. When the wire is advanced so as to withdraw the protective sheath, the snare is said to be open. When the wire is retracted back into the sheath, the snare is said to be closed.

Figure 12B.2 shows the commonest shape of snare used. However, more ingenious shapes are now also available to facilitate the capture of the polyp and prevent slipping. These types of snares are named according to their shape (e.g. oval, crescent, hexagonal, etc.). Figure 12B.3 shows some of these snares.

In both instances, the forceps are attached to a source of electrical current, the diathermy unit. It is essential that the forceps are electrically insulated and the patient is 'earthed' via the self-adhesive electrical plate attached to the patient's skin, usually the upper outer quadrant of the patient's buttock or thigh (Chapter 18). This must be done **before** the forceps or snare are used.

12B.4   HOT BIOPSY POLYPECTOMY

This technique is used for small (< 8 mm) generally sessile polyps. It enables the polyp to be completely removed and its base ablated in a 'biopsy' fashion. The polyp can be subsequently retrieved in the same action and sent for histology.

Plates 19 and 20 show this technique. In Plate 19 the polyp is grasped in the jaws of the forceps, the endoscopist carefully ensuring that it is

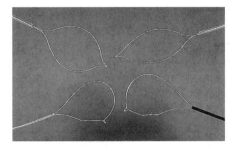

Fig. 12.B3   Different shapes of snare

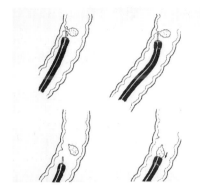

Fig. 12.B4   Snare excision   **Fig. 12.B5**   Piecemeal resection

the polyp only which is grasped and not also the surrounding intestinal mucosa. Once grasped, the polyp is lifted away from the wall of the tract and an electrical current is applied to the forceps. The polyp is now carefully observed. A whitish area begins to appear at its base. When this is some 1–2 mm wide the current is switched off and the polyp pulled off its base; it can now be retrieved through the endoscope and sent for histology. Plate 20 shows the coagulated base of the polyp. Before the endoscope is withdrawn the area is checked to ensure that there is complete coagulation and no other damage to the intestinal mucosa.

12B.5   SNARE POLYPECTOMY

This technique is used in the removal of pedunculated or larger sessile polyps. Here the loop of wire is placed over the polyp and slowly closed, capturing the polyp. An electric current is then applied to the snare. Current transfer to the polyp causes a considerable amount of heat to be generated to the narrowest part of the polyp. This, together with the 'guillotine effect' when the snare is closed, causes it to separate from the mucosa. Figure 12B.4 shows this; Plates 21–27 show the technique in more detail.

Plates 21–24 show the initial good visualization of the polyp. This preliminary visualization is important to ensure a good position is obtained to facilitate safe polypectomy. The snare is manipulated over the polyp and slowly closed around its base. When ready, the endoscopist will pull the polyp away from the surrounding walls to ensure no other tissue is trapped and no other contact with the intestinal mucosa is made by the polyp. This prevents 'leakage' of current to other areas of the intestinal mucosa and therefore injury to it. It also prevents the current travelling deeper into the layers of tract, which may cause bleeding, tissue necrosis and even perforation of the intestine. Plates 25 and 26 illustrate this technique. Before retrieval of the polyp the 'site' of removal is checked for damage and bleeding (Plate 27).

Sometimes polyps are large or have thick stalks; here there is a great risk of bleeding following polyp removal. If this is the case then the endoscopist may decide to remove the polyp piece by piece. This often referred to as 'piecemeal' polypectomy (Fig. 12B.5). Sometimes the endoscopist may remove part of the polyp and then remove the rest at a later date.

12B.6   THE ROLE OF THE ENDOSCOPY NURSE ASSISTING POLYPECTOMY

The role of the nurse assisting with polypectomy is very important. Safe and successful polypectomy, as well as relying on the skill of the endoscopist, also relies on the skill and co-ordination of the nurse assisting. The nurse must ensure that prior to polypectomy the equipment is correctly set up and is functioning: the jaws of the forceps must open and close freely without sticking; the snare must retract well into the sheath and open easily.

During the procedure the nurse must be fully attentive and listen carefully for the endoscopist's instructions with regards to opening and closing of the forceps and snare; this is especially important if video endoscopes are not used. Video endoscopy has greatly improved the co-ordination between endoscopist and assistant. With experience, the nurse can actively assist with the positioning of the forceps and snare to facilitate the polypectomy. The nurse is also responsible, once the polyp is retrieved, for depositing it into a receptacle with a preservation fluid and labelling it.

12B.7   RETRIEVAL FOLLOWING POLYPECTOMY

Polypectomy by hot biopsy usually requires no additional equipment to retrieve the polyp. The polyp is grasped firmly in the jaws of the forceps and they are withdrawn together through the endoscope.

Snare polypectomy often requires additional equipment to retrieve the polyp. When the polyp is snared, the closure of the snare may be enough to keep the polyp grasped. However, its retrieval means that the whole endoscope then has to be removed from the patient as the polyp is generally too large to be withdrawn through the endoscope without risking losing the polyp in the biopsy channel.

Often also the polyp breaks free from the snare as the snare is closed. Here the polyp can be removed either by 'sucking' it against the tip of the endoscope and then withdrawing it or by using a pair of grasping forceps. Suction risks the polyp being sucked into the channel of the endoscope where it may stick and block the channel. This can cause damage to the polyp and may produce a poor specimen for histology and ultimately polyp identification.

The polyp can be gently retrieved with grasping forceps. Figure 12B.6 illustrates a pair of three-pronged grasping forceps. The retrieval of a polyp by this method requires patience, skill and co-ordination on the part of the endoscopist and nurse assistant. The prongs are contained within a sheath, and once the polyp is found the forceps are slowly opened, releasing the prongs. Once the polyp is within the centre of the prongs they are slowly closed around the polyp, so grasping it. The endoscope is then removed whilst the forceps remain in the channel.

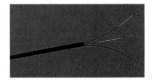

Fig. 12.B6   Three-pronged grasping forceps

Sometimes polyps are lost, however, being taken further into the tract by air and intestinal movements. If in the large intestine, the patient may need to be admitted and an enema given to facilitate evacuation of the polyp. This will involve collection of the patient's stool and the nurse sifting through the stool in search of the polyp!

12B.8   CARE OF THE PATIENT REQUIRING POLYPECTOMY

Some patients may come to the endoscopy unit with the knowledge that they have a polyp and they have come specifically for its removal. However, polyps are often an incidental finding to other investigations. Whatever the case, it is important that the nurse is sensitive to the patient's need for information and explanation. It is particularly important to clarify the patient's understanding of the word 'polyp'. This will depend on the patient's previous experiences; to some it may mean something innocent but to others it may mean something more sinister, such as: 'My mother had a polyp; it turned out to be a cancer!' Therefore it is essential that careful explanation is given about the reasons for polypectomy, what the procedure involves and what to expect afterwards (section 12B.9).

Careful pre-endoscopy assessment is important. One of the greatest risks following polypectomy is bleeding. Therefore a careful history needs to be gained to ensure assessment of this risk. Has the patient any disorders of the blood? Is there any known liver disease? Is the patient on medications that reduce the clotting time (e.g. warfarin, dipyridamole (Persantin), aspirin)? If this is the case then arrangements should be made to check the patient's clotting times **prior to** endoscopy and polypectomy.

The patient will need support and encouragement during polypectomy. It may be helpful to the patient to see the procedure if video endoscopes are used, therefore they should be offered that choice. Polypectomy can often be difficult and the examination may be long and require lots of air to ensure good visualization. The build-up of air may cause discomfort and distress to the patient. The nurse is vital at this time, providing continuous support by talking through what is happening, helping the patient to relax and therefore preventing sudden body movements and loss of polyp position. The patient needs to know that 'things are okay' especially if it is a difficult polypectomy.

If the patient is sedated then careful monitoring of oxygen saturation and pulse is important. Prolonged polypectomy and air insufflation may induce vasovagal effects on the cardiovascular system; therefore any changes to vital signs must be reported to the endoscopist. This is particularly important because of the risk of perforation during polypectomy.

Safety of the patient is paramount when using diathermy (Chapter 18). The patient must be attached to the diathermy unit via an earth plate. This is attached to the patient's skin, usually on the upper thigh or buttock. Again this process should be fully explained to the patient.

Following polypectomy the patient may wish to know exactly what has been done and what is to happen next, especially if he or she has been sedated. Time taken by the nurse to explain is important, and to answer questions, such as: Would the patient like to see the doctor?, What did they find?, When will I get the results? etc. As well as answering these questions, it is helpful to provide simple written instructions that give advice such as how to look for signs of complications and a contact number for the department in case of any queries. Figure 12B.7 is an example of such a form.

12B.9 COMPLICATIONS OF POLYPECTOMY

The main risks following polypectomy are those of bleeding and perforation. It is important that the site of resection is inspected soon

---

DISCHARGE FORM

Following your examination you have undergone **POLYPECTOMY**.

This means that a small piece of tissue, often resembling the shape of a 'lollipop', has been removed from your bowel. This will be sent away for further inspection under a microscope to find out what it is. You will be given an appointment to see your consultant before you leave so that the results can be given to you.

Following this procedure you may notice some bleeding and spotting of blood when you next go to open your bowels.

DO NOT WORRY! This is normal and should subside over the next few days. If it does not and the bleeding becomes profuse, please contact your doctor so he can check you over. If you have difficulty contacting your doctor do not hesitate to call this department at the number below. We will be happy to deal with any questions or worries.

IMPORTANT
If at any time when you leave the department you become unwell, feel 'hot and cold', feel as though your heart is racing, have severe tummy pains and feel sick, please contact your doctor immediately.

If you do have any questions or worries please call us on: . . . .

Fig. 12.B7 An example polypectomy discharge form

after polypectomy. If oozing or bleeding is occurring, then the hot biopsy forceps or snare may be placed on to the bleeding point and the electrical current used to coagulate the bleeding point. Sometimes injection into the excised base with a sclerosing agent is used.

Perforation of the bowel may not be immediately apparent. It may be only later during recovery that the patient begins to feel unwell, with raised temperature, tachycardia, abdominal pain and rigid abdomen. Therefore it is important that the patient, when discharged home, is aware of these symptoms so that he or she can seek medical attention quickly.

12B.10 POLYP LIGATION PRIOR TO POLYPECTOMY

Because of the risks of haemorrhage and perforation, especially in 'high-risk' patients, a ligation device called an 'Endo-loop' has been developed (Olympus). The principle is to apply a nylon 'tie' to the base of the polyp. The loop of nylon is similar in shape to a snare. Tightening of the loop causes strangulation of the polyp, inhibiting its blood circulation. Figure 12B.8 shows the tip of the ligating device.

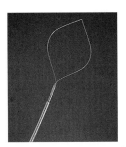

Fig. 12.B8 A polyp ligation device

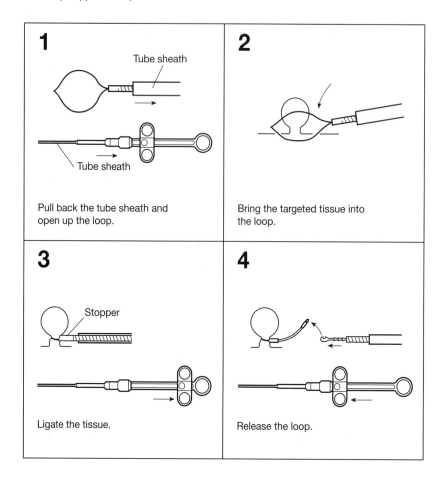

1

Tube sheath

Tube sheath

Pull back the tube sheath and open up the loop.

2

Bring the targeted tissue into the loop.

3

Stopper

Ligate the tissue.

4

Release the loop.

Fig. 12.B9   A simple ligation procedure

Plate 28 shows the loop being placed around a polyp prior to formal polypectomy. Polypectomy is then performed above the loop, leaving the polyp stump 'ligated' as in Plate 29. Figure 12B.9 shows the Endo-loop device in diagrammatic form; it is enclosed by a sheath. To all intents and purposes it resembles any other snare device and is passed through the operating channel of the endoscope in the same way. However, the sheath is not retracted by the handle of the device. To expose the Endo-loop ready for use, the shaft of the sheath is held firmly and pulled towards the handle. The loop is placed over the target polyp and the handle pulled in a direction away from the shaft towards the thumb. This causes the loop to close and tighten around the polyp. The loop is then closed against a silicone rubber stopper. Once tight, the handle of the device is pushed all the way forward towards the shaft. This releases the loop from the sheath, leaving the polyp ligated.

This device is being currently introduced and trialled by endoscopists throughout the country and their results and experiences of the use of this device are eagerly awaited.

12B.11 CONCLUSION

Polypectomy is a very common and 'routine' procedure during endoscopy. Yet the consequences for the patient can be fatal owing to the risks of bleeding and perforation. This chapter has highlighted the two basic techniques used for polypectomy. There are variations that have developed around these as endoscopists have become more skilful and innovative in tacking that 'tricky' polyp. The nurse's role in the assistance of polypectomy and the support and care of the patient cannot be overestimated. Polypectomy is very much a partnership between endoscopist and nurse assistant. Good co-ordination of skills will result in safe and effective polypectomy. Support of the patient before, during and after is essential in order to ensure that the patient is informed of what is happening and to gain trust and co-operation during a procedure that can often be a lengthy one.

BIBLIOGRAPHY

Cotton, P.B. and Williams, C.B. (1990) *Practical Gastrointestinal Endoscopy*, 3rd edn, Blackwell Scientific Publications, Oxford.

Geenen, J.E., Fleischer, D.E. and Waye, J.D. (1992) *Techniques in Therapeutic Endoscopy*, Gower Medical Publishing, London.

Hachisu, T., Yamada, H. and Hamaguchi, K. (1995) Effectiveness of a ligating device for endoscopic surgery. *Diagnostic and Therapeutic Endoscopy*, 2, 47–52.

Jones, D.J. and Irving, M.H. (eds) (1993) *ABC of Colorectal Diseases*, BMJ Publishing Group, London.

Keighley, M.R. and Williams, N.S. (1993) *Surgery of the Anus, Rectum and Colon* (2 vols.), Baillière Tindall, London.

Otto, P. and Klaus, E. (1979) *Atlas of Rectoscopy and Colonoscopy*, Springer-Verlag, New York.

Ravenscroft, M. and Swan, C. (1983) *Gastrointestinal Endoscopy and Related Procedures*, Chapman & Hall, London.

Endoscopic ultrasound 13

Sally Norton and Derek Alderson

13.1 INTRODUCTION

Endoscopic ultrasound (EUS, echoendoscopy) was first introduced in 1980 and is now an established technique in several countries, including the USA, Japan and parts of Europe. However, it has only recently started to gain acceptance in the United Kingdom. It utilizes a small, high frequency transducer (7.5 or 12 MHz) incorporated in the tip of an endoscope to visualize the gastrointestinal tract and associated organs. Although the higher frequency of the transducer means a smaller depth of penetration, the resolution is much better than conventional ultrasound as there is no intervening bowel gas or bone to impair images, allowing visualization of structures and lesions as small as 2–3 mm in diameter.

There are two commercially available designs at present. A radial-scanning echoendoscope gives a 360° image orientated perpendicular to the long axis of the instrument. A balloon at the tip of the endoscope is inflated with water to provide an interface between the transducer and the gut wall, which is essential for clear images (Fig. 13.1).

Linear-scanning echoendoscopes produce a sector image, similar to that seen in conventional ultrasound, which is orientated parallel to the long axis of the scope. Although the more limited field of scanning can make orientation difficult, it is easier to perform guided fine-needle aspiration with linear than with radial scanners.

Miniprobes are small (3 mm diameter) ultrasound probes that can be passed through the accessory channel of a conventional endoscope. They operate at a higher frequency (30 MHz) and consequently have a smaller range. They are useful in the evaluation of stenotic oesophageal tumours and can be passed into the ductal system to assess lesions of the pancreas and biliary tree.

Practical Endoscopy Edited by M. Shephard and J. Mason. Published in 1997 by Chapman & Hall, London. ISBN 0 412 54000 2

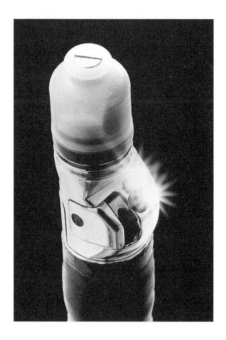

Fig. 13.1   (a) Tip of radial-scanning echoendoscope

13.2   BASIC TECHNIQUE

Endoscopic ultrasound is carried out in much the same way as standard endoscopy. It is performed as an outpatient procedure with the patient starved for 6 hours prior to upper gastrointestinal EUS or following the appropriate bowel preparation for lower gastrointestinal EUS. Anaesthetic throat spray and intravenous sedation make the larger EUS gastroduodenoscope easier to tolerate but sedation may not be necessary for anorectal procedures. Antiperistaltic drugs may also be useful in some situations. Standard endoscopy is often performed immediately prior to EUS of the oesophagus, especially if a stenotic lesion is known to be present.

If the stenosis is tight enough to prevent passage of the echoendoscope there are four options. First, EUS can be performed to the level of the obstruction, which may provide sufficient information to guide treatment, especially in the case of an obviously inoperable tumour. Secondly, dilatation can be performed immediately before the EUS examination. Although several centres follow this method with few reported complications there remains the risk of perforation. Perhaps safer is the third option – gradual dilatation over a few days preceding EUS. Finally, if the miniprobe is available it will pass through all but the tightest stricture without the need for dilatation.

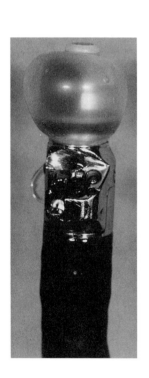

Fig. 13.1   (b) Balloon partially inflated (reproduced with permission from Olympus UK)

Special care must be taken with initial intubation of the oesophagus and in manipulation of the echoendoscope within the duodenum owing to the rigid tip of the scope that houses the transducer and can rarely cause trauma, especially in the elderly.

13.3   ENDOSCOPIC ULTRASOUND OF THE OESOPHAGUS

Endoscopic ultrasound is superior to both computed tomography (CT) and conventional ultrasound in the local staging of oesophageal tumours at the tumour (T stage) and lymph node (N stage) levels. The high resolution enables differentiation between the layers of the gut wall, which show up as alternating echo-dense and echo-poor images (Fig. 13.2). EUS can therefore be used to stage oesophageal tumours accurately based on depth of invasion (Fig. 13.3).

Local spread can be assessed using the 7.5 MHz frequency, which allows visualization of strictures within a 5 cm radius of the transducer. Hence involvement of the pericardium, aorta and bronchi can all be determined. Valuable information on the presence of lymph nodes in the paraoesophageal region or around the coeliac trunk can also be obtained with EUS. Several features have been identified that help distinguish involved from non-involved nodes, including size, shape, echogenicity and homogeneity (Fig. 13.4). Using these criteria, accuracy rates of up to 80% have been reported. Advances in the technique of EUS-guided fine-needle aspiration should make assessment of suspicious lymph nodes even more accurate.

EUS is unable to exclude haematogenous metastases, particularly in liver or lungs, although sometimes metastases can be identified in the left lobe of the liver. Distant spread can usually be diagnosed on CT or conventional ultrasound and chest radiography.

EUS also has a role in non-malignant conditions. Varices can be demonstrated and the response to sclerotherapy monitored. The evaluation of benign oesophageal tumours and motility disorders such as achalasia and scleroderma is also possible.

13.4   ENDOSCOPIC ULTRASOUND OF THE STOMACH

The principles of EUS of the stomach are essentially the same as those of scanning the oesophagus, and staging of gastric malignancies is performed in a similar way. The images obtained can be improved by filling the gastric lumen with water, which also serves to open out the mucosal folds. EUS is very useful in the diagnosis of thickened gastric folds or discrete submucosal lesions, as seen in barium studies or at endoscopy when multiple biopsies can often be negative in the presence

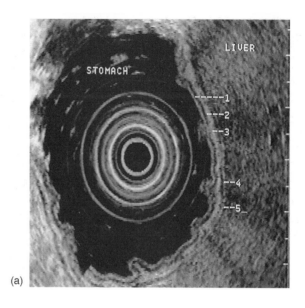

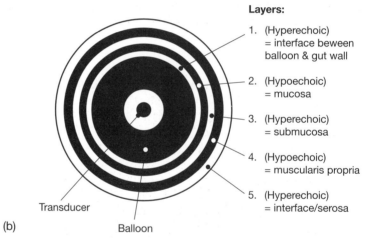

Fig. 13.2   (a) Normal gastrointestinal wall, five-layer image; (b) diagram of normal five-layer image

of an apparently normal mucosa. It may demonstrate an extraluminal structure compressing the gastric wall or reveal an intramural lesion such as a leiomyoma (Fig. 13.5). Infiltrating carcinoma and early lymphoma can also be seen. The diagnosis may be further elucidated by EUS-guided biopsy when intramural vascular structures can be avoided as a result of the real-time ultrasound characteristics.

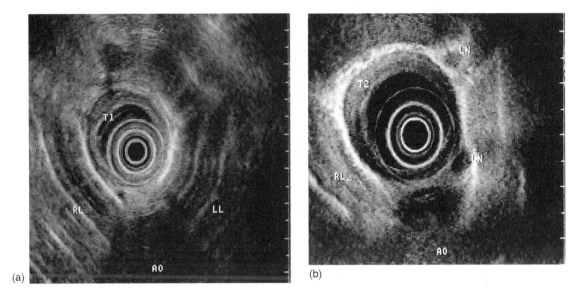

Fig. 13.3 (a) T1 oesophageal tumour; (b) T2 oesophageal tumour (T1, T2 = tumours; RL = right lung; LL = left lung; AO = aorta; LN = lymph node)

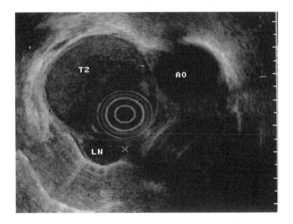

Fig. 13.4 Malignant paraoesophageal lymph node (LN) (T2 = tumour; AO = aorta)

EUS seems highly accurate in assessing depth of invasion and lymph node status in gastric lymphoma. It is much more accurate than endoscopy in assessing surface extension; however, there is some evidence that EUS tends to underestimate the extent of spread in low-grade cases when compared with resection specimens.

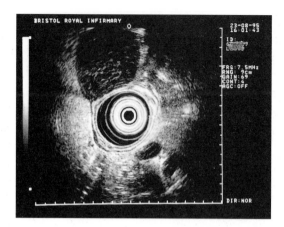

Fig. 13.5 Leiomyoma of stomach clearly seen arising from fourth hypo-echoic (muscle) layer

13.5 ENDOSCOPIC ULTRASOUND OF THE PANCREAS

Pancreatic carcinoma is rarely detected early enough to be operable. Even in those patients who undergo surgery, previously unrecognized vascular involvement can result in an 'open and close' procedure. It is important, therefore, to identify accurately those patients in whom surgery is likely to be beneficial. EUS is the most sensitive modality for the identification of small pancreatic tumours, and unlike CT and magnetic resonance imaging (MRI), can reliably detect tumours of < 2 cm. It may be particularly useful in patients with negative CT scans but raised levels of tumour markers. It is also highly accurate in the detection of portal venous invasion, showing involvement even when angiography reveals no abnormality. Pancreatic endocrine tumours are much less common than carcinomas and are often very difficult to localize when suspected on clinical and biochemical grounds. Conventional ultrasound and CT have a failure rate of 50–80% and angiography has one of 30–50%. EUS, however, has been shown to detect 85% of tumours not visible with conventional imaging including MRI and scintigraphy (Fig. 13.6).

As well as its use in the investigation of pancreatic malignancy, EUS can demonstrate benign conditions such as pancreatitis and its complications. Several features suggestive of chronic pancreatitis can be identified even when other tests have been negative or inconclusive. These may include hyperechoic foci and small cystic abnormalities scattered throughout the gland, ductal enlargement and the presence of stones and proteinaceous plugs within the ducts (Fig. 13.7). EUS does not, however, reliably differentiate focal chronic pancreatitis from carcinoma.

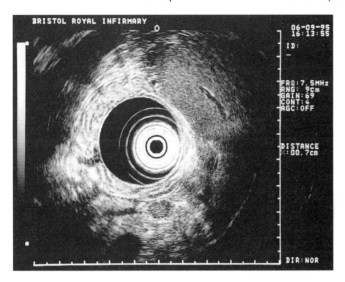

Fig. 13.6   0.7 cm neuroendocrine tumour of the pancreas (between crosses)

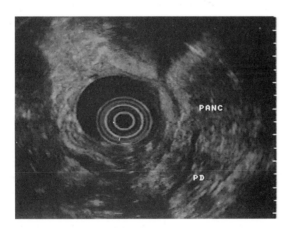

Fig. 13.7   Heterogeneous structure with echogenic foci and dilated, irregular duct in chronic pancreatitis (PANC = pancreas; PD = pancreatic duct)

13.6   ENDOSCOPIC ULTRASOUND OF THE BILIARY TREE AND AMPULLA OF VATER

EUS accurately stages tumour invasion in over 80% of proximal and distal common bile duct cancers although nodal staging is less accurate. As well as using the standard echoendoscope, the 30 MHz ultrasound

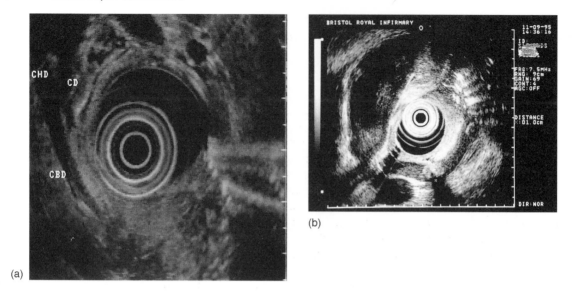

Fig. 13.8 (a) Normal biliary tree (CHD = common hepatic duct; CBD = common bile duct; CD = cystic duct). (b) Gall bladder and dilated bile duct with two duct stones (note acoustic shadowing)

miniprobe can be passed down the biopsy channel of a duodenoscope into the ductal system to produce high-resolution images of the bile duct wall and the adjacent structures.

EUS is better than conventional ultrasound at identifying stones within the common bile duct and can even identify stones missed on ERCP. Unlike ERCP, EUS is non-invasive and with no risk of pancreatitis or cholangitis. Consequently it may have a useful role in excluding ductal stones prior to laparoscopic cholecystectomy in non-jaundiced patients (Fig. 13.8).

Ampullary tumours are also easily assessable by EUS and can be reliably distinguished from pancreatic head carcinomas invading the ampulla.

13.7 ENDOSCOPIC ULTRASOUND OF THE COLON, RECTUM AND ANUS

As in the upper gastrointestinal tract, EUS can be used for accurate staging of colon, rectal and anal cancers. Intrarectal ultrasonography is carried out with short rigid endoprobes to give accurate information on spread and resectability in low-sited tumours. EUS clearly identifies when local treatment is likely to be sufficient in villous tumours. It is also useful in the investigation of suspected postoperative recurrence. Again the technique may be limited by the presence of stenosis.

EUS can demonstrate the components of the anal sphincter complex and has a valuable role in the investigation of incontinence.

13.8 CONCLUSION

EUS is clearly superior to other imaging modalities in tumour and nodal staging of most gastrointestinal cancers. By clearly demonstrating advanced tumours of the oesophagus, it prevents unnecessary operations. In future it may be important in the identification of patients in whom preoperative chemotherapy may be beneficial and in monitoring the response to such treatment. The accuracy of EUS in the assessment of oesophageal tumours makes it possible to tailor treatment in each individual with a real potential to influence mortality. It now seems appropriate that every patient with oesophageal cancer in whom surgery is a possibility should undergo EUS prior to a final decision on treatment.

In the assessment of the pancreas, EUS will occasionally provide additional information when a lesion has been clearly identified on CT imaging but is most useful when CT is equivocal or shows no lesion despite a clinical suspicion of pancreatic disease. It is invaluable in the location of endocrine tumours. EUS may be helpful in providing diagnoses when ERCP is technically impossible or contraindicated, and in establishing the nature of ductal obstruction seen on ERCP.

It also appears to have high accuracy in assessing bile duct tumours and can detect cholelithiasis not visualized at ERCP.

EUS is not difficult to perform but image interpretation requires considerable experience, as in conventional ultrasound. It is important to determine the precise role and particularly to see if patient outcome is improved as a result of more accurate assessment; for this, large studies are needed. For these reasons, EUS should be confined to centres with a sufficient throughput of gastrointestinal pathologies where EUS may be helpful.

Future advances in the field of endoscopic ultrasound will be due largely to the availability of better instruments. EUS technology is expanding rapidly with ever more sophisticated echoendoscopes being developed that combine the best features of the radial and linear echoendoscopes, with colour Doppler and improved fine-needle aspiration capability. In addition there will be further miniaturization to facilitate endoscopic access.

BIBLIOGRAPHY

Caletti, G., Odegaard, S. and Rosch, T. (1994) Endoscopic ultrasonography: a summary of the conclusions of the working party, tenth world congress of gastroenterology Los Angeles, California, October 1994. *Am J Gastro-enterol*, **89**(8), S138–43.

Muller, M.F., Meyenberger, C., Bertschinger, P., Schaer, R. and Marincek, B. (1994) Pancreatic tumours: evaluation with endoscopic US, CT and MR imaging. *Radiology*, **190**, 745–51.

Natterman, C., Goldschmidt, A.J.W. and Dancygier, H. (1993) Endosono-graphy in chronic pancreatitis – a comparison between endoscopic retro-grade pancreatography and endoscopic ultrasonography. *Endoscopy*, **25**, 565–70.

Palazzo, L., Roseau, G., Gayet, B. *et al.* (1993) Endoscopic ultrasonography in diagnosis and staging of pancreatic adenocarcinoma. *Endoscopy*, **25**, 143–50.

Palazzo, L., Roseau, G., Ruskone-Fourmestraux, A. *et al.* (1993) Endoscopic ultrasonography in the local staging of primary gastric lymphoma. *Endo-scopy*, **25**, 502–8.

Rosch, T., Lorenz, R., Braig, C. and Classen, M. (1992) Endoscopic ultra-sonography in diagnosis and staging of pancreatic and biliary tumours. *Endoscopy*, **24**(1), 304–8.

Snady, H., Bruckner, H., Siegel, J. *et al.* (1993) Endoscopic ultrasonographic criteria of vascular invasion by potentially resectable pancreatic tumours. *Endoscopy*, **25**, 182–4.

Speakman, C.T.M., Burnett, S.J.D., Kamm, M.A. and Bartram, C.I. (1991) Sphincter injury after anal dilatation demonstrated by anal endosonography. *Br J Surg*, **78**, 1429–30.

Yasuda, K., Mukai, H., Nakajima, M. and Kawai, K. (1993) Staging of pancreatic carcinoma by endoscopic ultrasonography. *Endoscopy*, **25**, 151–5.

Zimmer, T., Zeigler, K., Bader, M., Hamm, B., Riecken, E.O. and Wiedenmann, B. (1994) Localisation of neuroendocrine tumours of the upper gastro-intestinal tract. *Gut*, **35**, 471–5.

Zuccaro, G. Jr and Sivak, M.V. Jr (1992) Endoscopic ultrasonography in the diagnosis of chronic pancreatitis. *Endoscopy*, **24**(1), 347–9.

Endoscopy in children 14

Huw R. Jenkins

14.1 INTRODUCTION

Following the introduction of flexible fibreoptic endoscopy in the 1970s in adult patients, increasing experience has been developed with the use of the technique in children. In the United States of America both upper and lower gastrointestinal tract endoscopy in children became established in the late 1970s and early 1980s, although in the United Kingdom the development of the subspecialty of paediatric gastro-enterology has been somewhat slower. However, there are now several established paediatric gastroenterology centres in Britain, all of which regularly perform endoscopies on children.

Over the last 10 years there have been impressive developments in the range of instruments available and several small-diameter endoscopes have been produced by commercial companies, allowing routine and therapeutic endoscopy even in the tiny newborn infant.

14.2 FACILITIES

It is very important that endoscopy in children, particularly that performed under sedation, is undertaken only in units experienced in dealing with children. At present routine upper and lower gastro-intestinal endoscopy in infants and children is often an outpatient procedure using parenteral sedation, and for this procedure to be undertaken safely, and in a satisfactory manner, there must be a well equipped 'child-friendly' endoscopy facility and paediatric-trained nursing and medical staff on hand. It has been suggested by the British Society of Paediatric Gastroenterology and Nutrition (a group affiliated to the Royal College of Paediatrics and Child Health) that endoscopy in children should be performed only in centres that can provide the above

Practical Endoscopy Edited by M. Shephard and J. Mason. Published in 1997 by Chapman & Hall, London. ISBN 0 412 54000 2

facilities, and only by those individuals who are performing at least 75 endoscopies per year on children. There thus should be at least one paediatric gastroenterology centre per region performing endoscopies in children.

If there is not a dedicated paediatric endoscopy suite, then an adult endoscopy suite should be modified to provide either a separate paediatric session or a dedicated paediatric area with trained children's nurses, and the provision of a play specialist to help prepare the children, with a variety of toys and suitable materials available.

Although most regions in Britain are now able to provide a paediatric gastroenterology service, the numbers of children requiring endoscopy in most units will inevitably be relatively small, and it is necessary to maintain a good relationship with colleagues working with adults, and to use their expertise (in conjunction with a paediatrician) for the rarer endoscopic procedures that require the particular skills that can only be learned in sufficient numbers in adult practice.

It is vital that adequate literature is produced outlining the procedure for children and their parents, and the provision of a play specialist to prepare the children is an ideal (Boatwright and Crummette, 1991). Booklets and leaflets are produced by several paediatric gastroenterology units, which are distributed and discussed in the outpatient clinic prior to the arrangement of the endoscopy, so that the child and his or her parents are prepared for the procedure. The success of a paediatric endoscopic procedure depends to a large extent on the empathy of staff working on the unit, and helpful information for endoscopy nurses dealing with children has been recently published (Walsh, 1995).

14.3 INTRAVENOUS SEDATION VERSUS GENERAL ANAESTHETIC

Although historically the majority of endoscopies in children were performed under general anaesthetic, it is now common practice for upper gastrointestinal endoscopies and colonoscopies to be performed under sedation in all but the youngest child or baby. Perhaps part of the reason why the procedure had previously been performed under general anaesthetic is that the endoscopist has usually been an adult gastroenterologist or adult surgeon with little experience of paediatric practice. However, there remain a number of children who still require general anaesthetic and it is important that the endoscopy unit has provision to provide the facilities for anaesthetic gases and that a trained paediatric anaesthetist is available for the procedure.

Most centres in Britain (and in the United States of America) use a combination of intravenous pethidine (1 mg/kg) and midazolam (0.1 mg/kg per dose) (or diazepam, 0.2 mg/kg per dose). It is vital that a pulse oximeter is used for each child and a trained nurse is able to watch carefully and monitor vital signs during the endoscopy. With adequate sedation it is very rare that endoscopy under sedation is not possible (Fig. 14.1), although it may be difficult to titrate the doses of sedation adequately enough for small neonates, and it is often safer to undertake the procedure in this situation under general anaesthetic.

It is only the older children who may be able to tolerate endoscopy with Xylocaine spray alone with no need for sedation (Fig. 14.2).

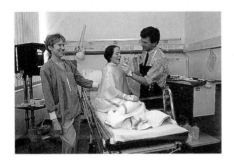

Fig. 14.1 After sedation, the relaxed patient tolerates the procedure easily

Fig. 14.2 The older patient may be able to tolerate the endoscopy following the use of a local anaesthetic spray

14.4 UPPER GASTROINTESTINAL ENDOSCOPY

14.4.1 INDICATIONS FOR UPPER GASTROINTESTINAL TRACT ENDOSCOPY

Indications for upper gastrointestinal tract endoscopy include:

- Recurrent abdominal pain and vomiting.
- Gastrointestinal tract haemorrhage.
- Dysphagia/foreign body ingestion/ingestion of caustic substances.
- Peptic ulcer disease/oesophagitis.
- ERCP.
- PEG placement.
- Biopsy of small intestine and stomach.
- Injection of varices.

The majority of upper gastrointestinal endoscopies are performed as investigative procedures to visualize the mucosa and, frequently, to obtain biopsy specimens. Increasingly endoscopy is the preferred route for obtaining small-intestinal biopsies to diagnose enteropathies such as coeliac disease or allergic enteropathy, although the use of Crosby or Watson capsules is still common in the youngest babies, as the latter technique can easily be performed under sedation whilst endoscopy in these small infants may require a general anaesthetic.

Therapeutic indications for the procedure include the injection of oesophageal and gastric varices, removal of foreign bodies, dilatation of an oesophageal stricture, ERCP and the placement of a percutaneous endoscopic gastrostomy (PEG). There is an increasing need for PEG placement in children and the procedure is usually undertaken under a general anaesthetic. The major indications are neurological problems, such as cerebral palsy, difficulties in swallowing and the need for supplemental feeds in children with particular nutritional and growth problems (e.g. cystic fibrosis) or those with the need for an unpalatable elemental diet for the management of specific bowel diseases (e.g. inflammatory bowel disease).

14.4.2 INSTRUMENTS

There are now available several slim instruments useful for paediatric practice and some of these are listed in Table 14.1. Paediatric instruments have been highly refined to provide excellent optical clarity and manoeuvrability, and the use of video fluoroscopy has improved the situation further. The oesophagus in the term infant measures 10 cm in length and 4 to 6 mm in diameter and, using the smaller paediatric endoscope, there is no problem with the passage of the instrument to the duodenum and no trauma sustained when used by an experienced

Table 14.1 Endoscopes available for childhood procedures

Make & model	Diameter (mm)	Biopsy channel (mm)	
Olympus GIF–N30 Gastroscope	5.3	2.0	
Olympus GIF–XP20 Gastroscope	7.9	2.0	Used for most routine paediatric endoscopies
Pentax EG–2400	7.9	2.2	
Olympus GIF–PQ20 Gastroscope	9.0	2.8	Suitable for most therapeutic procedures
Pentax FG–27X	9.0	2.8	
Olympus PJF–7.5 Duodenoscope	7.5	2.0	Suitable for ERCP

paediatric endoscopist. Older children are able to tolerate the procedure using the larger diameter endoscopes.

14.4.3   PREPARATION

Most endoscopies in children are performed on an outpatient or day-case basis, preferably early in the morning to minimize the need for starvation and to allow the child to recover from the sedation. Adequate preparation and explanation are the keys to success and the time given to a sensitive explanation of the technique and child-friendly explanatory leaflets are vital in this regard (Geeze, 1994; Walsh, 1995). It is helpful if the older child is able to look around the unit beforehand and that there is no rush on the day of the procedure. A children's trained nurse or play specialist will help to allay many of the child's fears and it is important for them to have time to articulate their particular worries and fears, which are usually unfounded. Most units will use a local anaesthetic cream to minimize problems with venous access, and any bloods that need to be taken (e.g. for *Helicobacter pylori* antibody) can be taken immediately prior to the administration of sedation. Written consent from parents is obtained either at a prior outpatient visit or when the family arrives at the endoscopy unit. In addition it is helpful, but not mandatory, for older children (age 10 years and above) to give their own consent in addition to written parental consent.

14.4.4   COMPLICATIONS

Upper gastrointestinal endoscopy is a safe procedure in children, although there are several, rare reported complications (Caulfield *et al.*, 1989) such as phlebitis and, even rarer, transient respiratory arrest and bronchospasm following sedation. With the provision of both trained paediatric medical and nursing staff and the use of pulse oximetry it should be possible to reduce the risk of respiratory embarrassment even further. Certainly vagal stimulation or airways compression and brady-cardia may occur in young infants and it is for this reason that a general anaesthetic is often used for very small children.

14.5   COLONOSCOPY

Since the late 1970s flexible colonoscopy has become an established procedure in the diagnosis, evaluation and treatment of large-bowel disease in paediatric patients, and the number of procedures continues to increase.

14.5.1   INDICATIONS/CONTRAINDICATIONS

Indications for colonoscopy include:

- Investigation of rectal bleeding.
- Investigation of diarrhoea.
- Detection of inflammatory bowel disease.
- Detection of polyps (including screening for familial polyposis).
- Polypectomy.

The most common indications for colonoscopy in children are occult rectal bleeding and chronic diarrhoea of unknown cause. In addition, colonoscopy may be performed for evaluation of possible inflammatory bowel disease or for screening for familial adenomatous polyposis, and in paediatric practice colonoscopy has largely superseded barium enema as the investigation of choice to investigate the large intestine. It is of particular value for possible mucosal disease, when biopsies can be taken, and in the case where polypectomy may be performed at the same time as colonoscopy, saving the child an anaesthetic and laparotomy. Furthermore, polyps causing isolated rectal bleeding may be found in the more proximal colon and experience has shown that total colonoscopy (rather than limited sigmoidoscopy) is wise and rewarding in any child with persistent or intermittent rectal bleeding (Habr-Gama *et al.*, 1970; Latt *et al.*, 1993). Though diagnostic colonoscopy is the usual reason for investigation, therapeutic colonoscopy is sometimes necessary to snare polyps, and to treat bleeding lesions of angiodysplasia with cautery. In addition it is sometimes possible to dilate strictures of the sigmoid and rectum, and also to remove foreign bodies.

Any contraindications are relative and, if it is possible that a perforated viscus is present or if there is evidence of severe colitis, the procedure may be dangerous because of the risk of perforation, bleeding or bacteraemia.

14.5.2   INSTRUMENTS

Paediatric colonoscopes are available from manufacturers (Olympus and Pentax) and video colonoscopes with a diameter of 11.5 mm and a biopsy channel of 2.8–3.5 mm provide excellent optical clarity and adequate mucosal biopsies.

14.5.3 PROCEDURE

Bowel preparation

Many paediatric colonoscopists recommend a liquid diet for 48 hours before the procedure and in the child with diarrhoea this is often the only preparation necessary (Steffen *et al.*, 1989). We have found for children without diarrhoea that a combination of dietary measures and laxatives given at home (Fig. 14.3) provides excellent bowel preparation in over 95% of patients. Other centres employ the lavage method of colon preparation in which relatively large volumes of balanced electrolyte solutions (e.g. Kleen-Prep) are ingested although, to achieve the volume necessary, the solution may have to be administered via a nasogastric tube. Alternative regimens have been recently suggested (Abubakar *et al.*, 1995) and, whichever regimen is used, it must be acceptable to the child and the nursing staff, and should require the minimum duration of admission to hospital.

Consent is usually obtained 2 days prior to the procedure, when the child and family may be seen as an outpatient to give the necessary dietary advice and laxatives for bowel preparation. At the same time, as for upper gastrointestinal endoscopy, adequate explanation and the use of leaflets can be very helpful.

Sedation and technique

The vast majority of colonoscopies in children are performed under sedation. Most paediatric centres use a combination of intravenous pethidine (1 mg/kg) and midazolam (0.1 mg/kg per dose) or Diazemuls (0.2 mg/kg per dose). It is the experience of some endoscopists that addition of an oral premedication (e.g. chlorpromazine 2 mg/kg per dose up to 60 mg) may also be useful 2 hours prior to the procedure. It is very rare that the procedure has to be abandoned because of discomfort, although general anaesthesia may be necessary in a small proportion of patients. Colonoscopy can be performed in most children without trauma to the bowel when sedation and nursing support are adequate, and the thin abdominal wall in children usually makes fluoroscopy unnecessary because transillumination may easily identify the tip of the endoscope within the colon. Children are normally placed in the left lateral decubitus position and the experienced paediatric endoscopist should be able to reach the caecum in at least 90% of examinations (Williams *et al.*, 1982; Hassal, Barclay and Ament, 1984).

BOWEL PREPARATION

On admission or arrival at the unit 2 days before colonoscopy.

1. Check patient and obtain consent.
2. Check full blood count, platelets and clotting.
3. Confirm time of colonoscopy and write up sedation for a time 2 hours precolonoscopy (see below).
4. Dietitian to see child and advise regarding low-residue diet from 48 hours till 24 hours before colonoscopy – thereafter clear fluids only.
5. Prescribe laxatives as below.
6. Arrange for admission the evening before for colonoscopy (nil by mouth from midnight). Child can go home after the procedure, when alert.

Bowel preparation:

2 days before colonoscopy: 2 pm   Sodium picosulphate elixir
Day before colonoscopy: 11 am Sodium picosulphate and Senokot elixirs
                              6 pm   Sodium picosulphate elixir
Day of colonoscopy: 7 am   Rectal washout if necessary

Encourage child to drink **large** volumes of clear fluid in addition.

Dose (each dose as above)	Sodium picosulphate (mg)	Senokot (ml)
12+ years	10 (10 ml)	60
8–12 years	10 (10 ml)	50
5–8 years	5 (5 ml)	40
2–5 years	2.5 (2.5 ml)	30
Below 2 years, rectal washout alone may be sufficient		

Sedation: Chlorpromazine 2 mg/kg oral 2 hours precolonoscopy. Insert IVI and Hepsal the line (for pethidine/midazolam) on morning of colonoscopy.

Fig. 14.3   Bowel preparation procedure for children undergoing colonoscopy

14.5.4 COMPLICATIONS

Reports of 1425 colonoscopy procedures document the effectiveness and lack of complications following the procedure in children (Habr-

Gama *et al.*, 1970; Williams *et al.*, 1982). Bleeding is reported but transfusion is rarely, if ever, required even for bleeding after poly-pectomy (Habr-Gama *et al.*, 1970). Bacteraemia is seldom a problem in children and, although rare, perforation of the colon related to polyp removal has been reported (Caulfield *et al.*, 1989; Steffen *et al.*, 1989). It is very important to minimize abdominal discomfort and distension secondary to air insufflation by suctioning during withdrawal of the instrument.

14.6 CONCLUSIONS

Over recent years paediatric endoscopy has become increasingly avail-able in several regional centres, and is now an established technique for the investigation and treatment of paediatric gastrointestinal disease. There is now little or no place for the enthusiastic 'amateur' paediatric endoscopist, and paediatric endoscopies should usually be undertaken in designated paediatric gastroenterology centres, with the provision of an adequate children's endoscopy suite (or certainly separate lists) and appropriately trained staff.

REFERENCES

Abubakar, K., Goggin, N., Gormally, S., Durnin, M. and Drumm, B. (1995) Preparing the bowel for colonoscopy. *Arch Dis Child*, 73, 459–61.

Boatwright, D.N. and Crummette, B.D. (1991) Preparing children for endo-scopy and manometry. *Gastroenterol Nursing*, 13, 142–5.

Caulfield, M., Wy Mie, R., Sivak, M.V., Michener, W. and Steffen, R. (1989) Upper gastro-intestinal tract endoscopy in the paediatric patient. *J Pediatr*, 115, 339–45.

Geeze, M.A. (1994) Pediatric out-patient upper endoscopy: perioperative case management. *Seminars in Perioperative Nursing*, 3, 27–39.

Habr-Gama, A., Alves, P.R.A., Gara-Rodrigues, J.J., Teixeria, M.C. and Bar-bieri, D. (1970) Pediatric colonoscopy. *Dis Colon Rectum*, 22, 530–5.

Hassal, E., Barclay, G.N. and Ament, M.E. (1984) Colonoscopy in childhood. *Pediatrics*, 73, 594–9.

Latt, T.T., Nichol, R., Domizio, P., Walker-Smith, J.A. and Williams, C.B. (1993) Rectal bleeding and polyps. *Arch Dis Child*, 69, 144–7.

Steffen, R.M., Wy Mie, R., Sivak, M.V., Michener, W.M. and Caulfield, M. (1989) Colonoscopy in the pediatric patient. *J Pediatr*, 115, 507–14.

Walsh, S. (1995) 'Oh no, the patient is six, not sixty': the paediatric endoscopy patient. *Gastroenterol Nursing*, 18, 57–61.

Williams, C.B., Laage, N.J., Campbell, C.A. *et al.* (1982) Total colonoscopy in children. *Arch Dis Child*, 57, 49–53.

Flexible bronchoscopy, thoracoscopy and endoluminal brachytherapy

15

Marlene Littlewood, M.F. Bone and D. Morgan

15.1 INTRODUCTION

Bronchoscopy using a flexible endoscope is within the remit of most endoscopy units as space and expense requires a sharing of disciplines. Over the last 25 years, advances in fibreoptic and more recently video endoscopy have improved the diagnosis of diseases of the respiratory tract. The procedure can be undertaken with local, instead of general, anaesthesia and is generally well tolerated by the patient. Biopsies may be taken with this technique and there have been advances in the processing of pathology specimens producing a high degree of diagnostic accuracy. Rigid bronchoscopy is still required for certain patients and is usually performed in the operating theatre under general anaesthesia, but this is now a rare procedure except in specialist units.

The use of a flexible endoscope allows for greater flexibility and mobility in attaining views of the more narrow bronchi and has been shown to be extremely useful in obtaining specimens from specific areas of the bronchial tree, and allows washings to be obtained from more peripheral areas.

These advances have meant that bronchoscopy is increasingly being carried out as an outpatient procedure, and investigation time has been speeded up. Most 400–600 bed general hospitals cater for approximately 10 procedures per week over two sessions (Collins, Dhillon and Goldstraw, 1987).

Practical Endoscopy Edited by M. Shephard and J. Mason. Published in 1997 by Chapman & Hall, London. ISBN 0 412 54000 2

15.2   ANATOMY AND RELATED PHYSIOLOGY

This section deals with the features of the respiratory system that are felt to be essential to nurses and other practitioners involved in flexible bronchoscopy and thoracoscopy.

Respiration is the process by which oxygen is transferred from the atmosphere to the tissues, and carbon dioxide (CO_2) is excreted from the tissues into the surrounding air. During this process, water vapour is also excreted from the body.

Respiration comprises essentially two processes (Fig. 15.1):

1. *External respiration*; the transfer of oxygen from inhaled air into the bloodstream, and carbon dioxide from the bloodstream to the air.
2. *Internal (tissue) respiration*; the transfer of oxygen from the bloodstream to tissue cells and carbon dioxide from the cells to bloodstream.

For these two processes to occur there must be adequate lung ventilation (breathing) and blood flow between tissues and lungs (circulation). There must also be adequate lung area available for gaseous transfer, and diseases which decrease this area (such as bronchitis and emphysema) lead to a ventilation/perfusion mismatch resulting in inadequate oxygen reaching the tissues and carbon dioxide being retained in the circulation.

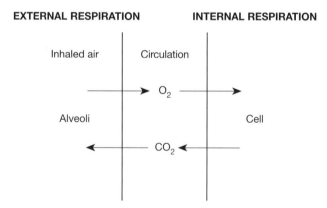

Fig. 15.1   Relationship between external and internal respiration

15.2.1   ANATOMY OF THE RESPIRATORY TRACT

The respiratory tract consists of the following structures:

nasal cavities
pharnyx
larynx
trachea
bronchi
bronchioles
alveoli (air sacs)

Nasal cavities

The nose should be considered as the entrance to the lungs, and has the very important function of moistening and warming air as it is inhaled. The anterior nares (nostrils) form the entrance to the nasal cavities (Fig. 15.2), and contain small hairs, which act to filter dust from the inhaled air. The nasal cavities are separated into left and right by the nasal septum. This may be deviated to either side either naturally or owing to trauma, and can make the passage of a bronchoscope very difficult or impossible. Each nasal cavity is lined by a mucous membrane of ciliated columnar epithelium and has a rich blood supply, which makes it liable

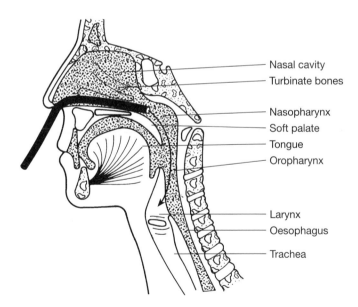

Fig. 15.2   Anatomical relationships during passage of fibreoptic bronchoscope nasally into the trachea

to haemorrhage. The surface area of this membrane is increased by three turbinate bones (upper, middle and lower), which project inwards from the lateral wall, and allow adequate moistening and warming of the inhaled air. Thickening of these bones may also impede the passage of a bronchoscope. The maxillary, frontal, ethmoid and sphenoid air sinuses all connect to the nasal cavities, and the nasolacrimal duct runs between the conjunctival sac of the eye and the nasal cavity, allowing tears to pass into the nose.

Pharynx

The pharynx may be divided into two areas:

nasopharynx
oropharynx.

The nasopharynx lies directly behind the nasal cavities and above the level of the soft palate. The left and right pharyngotympanic (Eustachian) tubes open on to its lateral walls, and the nasopharyngeal tonsils (adenoids) form its posterior wall.

The oropharynx is continuous with the nasopharynx and is that area below the level of the soft palate adjoining the buccal cavity (mouth) anteriorly. The tonsils form its lateral walls. Below, the larynx lies anteriorly with the oesophagus in a posterior and slightly inferior (lower) position.

Larynx

The larynx is situated in the midline between the pharynx above and the trachea below at the level of the fourth to sixth cervical vertebrae. The oesophagus lies posteriorly. The larynx forms part of the air passage, but its structure is modified to allow vocalization.

The larynx consists of a box-like framework of hyaline cartilages:

1. The thyroid cartilage.
2. The cricoid cartilage.
3. Two arytenoid cartilages.
4. The epiglottis.

The cricothyroid membrane lies between the cricoid and thyroid cartilages and is the preferred site for emergency tracheostomy and for local anaesthesia of the respiratory tract prior to bronchoscopy (section 15.3.4). The lobes of the thyroid gland lie lateral to the midline anteriorly over the thyroid and cricoid cartilages, and hypertrophy of this gland may complicate or contraindicate the use of this injection.

The vocal cords are fibroelastic bands of tissue extending between the thyroid cartilage anteriorly and the arytenoid cartilages posteriorly, and muscles attached to the latter cause these cartilages to rotate and alter the pitch of the voice. The nerve supply to these muscles is from the right and left recurrent laryngeal nerves. The left nerve passes downwards into the thorax and loops around the aorta before ascending to the larynx. For this reason, thoracic tumours involving this nerve cause a left vocal cord palsy, which may be seen bronchoscopically during intubation if the patient is asked to say 'E'.

The epiglottis is a flap of fibroelastic cartilage situated anteriorly between the upper opening of the larynx and the base of the tongue. Its function is to prevent food entering the larynx during the act of swallowing.

Trachea

The trachea is approximately 12 cm (5 inches) in length with a diameter of about 2.5 cm (1 inch). It lies in the midline and runs from the level of the seventh cervical to the fourth thoracic vertebra, where it divides into the right and left main bronchi at the carina. The carina is usually a sharp ridge with the right main bronchus running more vertically than the left, making it the most common site for inhaled foreign bodies to lodge.

Infiltration by a tumour of the lymph glands in this area may cause the carina to become flattened and/or distorted and is an important factor in the assessment of operability during bronchoscopy. Tumours within 2 cm of the carina are not considered suitable for surgical resection. The trachea consists of a series of C-shaped cartilaginous rings connected by fibrous tissues, with the opening of the 'C' lying posteriorly over the oesophagus. The cartilaginous rings keep the airway permanently open, and this structure continues into the bronchi.

Bronchi and bronchioles

The left and right main bronchi pass to the corresponding lung and divide into smaller bronchi in a manner similar to that of the branches of a tree (Fig. 15.3). Their structure is similar to that of the trachea except that involuntary muscle is present in their walls, and the smallest branches have no cartilaginous rings and are termed bronchioles. The involuntary muscle is responsible for the spasm found in asthma as contraction of this muscle causes narrowing of the bronchi and bronchioles, making passage of air more difficult.

Alveoli

Alveoli are irregular sac-like air pockets found at the end of each terminal bronchiole. The walls of the alveoli consist of a single layer of flattened epithelial cells surrounded by a network of capillaries.

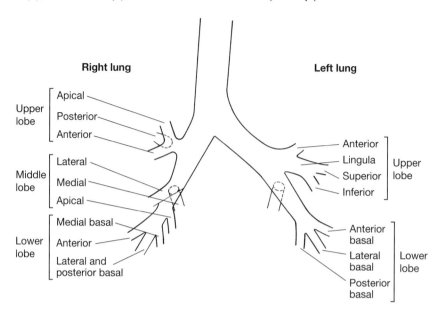

Fig. 15.3 Anterior view of bronchial tree showing lobar and segmental divisions

15.2.2   THE LUNGS AND PLEURA

The lungs are a pair of conical-shaped organs that occupy the greater part of the thoracic cavity. The area between the lungs is called the mediastinum and contains the heart, major blood vessels, oesophagus and trachea. Each lung is divided into lobes – three on the right and two on the left. The surface of the lungs is covered by a serous membrane called the pleura; another layer of pleura covers the costal surface of the thoracic cavity. These two layers are called the visceral pleura (covering the lungs) and the parietal pleura (covering the costal surface and upper surface of diaphragm). These two layers are normally in contact with each other and secrete a small amount of serous fluid, which acts as a lubricant and allows the two layers to glide smoothly over each other as the lungs expand and contract during breathing. Diseases associated with the pleura can cause the lining to become inflamed, causing pain (pleurisy), or separated by fluid (pleural effusion) or air (pneumothorax).

The structure of the lungs consists of the bronchi, bronchioles and alveoli, supported in a framework of fibrous tissue containing blood vessels and lymphatics. The 'hilum' is the term used to describe the area where the main bronchus, blood vessels and lymphatics enter each lung from the mediastinum. It contains a number of lymph glands, and in diseases such as tuberculosis and cancer these glands become enlarged and this may be seen bronchoscopically as distortion of the airway owing to external compression.

15.2.3 RESPIRATORY MOVEMENTS

There are two specific respiratory movements:

1. Inspiration (breathing in).
2. Expiration (breathing out).

The mechanism is as follows. The thoracic cavity is best regarded as an enclosed box that can alter in size. During inspiration, the ribs move upwards, increasing the size of the thoracic cavity. This has the effect of reducing the air pressure in the lungs below that of the atmosphere so that air is drawn into the lungs which expand to fill the space. During expiration, the intercostal muscles and diaphragm relax and this, together with the natural elasticity of the lungs, forces air outwards.

Emphysema destroys the elasticity of the lungs and makes expiration difficult leading to floppy airways that collapse easily. Expiration is also difficult in bronchial asthma, but this is caused by the increased air resistance caused by bronchospasm and inflammation in the small airways. In this situation, the muscles of the neck and shoulders may be used to aid respiration; these are the trapezius, sternomastoid and scalene muscles, which are often termed the accessory muscles of respiration. Continuous use of these muscles cause them to enlarge (hypertrophy) and become more prominent.

The healthy adult takes 14 to 18 breaths per minute. In children, the younger the child the higher the rate, and infants approach 40 breaths per minute.

15.2.4 CONTROL OF RESPIRATION

The respiratory centre is a collection of nerve cells situated in the medulla oblongata at the base of the brain that are responsible for the control of the respiratory muscles. This control is affected by a number of factors and is best shown diagrammatically (Fig. 15.4).

Higher centres

Although breathing is largely involuntary, it is possible for a person to control their rate of breathing consciously. Emotion and sexual excitement also affect this as a result of impulses from the cortex of the brain.

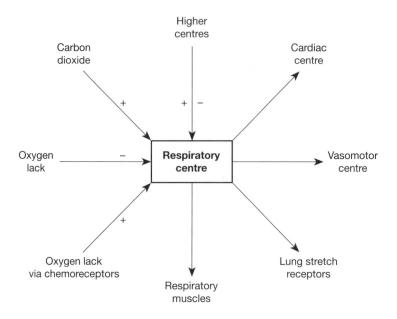

Fig. 15.4   Factors affecting the control of respiration

Carbon dioxide

An increased level of carbon dioxide in the blood causes increased respiration. Conversely, a decreased level inhibits respiration. Patients with chronic respiratory disease such as bronchitis have often had a high level of carbon dioxide in their blood for a number of years and this causes the respiratory centre to become insensitive to this stimulus. In these patients it is the lack of oxygen that stimulates respiration (see below). Oxygen should always be given with care to this group of patients as excess will remove their respiratory 'drive' and they will stop breathing.

Oxygen

A lack of oxygen in the blood has a direct effect on the respiratory centre, depressing the respiratory rate. However, this is compensated for by chemoreceptors closely associated with the carotid arteries and the aorta (carotid and aortic bodies), which respond to a lack of oxygen and stimulate the respiratory centre to increase the rate of breathing.

Lung stretch receptors

Special fibres (Hering–Bruer fibres) situated in the interstitial tissue of the lungs are stimulated when stretched during inspiration, and when the lungs are fully inflated the respiratory centre is inhibited by signals from these fibres via the vagus nerve, resulting in expiration.

Effect on other systems

The respiratory centre is situated in close proximity to the cardiac and vasomotor centres, which control heart rate and blood pressure respectively, and stimulation of the respiratory centre causes an increase in both.

15.3 BRONCHOSCOPY

15.3.1 INDICATIONS

Indications for bronchoscopy include the following:

1. *Investigation of symptoms such as persistent cough, wheeze, dyspnoea, chest pain, haemoptysis, finger clubbing, and weight loss.*
2. *Investigation of abnormal chest X-ray.*
3. *X-ray may show shadowing, collapse of lung or cavitation.*
4. *Haemoptysis*; this can be the first indication of any ill health problems and very frightening to patients. Bronchoscopy within 48 hours of bleeding often allows identification of bleeding source.
5. *Unresolved pneumonia*; when courses of antibiotics and other treatments have not been beneficial an underlying cause may be suspected.
6. *Hoarseness of voice*; probably vocal cord paralysis due to recurrent laryngeal nerve palsy.
7. *Cough/wheeze*; as coughing is a normal defence mechanism to clear the airways other features have to be present to indicate bronchoscopy (e.g. history of smoking or chronic bronchitis where the pattern of coughing has changed).
8. *Suspected lower airways disease*; expectorated specimens become contaminated passing through the upper airways, making diagnosis inconclusive, but collecting mucus trap specimens at bronchoscopy prevents contamination and helps to clear the airway.
9. *Obstruction*; inhalation of foreign bodies (e.g. peanuts) can cause airway obstruction and require removal. This can be achieved with the passage of a Dormier basket via the biopsy channel of the bronchoscope (Fig. 15.5). Haemoptysis of any severity can also cause obstruction.

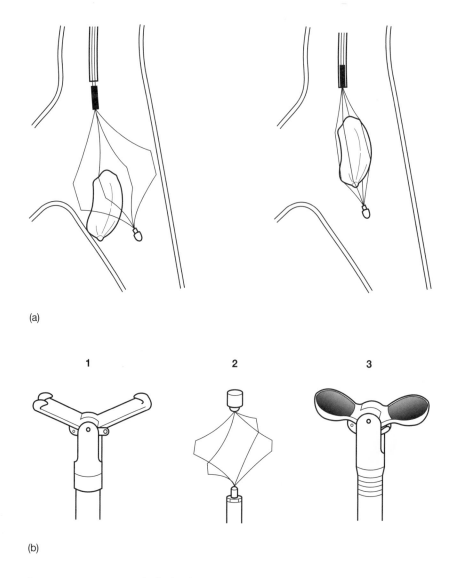

(a)

(b)

Fig. 15.5 (a) An inhaled object such as a peanut can be removed endoscopically using a Dormier basket. (b) Types of foreign body removal accessories available for bronchoscopic use: (1) rat-toothed grasper; (2) Dormier basket; (3) rubber-cupped forceps

15.3.2 DEPARTMENT LAYOUT

Most units involved with providing a bronchoscopy service vary in their layout owing to working area available and the geography of their placement within the hospital complex. Good signposting for easy accessibility is essential.

The following are required:

- A preparation room for preprocedure assessment and premedication.
- An endoscopy theatre room equipped for the procedure.
- A recovery room.

All these rooms require oxygen, suction, resuscitation equipment and a nurse-call system.

15.3.3 EQUIPMENT REQUIREMENTS

1. *Preprocedure*; A nebulizer and local topical anaesthesia.
2. *Procedure*; A variable-height trolley (a theatre table is an unnecessary expense).

    An endoscopy workstation trolley housing:
    - the light-sources
    - hanger for bronchoscope
    - small- and large-channel bronchoscopes (Fig. 15.6)
    - biopsy forceps of various shapes and sizes appropriate to scope channel size
    - cytology brushes
    - mucus traps
    - injector needle (sheathed)
    - sterile saline and syringe (20 or 50 ml) to obtain washings.

    Small trolley containing: specimen pots, tissue cassettes (for biopsy tissue), labels, suction catheters, oxygen cannulae (nasal or oral), mouthguard for difficult intubation when the nasal passage is inadequate.

    Tray for sedation: Venflons, syringes, needles, sterets, tape and a sharps box.

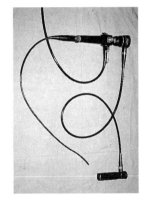

Fig. 15.6 Fibreoptic bronchoscope with camera attachment

For patient safety

An oximeter is needed to monitor oxygen levels from preprocedure to recovery stage. Oxygen therapy should be given throughout the procedure and a Venflon sited to allow venous access at all times.

For staff safety

A gown, face visor or glasses and mask and a pair of gloves are to be worn when assisting at bronchoscopy to protect from spray from

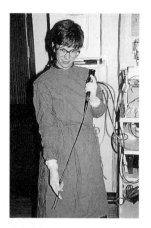

Fig. 15.7 Protective clothing worn by medical and nursing staff during bronchoscopy

coughing and whilst specimen taking (Fig. 15.7) (Woodcock and Campbell, 1989).

If powdered gloves are used by the bronchoscopist the powder must be washed away as it can contaminate specimens with the starch granules contained within the powder.

Staff requirements

Staffing requires at least two endoscopy-trained nurses: one to assist the bronchoscopist and one to monitor and assess the patient throughout the procedure. A third trained nurse is required for recovery of the patient in the recovery room when oxygen, suction and an oximeter should be available.

15.3.4 PREPARATION

Patient preparation

Many patients are understandably anxious about having a bronchoscopy, and much of this anxiety can be alleviated by giving the patient adequate information about the procedure.

Inpatients can be visited on the ward by a unit nurse who can explain the procedure and answer any questions. The patient's understanding of the procedure is thereby improved and this helps allay anxiety, which in turn aids recovery (Bysshe, 1988).

Outpatients often have to consent to the procedure without, in most cases, having the advantage of talking to unit staff. If the patient is seen by the doctor in the outpatient department then the procedure can be explained and adequate information given to allow consent to be obtained. However, if abnormal findings on a routine chest X-ray or a sudden onset of haemoptysis occur a patient may be referred direct to the bronchoscopy list with little knowledge of the procedure.

A letter of appointment explaining the date, time, place and instructions for preparation can be combined with a booklet or leaflet that explains clearly but simply the procedure to be undertaken with a contact telephone number for any queries. There are company-produced booklets provided free for this purpose. A collaboration of the unit team can produce a more personalized booklet or leaflet. Such literature enables patients to read all the instructions in the privacy of their own home with time to think of questions they can ask on their arrival for their appointment.

On arrival at the unit both patient and their escorting relative or friend should be greeted in a warm friendly way to help allay anxiety. Any procedure that overruns its scheduled time will cause a delay to others following them and the person greeting the arrivals should make them aware of any time delay, because the already nervous person will become more anxious whilst waiting.

Consent

Prior to obtaining consent, patients should be given sufficient information about the procedure, including potential complications and risks, to allow them to make an informed decision (Chapter 5). Although it is the responsibility of the person carrying out the investigation to do this, the endoscopy assistant has a responsibility to ensure this is done.

Nursing documentation

Recording is important and should include assessment, planning and implementation of care, evaluation of care and discharge requirements.

Nursing assessment during preparation should include previous medical history, relevant treatment or medication, blood pressure and any implants which may affect care.

The removal of glasses and dentures should be noted and patients informed of their safe keeping.

Some units still require patients to wear special 'hospital' gowns, but this is generally unnecessary unless X-ray screening is required. Most units only require the removal of heavy outer garments.

Patients with reversible airways disease controlled by bronchodilator therapy may require to take this prior to the procedure.

Preprocedure preparation

There are several ways to prepare a patient prior to bronchoscopy.

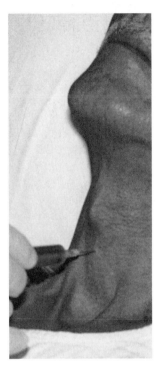

Fig. 15.8 The cricothyroid injection

1. *Nebulization of topical anaesthesia*; 10 ml of 4% lignocaine, to help reduce the cough reflex. Instillation of local anaesthetic gel into the nasal passages using a cotton bud is very effective.
2. *Cricothyroid injection*; lignocaine 4%/4 ml is injected through the cricothyroid membrane (Fig. 15.8), which causes transient vigorous coughing but provides good analgesia. This can be a little frightening initially for the patient.
3. *Premedication with drugs*; atropine and opiates are used by some centres.
4. *Topical spray*; the mouth and pharynx are sprayed with local topical anaesthesia spray, which takes time to reach optimal effect.
5. *Topical application during procedure*; aliquots of 1–2 ml of lignocaine 2% solution through the biopsy channel of the scope allow effective analgesia with the advancing scope to the larynx and trachea. Lignocaine 4% is used for the vocal chords in 2 ml amounts.

Toxic reactions to lignocaine are rare but early signs are tremors, dizziness, talkativeness and sedation.

Sedation

Intravenous sedation of midazolam 2.5–5 mg is an average dose, depending on the age and size of patient. Diazepam or Diazemuls 5 mg may be a choice in some centres.

As sedation can depress respirations, patients at risk with respiratory impairment may not be sedated, although venous access should be maintained in case of emergency.

If respiratory depression becomes a problem then flumazenil can be given as a reversal agent to midazolam.

15.3.5   PROCEDURE

The patient is put either in a semirecumbent position on the trolley with the bronchoscopist positioned behind their head or in a sitting-up position with the bronchoscopist at the side, facing the patient, enabling easier rapport. Some bronchoscopies are performed with the patient sitting in a chair (a dental-style chair is useful) and the doctor facing them.

The nurse assistant will attach the oximeter to obtain base readings and attach a nasal oxygen cannula in the opposite side to the scope insertion.

Once local analgesia is applied to the nasal passages the scope is passed via the nose (or mouth, if necessary) into the oropharynx and a view of the epiglottis and vocal cords is obtained. The patient may be asked to say 'E' to see the movement of the cords, followed by local anaesthesia of the cords. Once through the cords, visualization of the trachea and lobes of the lung can take place, allowing a specimen to be obtained, if necessary.

If a lesion is seen and accessible then tissue biopsies can be taken using various forceps (Fig. 15.9). Cytology brushings can be an alternative if access is limited to forceps. Cytology brushings cover a wider area and obtain good cell samples. Mucus traps, used either one at a time or in pairs, allow washing of airways and alveoli (Fig. 15.10).

TIP

If 1:1000 adrenaline (ephedrine) in 5 ml of molar (1 mol/l) saline is introduced via the bronchoscope on to vascular tumour tissue prior to biopsy then this reduces haemorrhage from biopsy and allows a clear view throughout the procedure.

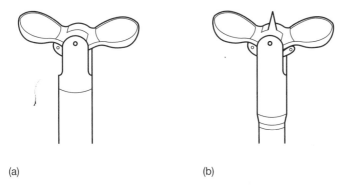

(a)   (b)

Fig. 15.9 Biopsy forceps used in bronchoscopy: (a) standard; (b) ellipsoid with spike

The nurse assistant monitors the patient and gives reassurance to allay anxiety, records all observations and maintains a safe airway. The second nurse assists with specimen taking and labelling, and disposal and cleaning of used equipment.

Care of specimens

All specimens should be handled with care to avoid contamination both of contents and of handlers. All should be labelled correctly and a record made in either a special record book or the day-procedure ledger. Biopsy specimens need to be handled very carefully when removing them from the forceps to a holder of choice (e.g. a tissue cassette). Using a needle can be dangerous as the specimens are small and can fragment. A small plastic pipette can be used for this.

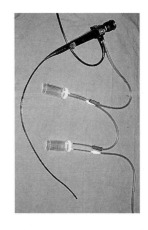

Fig. 15.10 The use of two mucus traps in series helps prevent specimen loss

Cytology specimens require the brush head to be swept along the microscope slide and placed in a container (Fig. 15.11). Trap specimens are useful because the trap, attached between the scope and the suction by tubing, allows aspiration washings to collect the material dislodged by brushing. These traps need to be sealed before sending to the laboratory.

Specimens with a high risk of infection transmission (e.g. TB, HIV) should be properly labelled with a clear warning.

Recovery

Patients may need oximetry and oxygen therapy extended into the recovery phase with observation and monitoring by a trained recovery nurse.

If bleeding occurred following biopsy then the patient may need to lie on the affected side to reduce the risk of blood entering the unaffected

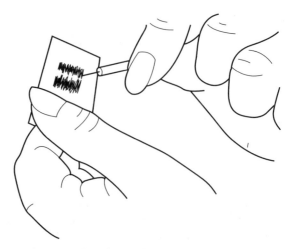

Fig. 15.11   Transferring a brush cytology specimen to a slide

side and to aid good respiration. Once recovered the patient is able to sit in a chair and be spoken to by the bronchoscopist. A relative or friend needs to be present as the sedation gives an amnesic effect. Perhaps speaking to the patient at a later date in clinic may be preferred but just a simple chat at the end of the procedure for reassurance from the doctor will allay some anxiety.

Most people worry about the results of the test so a date for the next appointment when specimen results will be known is important. After-care instructions should be given also, and any other investigation appointments made.

15.3.6 COMPLICATIONS

Haemorrhage

This can be arrested by application of adrenaline 1:10 000 directly through the biopsy channel of the scope or by direct injection via the biopsy channel with the passage of the injector needle (see also the 'Tip' in section 15.3.5).

A balloon catheter can also be passed through the scope channel and, on inflation, pressure is applied to the bleeding area.

A heater probe can be applied in the same way and diathermy current applied to cauterize the bleeding area. This is similar to the bipolar diathermy probe used to achieve haemostasis in the gastrointestinal tract.

Respiratory depression

This may be caused by oversedation and the following reversal agents should be readily available:

- Flumazenil for midazolam and other benzodiazepines.
- Naloxone for opioids.

Oxygen therapy and oximetry are mandatory, and resuscitation equipment should be readily available.

Infection

It is possible to transmit infection from patient to patient via an endoscope. Therefore strict codes of cleaning and disinfection need to be adhered to in line with national and local policy.

15.3.7 TRANSBRONCHIAL BIOPSY (TBB)

Diffuse lung disease can be investigated with radiologically supported bronchoscopy.

A bronchoscopy with screening allows biopsy specimens from the periphery of the lungs not visible with the scope alone. Screening allows vision to guide the forceps to obtain specimens. Many units now carry out this procedure without radiological screening, but in all cases a chest X-ray is required afterwards to check for pneumothorax. Transbronchial biopsy should **never** be taken from both left and right lungs on the same occasion because of the danger of producing a bilateral pneumothorax.

Interstitial lung disease, pulmonary metastases, lymphangitis carcinomatosa and lymphomatous infiltration of the lung are conditions where TBB is helpful to aid diagnosis.

Complications of TBB

Complications include haemorrhage and possible pneumothorax. X-ray of the chest is routinely performed after TBB to check for pneumothorax as outlined above.

15.3.8 THERAPEUTIC BRONCHOSCOPY IN VENTILATED PATIENTS

Bronchoscopy clearance of retained scretions in critically ill patients is very useful as cough reflexes are depressed and airway clearance is difficult.

15.4 THORACOSCOPY

Thoracoscopy is a procedure that enables examination of the pleural space and the obtaining of pleural biopsies or drainage of pleural effusion with direct vision.

Usually it is performed under general anaesthesia by a chest surgeon using a rigid scope. It can also be performed using local anaesthesia and intravenous sedation.

Chest physicians familiar with bronchoscopy have adapted the bronchoscope for use in thoracoscopy. Some centres have a semiflexible thorascope for this procedure (Fig. 15.12). This has a rigid proximal insertion tube with a flexible, controllable distal tip.

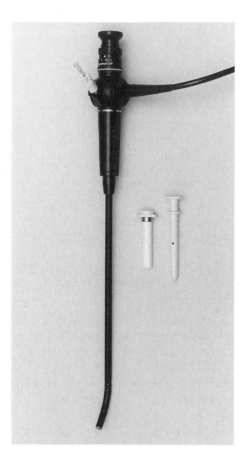

Fig. 15.12 Flexible thoracoscope (Olympus) showing rigid proximal shaft and flexible distal tip. The irrigation device is *in situ*, inserted through the biopsy channel allowing the lens to be cleaned. The trocar and cannula are used for insertion

This procedure can be performed within the endoscopy suite using aseptic techniques and the same staff requirements as for bronchoscopy.

15.4.1 EQUIPMENT REQUIRED

Equipment needed includes a trolley containing:

- A chest drainage set containing a trocar and cannulae of adequate size to enable free passage of the scope, and a chest drain catheter of choice.
- Chest catheter, sterile suction tubing, sterile gauze, swabbing solution of choice, syringes and needles, xylocaine 2%, sutures.
- A large-channel bronchoscope or thoracoscope.
- Sterile biopsy forceps.
- A light-source or video processor.
- Suction and oxygen supply.
- Sterile gowns and gloves for the endoscopist and nurse assistant.

For patient safety

A cardiac monitor is needed to observe any arrhythmias as insertion into the chest cavity can give vagal stimulation and cause a collapsed state. An oximeter should also be available to monitor pulse and oxygen levels as sedation can depress respirations and impair oxygen levels.

15.4.2 PROCEDURE

The patient is placed in a lateral position with the pleural space for examination uppermost. A pillow in front of the chest with the patient's arms around it in a 'hugging' position is quite comfortable. IV access is obtained and sedation given, usually 2–5 mg of Hypnovel and 50 mg of pethidine. If preferred the pethidine can be given intramuscularly 1 hour before the procedure as a premedication, negating its use as sedation.

The cardiac monitor and oximeter are attached to the patient to record vital signs and maintain continual visual assessment. Once the patient is positioned for maximum safety and comfort then the cleansing and draping of the skin can begin to required aseptic techniques.

Local anaesthesia (xylocaine 2%) is injected into the incision site and an E11 bladed knife is used to puncture the incision site to allow insertion of the trocar and cannula. The trocar is removed and the bronchoscope or thoracoscope inserted through the cannula into the pleural space.

Biopsies or pleural fluid can be obtained by direct vision and sent for cytological, histological or bacteriological inspection. If using a video or fibreoptic-adapted scope, hard-copy photographs or video recordings can be taken of the pleural space allowing further review between specialists or audit sessions.

Once the examination is completed the scope and trocar are removed and an intercostal drain inserted through the same incision, which is sutured in place before attachment to an underwater seal. This remains in place for approximately 48–72 hours.

Patients with a malignant pleural effusion may require a chemical pleurodesis – the insertion of iodinized talc with an insufflator. This is an inexpensive way to obliterate the pleural space and give symptomatic relief.

15.4.3   COMPLICATIONS

Complications of thoracoscopy include:

- Pneumothorax.
- A chemical pleurodesis (can be useful in some cases).
- Pleural oedema (a rare complication).
- Respiratory depression due to sedation.

15.5   ENDOLUMINAL BRACHYTHERAPY

Direct application of radioactive materials to tumours, or their close vicinity, is one of the oldest forms of radiotherapy, but such treatment in the past inevitably exposed medical and other staff to the ionizing radiation emitted by these materials. Modern technology is able to overcome this problem by the use of sources that are mechanically introduced to the desired site by microprocessor-controlled machines operated from a safe distance, usually from outside a protected room. Various tumour sites are treated in this way, each requiring a specific type of applicator to be applied or introduced prior to the treatment. Treatment is planned by taking radiographs with the applicator *in situ*. The relationship of the tumour to the applicator can then be accurately determined, and the dose and area to be treated programmed into the microprocessor.

The patient is then taken to the treatment room and connected to the processor. This process is known as 'afterloading'.

Many of the symptoms of incurable lung cancer are attributable to endobronchial disease. Such symptoms include haemoptysis and cough and, with the tumour significantly occluding major airways, breathlessness. If the endobronchial disease can be reduced or ablated, then symptomatic improvement can be achieved. Endoscopic debulking of tumours has often been done, and is not new. The problem has usually been that regrowth is rapid and the benefit of debulking is usually only transient. Eradication of endobronchial disease by lasers is a more modern approach; the problem of fairly rapid regrowth applies here as well, however.

The development of afterloading radiotherapy equipment has opened up a new and interesting approach to endobronchial tumour ablation.

The technique of endoluminal brachytherapy used in the author's unit, and at many others, is as follows. The endobronchial disease is visualized by a fibreoptic bronchoscope, and a special catheter is passed through the suction channel of this.

Note: Because of the diameter of the blind-ended catheter used in this treatment, a 2.3 mm or larger channelled bronchoscope must be used.

The distal end of the catheter is sealed, and the aim is to push the tip of the catheter well beyond the tumour until it enters a minor bronchiole that will not allow it to pass any further (the external diameter of this catheter is approximately 2 mm (6 Fr)). The bronchoscope is then withdrawn over the catheter, which should not be displaced while this is done. Then, through the open, proximal end of the catheter a special marker wire is passed. This wire has expanded portions at 1 cm intervals from the distal end backwards for 26 cm. A plain X-ray is taken with this marker wire in place (Fig. 15.13). The bronchoscopist then identifies on the X-ray where the tumour is in relation to the points

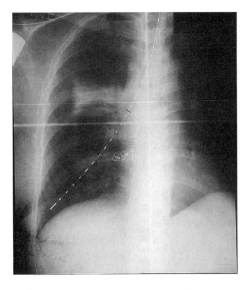

Fig. 15.13 Chest X-ray of patient with wire marker passing through site of tumour (in previously irradiated lung)

of the marker wire, and the marker wire is withdrawn, leaving the catheter where it was. The exact length of the catheter being known (either 100 or 150 cm), the distance of the tumour from the proximal, open end of the catheter is determined by the chosen marks, and it is a simple procedure to program the microprocessor-controlled afterloading device to propel the iridium pellet to the point at which the tumour mass is deemed to begin endobronchially and then at steps of 0.5 cm at a time to the far end. In general, the start and end positions will be chosen a centimetre or two either side of where the tumour is identified as having been, to allow a certain margin of error. In our unit we usually treat patients with a single such treatment delivering a fairly high dose; other centres prefer to repeat the procedure on several occasions, usually a week apart, delivering a smaller dose on each occasion. By convention, most centres using this treatment will specify dose at 1 cm from the central axis of the iridium pellet.

Iridium-192 has a half-life of 74 days, so the pellets need to be changed fairly frequently, usually about every 3 months. Even when reaching the end of its period of use, when the dose rate of emitted radiation is at its lowest, such treatments will rarely take more than half an hour to deliver. Patients are able to tolerate the fine catheter passing through the nostrils down into the trachea and bronchi for this period relatively well, almost without exception.

Relief of symptoms can often be quite dramatic with this treatment. How well it compares with external beam radiation is a matter that has been addressed in randomized controlled trials, and definitive results are still awaited. We have found it particularly useful in treating patients with recurrent disease who have already received external beam radiotherapy, when quite large volumes of lung or other chest structures have already received a considerable amount of irradiation in these circumstances, and the value of this approach is that further high doses of radiation are delivered to the tumour only and the immediately surrounding tissues. However, a number of centres have reported that death from catastrophic haemoptysis is seen occasionally following this form of treatment; it is not clear at present whether this mode of death, which is seen occasionally in any event in patients with lung cancer, is actually occurring more frequently as a direct result of the treatment.

In summary, this is an interesting, and technically elegant, form of palliative radiotherapy for endobronchial carcinoma, although its exact place in modern management needs to be clarified further.

15.5.1 OESOPHAGEAL TUMOURS

Brachytherapy can also be applied successfully to oesophageal tumours. The applicator can be introduced through the biopsy channel of a standard gastroscope, although this is technically more difficult because of the short length of the applicator in relation to that of the gastroscope.

If the 100 cm length catheter is used, then this must be 'lengthened' using a stiff stainless-steel guide wire (as would be used for oesophageal dilatation), which is inserted in reverse into the catheter and taped in place. This allows easy withdrawal of the bronchoscope without displacing the catheter. (The technique used is similar to the 'exchange' technique described in Chapter 11.)

If the 150 cm length catheter is used, then the guide wire is not needed.

REFERENCES

Bysshe, J.E. (1988) The effect of giving information to patients before surgery. *Nursing*, **13**(30).

Collins, J., Dhillon, P. and Goldstraw, P. (1987) *Practical Bronchoscopy*, Blackwell Scientific, Oxford.

Woodcock, A. and Campbell, I. (1989) Bronchoscopy and infection control. *Lancet*, July 29.

BIBLIOGRAPHY

Green, J.H. (1975) *An Introduction to Human Physiology*, 4th edn, Oxford Medical Publications, Oxford.

Sears, G. and Winwood, R. (1982) *Anatomy and Physiology for Nurses and Students of Human Biology*, 5th edn, Arnold, London.

Stradling, P. (1991) *Diagnostic Bronchoscopy*, Churchill Livingstone, Edinburgh.

Flexible cystourethroscopy 16

Jayne Mason

16.1 INTRODUCTION

The earliest endoscopy of the urinary tract was performed in the first decade of the nineteenth century, using reflected candlelight as a light-source. It was only around the late 1800s that cystoscopy was performed with the use of electric light and a lens system.

In 1954 Professor H. Hopkins introduced the rigid cystoscope, which contained a rod-lens. During the last 15 years, since the introduction of small-calibre choledochoscopes, the introduction of flexible cystoscopes has revolutionized the diagnosis and treatment of patients with urinary tract problems. The flexible cystoscope is efficient, safe and can be used in outpatients or within day-surgery units, using local rather than general anaesthetic.

Over the years the new improved optics and mechanical technology have been researched and designed to minimize patient trauma. A major factor in the design of the cystoscope has been the operability and the atraumatic insertion, with high-quality imaging that enhances the success of the urological endoscopic examination.

Flexible fibreoptic cystoscopes are designed with a slim insertion tube with a diameter of 4.9 mm (or 15 French), which can be used for both diagnostic and therapeutic procedures. The flexible slim insertion tube decreases the patient's discomfort on insertion and during the procedure. The angulation of the cystoscope allows the whole bladder to be viewed in less time than with a rigid scope, thus reducing the operating time.

16.2 INDICATIONS FOR FLEXIBLE CYSTOSCOPY

Cystoscopy is one of the most common urological procedures. It allows careful examination of the urethra and interior bladder.

Practical Endoscopy Edited by M. Shephard and J. Mason. Published in 1997 by Chapman & Hall, London. ISBN 0 412 54000 2

Many patients undergoing urological assessment are within an older age bracket. The most common indication for cystoscopy is haematuria or abnormal bleeding when passing urine, and frequent urinary tract infections. In around 80% of these patients the procedure is for diagnosis and no further procedure or follow-up is required.

16.2.1 DIAGNOSTIC CYSTOSCOPY INDICATIONS

Indications for diagnostic use of cystoscopy include:

- The evaluation of micro/macrohaematuria.
- Investigation of obstructive/irritative voiding symptoms.
- Bladder biopsy.
- Retrograde ureterography.

16.2.2 PROCEDURES WHICH CAN BE PERFORMED THROUGH THE CYSTOSCOPE

The following procedures can be performed in addition to diagnosis:

1. Fulguration using diathermy.
2. Balloon dilatation of urethral strictures.
3. The removal and insertion of ureteric stents.
4. Laser vaporization.

   Alternative uses include:
1. Inspection of conduit following diversion, removal of a stent and haematuria.
2. Cystoscopy via a suprapubic catheter to assist in following the course of the urethra.

Some patients undergoing flexible cystoscopy have been diagnosed with bladder tumours or warty lesions. These patients return for frequent cystoscopy checks to assess any regrowth.

16.2.3 ADVANTAGES OF FLEXIBLE CYSTOSCOPY

There are a number of advantages to cystoscopy over other surgical procedures:

1. The patients are able to tolerate the procedure much better.
2. The procedure can be undertaken in outpatients or day-surgery units.
3. There is less postoperative pain for the patients.
4. There is a shorter operating time.
5. There are no external wounds.
6. There is less disruption to home life.
7. It is performed under local rather than general anaesthetic.
8. The patients are able to go home after the procedure.
9. It carries less of a risk.

16.3 EQUIPMENT

Equipment needed includes the following:

- Flexible cystoscope (cleaned as per hospital policy).
- Light-source.
- Irrigation tube.
- Suction tubing.
- Suction machine.
- Sterile dressing pack (containing sterile drapes, swabs, receivers).
- Cystoscopy drape.
- Lignocaine gel 1%.
- Prepping water-based solution.
- Biopsy forceps.
- Specimen pots.
- Oxygen and patient mask.
- Waterproof pads.
- Penile clamp.

16.4 TECHNIQUE

The aim of flexible cystoscopy is for the procedure to be relatively painless and atraumatic for the patient. The procedure is carried out as a sterile procedure to avoid any cross-infection. All patients are carefully selected for the procedure and are prepared preoperatively. There is a need to avoid 'conveyer-belt clinics', and each patient should be treated as an individual and given a high standard of care. Time must be allocated for the local anaesthetic lubricant gel to take effect before commencing the procedure. In males, 10–20 ml of 1% lignocaine gel is used, and in females 3–5 ml of the same gel. In males a penile clamp may be used 5–10 minutes before passing the scope. Some patients may feel discomfort and require intravenous sedation such as Diazemuls. Informed consent needs to be obtained from the patient prior to the procedure. The patient is required to empty their bladder before the procedure. The solution used for preparing the area must be water-based aqueous Hibitaine, as alcohol or betatine solutions will damage the delicate mucous membrane.

16.5 POSTOPERATIVE COMPLICATIONS

As with any form of intrinsic procedure there is a risk of complications, including:

- Infection.
- Haemorrhage.
- Urine retention.
- Cardiovascular problems.
- Bladder perforation.

16.6 NURSING CARE

Both the psychological and physical preparations are very important for patients undergoing flexible cystoscopy. Due to the nature of the procedure both male and female patients will be embarrassed.

Patients who are well informed have a better postoperative recovery. Nursing staff working in areas where flexible cystoscopy is performed have a very important part to play in the case of these patients – to answer any questions, make the patients feel relaxed and consider the patient's dignity.

Many units have designed their own patient information leaflets for patients undergoing this procedure (e.g. Richards, n.d.). These leaflets are sent to the patients prior to having surgery. An example of areas that should be addressed is:

What is cystoscopy?

This investigation allows the doctor to view directly the inside of your urethra and bladder using a fibreoptic instrument known as a cystoscope.

What should you expect?

The nurse who has the responsibility for your care during your stay on the unit will do the formal admission and plan care to suit your needs. The admission will include questions about yourself and your past medical history and will be a time of 'getting to know you'. The nurse will ask you to change into a theatre gown in readiness for your procedure. We ask you to wear the gown in order to avoid any accidental soiling of your own clothing.

During the procedure

In the examining room you will be asked to lie flat on your back on a trolley. Occasionally you will be required to have your legs supported by stirrups. Be sure you are comfortable, and if not then inform the nurse or doctor who is looking after you.

The area between your legs will be washed with an antiseptic solution and a sterile drape put over to cover the area and your dignity. The local anaesthetic, which comes in the form of a gel, will be inserted into your urethra. This is relatively painless and the anaesthetic takes a few minutes to take effect. The doctor will then tell you when the procedure is going to start. The instrument will be placed gently into your urethra and the examination will commence. You may experience the sensation of wanting to pass urine and this is quite normal. The examination itself is not painful and routinely takes approximately 10–20 minutes. At no time will you be left alone. A nurse will sit with you throughout the procedure.

After the procedure

On return to the ward the nurse will assess your condition and you will be offered light refreshments. You may experience a sense of urgency to pass urine. This is quite normal and will ease over the next 24 hours.

Going home

We advise that you take the remainder of the day easy. You may experience a little bleeding on passing urine, but this should be no cause for concern. However, if the bleeding is excessive or prolonged you are advised to contact your own family doctor immediately.

16.7   POSTOPERATIVE INSTRUCTIONS

Before being discharged the patient should have passed urine, in order to assess any pain or bleeding.

The nurse must also explain to the patient that they will feel the need to pass urine frequently over the next 12–24 hours. The patient may feel a slight discomfort (stinging) for the first few times when passing urine.

If the patient does not pass urine within 6–8 hours of being discharged, they should be told to contact their family doctor immediately. On discharge the patient must drink plenty of fluids for the next 24 hours as this will encourage the production of urine.

16.8   CONCLUSIONS

In conclusion, flexible cystoscopy has become a valuable method to diagnose some of the most common causes of urinary tract diseases:

1. Haematuria – from the following causes:
   (a) Congenital.
   (b) Trauma.
   (c) Calculi.
   (d) Tumours.
2. Incontinence.
3. Urinary tract infections.
4. Renal failure.

This procedure can be undertaken using local anaesthetic lignocaine gel rather than a general anaesthetic. Therefore it can be undertaken in the outpatient department or day-surgery units.

The doctor needs to be trained in the use of fibreoptic cystoscopes. Good hand/eye co-ordination is required to give clear visualization of the urethra and bladder in order for the procedure to be atraumatic for the patient.

REFERENCES

Richards, D. (n.d.) *Understanding Your Cystoscopy*. [Patient information leaflet.] Day Surgery Unit, University Hospital of Wales, Heath Park, Cardiff.

Flexible hysteroscopy 17

Suresh Nair

17.1 INTRODUCTION

Visualization of the uterine cavity was first successfully accomplished by Pantaleoni (1869) who discovered a polyp causing menorrhagia and cauterized it with silver nitrate. However, it was not until uterine distension with carbon dioxide gas was developed by Rubin (1925) that hysteroscopy became a reliable procedure. A major obstacle to the widespread use of hysteroscopy was the lack of adequate illumination and the relatively large diameters of hysteroscopes, which could only be passed through widely dilated cervices.

Diagnostic hysteroscopy was greatly facilitated with the manufacture of smaller calibre rigid endoscopes. Furthermore, the markedly improved visualization resulting from internal light systems enabled the illuminating light to be carried from an adjacent light-source via a flexible conducting fibreoptic or fluid cable. The light passes through a system of rod-lenses without exposing the uterus to thermal injury. Flexible fibreoptic hysteroscopes with a 3.5 mm diameter have now been developed. The distal tip of these hysteroscopes are slender yet steerable and sufficiently malleable to negotiate through the narrow endocervical canal so that the uterine cavity can be visualized without the need for prior cervical dilatation. This has allowed painless atraumatic insertion of the flexible hysteroscope into the uterine cavity.

The major advantage of the flexible hysteroscope is that it can be used in an outpatient 'office' setting and its capacity of visualizing the cornua and uterotubal junction (Fig. 17.1). However, a significant disadvantage (aside from its greater cost), in comparison to the rigid system, is the fact that, because the image is made up of a composite of numerous smaller optical fibres, the view obtained of the uterine cavity is of an inferior quality compared with the rigid hysteroscope, which

Practical Endoscopy Edited by M. Shephard and J. Mason. Published in 1997 by Chapman & Hall, London. ISBN 0 412 54000 2

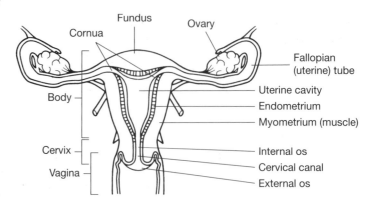

Fig. 17.1   Anatomy of the female reproductive system

can also attain an outer calibre of less than 4 mm. Currently, therefore, the rigid hysteroscope is also being widely used in the outpatient setting. There have been numerous reviews on the role of outpatient hysteroscopy (Hill, Broadbent and Magos, 1992) as well as the flexible hysteroscopic system. Lin *et al.* (1990) described their experience of more than a thousand patients using the diagnostic flexible 3.7 mm fibreoptic hysteroscope without the need for anaesthesia or prior cervical dilatation.

17.2   INDICATIONS/CONTRAINDICATIONS

17.2.1   INDICATIONS FOR FLEXIBLE HYSTEROSCOPY

The commonest indication for hysteroscopy is abnormal uterine bleeding. This can be divided into two broad categories, namely premenopausal and postmenopausal bleeding. Premenopausal bleeding includes menorrhagia, prolonged bleeding, intermenstrual and postcoital bleeding. In recent times, since endometrial ablation has become a fairly common hysteroscopic operative procedure, bleeding post-endometrial ablation can also be evaluated by outpatient diagnostic flexible hysteroscopy.

The other large category is that of postmenopausal bleeding. Outpatient flexible hysteroscopy is particularly useful when running a menopause programme as a prelude to starting hormone replacement therapy or to evaluate any abnormal uterine bleeding that may occur during the postmenopausal period whether or not the patient is on hormonal therapy.

Lesions such as submucous myomata, polyps, cystic hyperplasia with or without atypia and frank malignancy can be detected and directed biopsies taken to obtain histological confirmation. With regards to submucous myomata, outpatient flexible hysteroscopy can provide valuable information as to the site, size and extent to which the myoma is protruding through the myometrium into the uterine cavity. Hysteroscopy is presently so precise, especially when done by an experienced operator, that significant endometrial lesions should rarely be missed. Nevertheless, very early malignancy has on occasion gone undetected and hence this emphasizes the need for biopsies of any abnormal areas and also routine endometrial sampling. One must be reminded that malignancies have been missed by every technique used for evaluation of abnormal bleeding and that the best precaution is to use a combined approach (i.e. hysteroscopy and directed biopsy). This certainly has more specificity and sensitivity in comparison to blind curettage performed under general anaesthesia.

The investigation of amenorrhoea in the absence of any hormonal cause can be very expeditiously performed via flexible outpatient hysteroscopy. Evidence for Ashermann's syndrome, especially when there is a preceding typical history of postabortal or postpartum infection or curettage, or history of infertility, can be obtained through hysteroscopy. Subsequent intrauterine adhesiolysis can be adequately planned after the diagnostic hysteroscopy. Women with habitual abortion and infertility, especially where laparoscopy had been done but not hysteroscopy, and those for whom the hysterosalpingogram report was abnormal (i.e. intrauterine filling defects or septa), are ideally evaluated in an outpatient setting via flexible hysteroscopy.

When synechiae or septa are discovered at prior outpatient hysteroscopy, then definitive operative hysteroscopy can be planned at the time of laparoscopy and fertility evaluation done under general anaesthesia. Aside from intrauterine adhesions, cervical stenosis and adhesions, postendometrial ablation or postcone biopsy with resultant haematometra can be effectively drained under direct visualization using the flexible hysteroscope. The author has had occasion to drain haematometra using the flexible hysteroscope, especially if it is situated high into the cornua as a result of previous inadequate ablation of the cornua. However, this may not always be successful, especially if the adhesions are of a denser consistency. The author generally uses a fluid medium under low pressure so as to avoid 'pushing' the contents of the uterine cavity up through the tubes.

Simple operative procedures such as excision of small tubal, endometrial and endocervical polyps can usually be accomplished at the diagnosis of these lesions during fibreoptic hysteroscopy using flexible graspers and scissors. However, the author usually uses the hysteroresectoscope for larger, more complex synechiae or septa under general anaesthesia and glycine irrigation.

The removal of retained intrauterine devices or the recovery of 'fetal bone' – a very rare complication of a missed abortion – can be performed in an outpatient setting. In instances where the contraceptive device is firmly embedded in the myometrium, the hysteroresectoscope with the knife or needle electrode is required to dislodge it from the uterine cavity and this should be performed under laparoscopic guidance.

Outpatient flexible hysteroscopy is valuable following previous uterine surgery. This is best performed about 6 weeks after formal myomectomy involving the uterine cavity or surgery involving major uterine reunification. Although in effect fertility enhancing, such surgery can nevertheless induce intrauterine adhesions. This is also the case with intrauterine myoma resection, division of septa or synechiae. A second-look hysteroscopic evaluation can help to identify and deal with such adhesions.

17.2.2   CONTRAINDICATIONS TO FLEXIBLE HYSTEROSCOPY

Flexible hysteroscopy is a safe procedure but there are well-defined contraindications, which include:

1. *Infection*; hysteroscopy in the presence of vaginitis and cervitis can cause ascending endometritis, salpingitis and peritonitis. It is also inappropriate to perform hysteroscopy when there is a suspicion of pelvic inflammatory disease unless there is an intrauterine contraceptive device that needs to be removed. Preliminary antibiotic cover is then mandatory.
2. *Cardiorespiratory disease*; severe cardiorespiratory disease is a contraindication to outpatient procedures where vasovagal attacks, carbon dioxide embolism or even an acute myocardial infarct could occur. An operating theatre setting with all the requisite resuscitation equipment is the appropriate place to perform hysteroscopy in such patients.
3. *Pregnancy*; with the advent of high-resolution transvaginal sonography, there is little indication to perform hysteroscopy of the pregnant uterus unless it is to remove a retained intrauterine contraceptive device when the patient wishes to carry on with the pregnancy. However, the operator must be cognisant of the fact that carbon dioxide insufflation can cause retroplacental bleeding and placental separation and carbon dioxide embolization through the large dilated veins of the pregnant uterus. The author uses only molar (1 mol/l) saline for hysteroscopy of the pregnant uterus. Furthermore, the optic nerve of the fetus may be damaged by the

illuminating light after the 10th week of pregnancy, although there does not appear to be any danger before this stage (Taylor and Gordon, 1993).

4. *Uterine bleeding*; if fluid irrigation is used, moderate bleeding does not pose a problem to adequate visualization of the uterine cavity. If, however, there is heavy bleeding, this is best suppressed first to obtain a better subsequent view of the uterine cavity and also to prevent intravasation of distension media.

5. *Cervical carcinoma*; there is a definite risk of spread of cancer cells, especially during the passage of the hysteroscope, which may open up blood or lymphatic vessels and cause systemic dissemination of the malignancy (Siegler *et al.*, 1990).

17.3 NURSING CARE

Aside from the standard preparation and maintenance of flexible endoscopes addressed in Chapter 7 some general comments from the author's personal experience in organizing a diagnostic hysteroscopy set-up are described.

As most women are invariably anxious about the procedure, prior counselling and provision of details of what to expect go a long way to calm the patient sufficiently to make them more receptive to having the procedure done with local or no anaesthesia. A mild sedative or neuroleptanalgesia or a non-steroidal anti-inflammatory agent can be administered to minimize anxiety and discomfort from prostaglandin-induced cramps.

The scrub nurse in charge must ensure that all equipment and instruments are properly laid out. A well-trained team that understands the workings of all the equipment and maintains it carefully is critical to the successful progress of the diagnostic hysteroscopic procedure.

In present-day gynaecological practice, there is a plethora of optical and electronic equipment and instruments, with a wide variety of sheaths, telescopes and ancillary instrumentation. It is mandatory therefore for the nursing staff to be able to set up and assemble the compatible equipment and instruments quickly and efficiently. A system where compatible instruments are stored closely together in clearly labelled trays and compartments and ensuring adequate back-up replacements in the event of breakdowns is the only way to avoid costly delays.

Each endoscopist has subtle differences in requirements and styles. The idiosyncrasies of each surgeon should be duly recorded on a card or record book to ensure the availability of correct equipment for each procedure, be it in the operating theatre or outpatient setting.

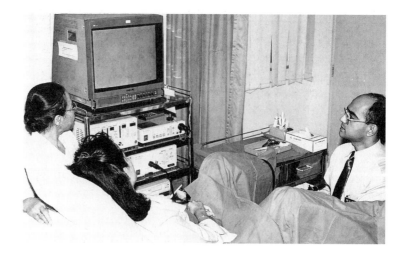

Fig. 17.2   The participation of the patient in flexible hysterectomy

Meticulous care and attention to gentle handling of equipment will ensure a lengthy life-span of endoscopic equipment and consistently good surgical results.

The nurse can also assist the surgeon to counsel the patient and explain the findings when he or she watches the monitor when hysteroscopy is performed in the conscious patient. A patient will generally feel much more at ease when her nurse and doctor are watching and explaining the findings on the monitor so that she can comprehend what is being done and obtain a keener insight into her problem, and how it will impact on her subsequent health (Fig. 17.2).

17.4   PROCEDURES

The first step in the procedure is to adequately expose the cervix and the external os. For this, a bivalve speculum is required that has a single hinge that can be disarticulated once the hysteroscope is in place, or a single-blade Sim's speculum, along with the single-toothed tenaculum for exposure of the cervix.

The cervix is cleansed with a mild antiseptic (e.g. 1% cetrimide), wiping away any cervical mucus that may be at the os. Very occasionally local infiltration of an anaesthetic (e.g. 1% lignocaine) paracervically is required, especially if larger bore hysteroscopes are used. But if the diagnostic flexible hysteroscope of 3.5 mm is used then this is rarely necessary. If there is acute anteflexion or retroflexion of the

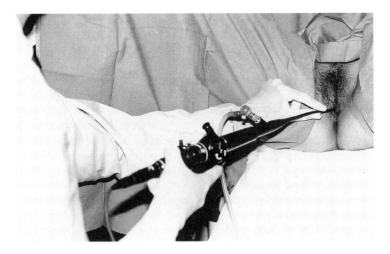

Fig. 17.3 Navigation of the flexible hysteroscope into the undilated endocervical canal

uterus and the operator experiences difficulty in negotiating the endo-cervical canal, then a single-toothed vulsellum can be applied to the anterior lip after infiltration with lignocaine to 'straighten' the canal; however, this is very rarely necessary as the flexible hysteroscope is very slender and malleable and in the majority of instances can be easily negotiated through the endocervical canal.

The fluid distending medium that can be used is 10% dextrose administered through a bottle suspended about 80 cm above the uterus and connected to the irrigation port of the hysteroscope via the standard intravenous infusion set. The efflux is collected into a container at the base of the table.

Another method of uterine distension is use of carbon dioxide gas via the hysteroflator. The flow rate is between 30 and 50 ml/min and the intrauterine pressure is monitored between 50 and 80 mmHg. Although carbon dioxide gas is satisfactory in most circumstances, fluid medium is valuable when bleeding occurs.

After entry into the uterus, all surfaces are inspected carefully. Most flexible hysteroscopes have a forward direction of view and hence the panoramic view of the endocervical canal, its glandular elements, the internal os and thereafter the entire uterine cavity is obtained in sequence. In the experience of the author the endocervical canal is best visualized at the time the hysteroscope is being withdrawn out of the uterus (Fig. 17.3).

Obvious macroscopic lesions such as polyps, septa, synechiae, myo-mata and tumours can be readily seen, but attention must also be given to the subtle changes that help to ascertain the stage of the menstrual cycle, the presence of endometritis or hyperplasia.

The virtue of the flexible hysteroscope is the fact that the cornua and the tubal ostia can easily be visualized by deflecting the tip. Minute details such as periostial contractions and ostial polyps can be studied in detail. These tiny polyps could also be removed atraumatically using fine flexible biopsy forceps; such forceps can also be used to obtain directed biopsies of lesions within the uterine cavity without needing to resort to curettage. If, however, curettage is performed then the slender Novak's curette or the various flexible outpatient endometrial samplers can be used (e.g. the Pipelle or the Z-sampler). Generally, the whole procedure takes between 5 and 10 minutes and will be lengthened only when still photography of interesting lesions is required.

The author is of the opinion that concomitant transvaginal sonography helps to determine any adnexal pathology and provide a precise picture of the disposition and flexion of the uterus and whether there are extracavitatory myomata (i.e. intramural, subserous) and also whether the submucous myomata detected on hysteroscopy has a significant intramural or transmural extent. Often when 'septa' are detected, transvaginal sonography might, in certain instances, help to differentiate the bicornuate uterus from the subseptate uterus with a median septum. The extent of the base of the septum can also be measured. This, however, must be further confirmed by hysterosalpingography or more definitively using concomitant laparoscopy done at hysteroscopic division of the septum.

17.5 EQUIPMENT

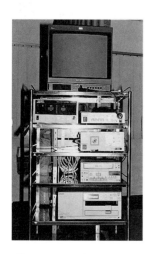

Fig. 17.4 The instrument cart

In the 'office' set-up, flexible hysteroscopy can be performed with the patient on the standard examination couch, which can be raised and tilted. Heel stirrups should suffice provided there is adequate capacity for adjustments for comfortable placement of the patient's legs at a sufficiently wide angle of abduction to allow good access.

The patient is positioned such that her head and bottom are slightly raised and the whole couch elevated to a comfortable level for the operator. To make efficient use of space, it is useful to have an instrument cart carrying the video monitor (450 lines resolution), the camera console with the lead cable to the camera head (carefully stowed away when not in use), the carbon dioxide hysteroflator with tubings and the light-source (150 watts is usually sufficient) (Fig. 17.4); the compact arrangement of monitor, hysteroflator, light-source and documentation equipment in one cart makes it more portable and uncomplicated to use. The monitor should be placed such that both the operator and patient can view it easily (Fig. 17.5). If this is not possible,

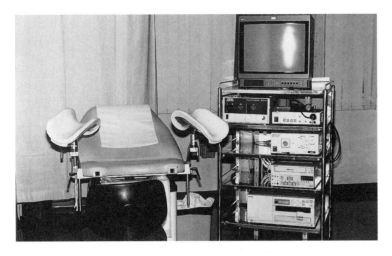

Fig. 17.5 The office 'set-up' for flexible outpatient hysteroscopy

then a second monitor could be made available for patient viewing. There should also be a sterile trolley for the basic dilatation and curettage instruments. A good vaginal light-source is essential for the preliminary preparation prior to hysteroscopy.

The flexible endoscopes that are generally available have an outer diameter of 3.5 mm and are capable of being bent in many directions. The distal tip can be deflected 160° upward or downward. The diagnostic hysteroscope has a 1 mm channel for delivery of distension media, whereas the operative flexible hysteroscopes have in addition an operating channel of 2 mm (Fig. 17.6)). These hysteroscopes, however, have an outer diameter of 4.8 mm. Long flexible instruments (i.e. scissors, biopsy forceps, grasping forceps) can be introduced through the operating channel to perform various procedures (Fig. 17.7).

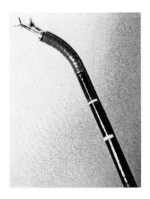

Fig. 17.6 The operating flexible hysteroscope, with additional channel for the passage of flexible instruments

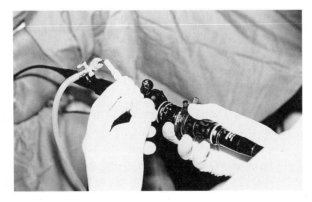

Fig. 17.7 The flexible biopsy forceps and graspers are used to take directed biopsies or retrieve intrauterine contraceptive devices

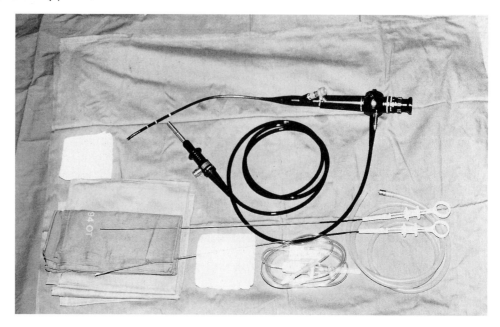

Fig. 17.8 A fibreoptic hysteroscope

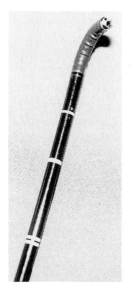

Fig. 17.9 The distal tip of the flexible hysteroscope

Most fibreoptic hysteroscopes are flexible through their whole length (Fig. 17.8); the light-cable is integrated to the hysteroscope's eye-piece as a single compact unit. However, in these the insertion tube may sometimes be difficult to control during the procedure. A fibrescope (e.g. Fujinon) with a soft flexible tip, rigid midsection and a flexible proximal portion with a distal 3.7 mm outer diameter and total length of 58 cm was therefore developed (Fuji Photo Optical Company). The proponents of this instrument find that the rigid midsection allows better and easier handling and positioning of the fibrescope (Lin *et al.*, 1990). The distal tip has a wide field angle (90 ° in air, 65 ° in 10% glucose), and a bending capacity of 100 ° up and 90 ° down (Fig. 17.9), enabling it to be negotiated through the endocervical canal and to visualize the uterine cornua. The flexible proximal part enables the endoscopist to attain a comfortable working position more readily.

Documentation and recording of the endoscopic findings have now become an integral part of this diagnostic process. It is therefore prudent to have a video recorder and a video printer for both teaching and patient-counselling purposes. As mentioned earlier, space for a transvaginal ultrasound machine is extremely useful, although not mandatory, as this can be done either prior to or after the hysteroscopy at a separate sitting.

17.6 COMPLICATIONS AND PRECAUTIONS

As with any invasive operative procedure, flexible hysteroscopy is a safe procedure when performed by a well-trained surgeon and for the appropriate indication. A good diagnostician will make a good endoscopic surgeon and there is no short-cut around this. Training is therefore just as important for the use of diagnostic hysteroscopy as for the more complex endoscopic surgical procedures if complications are to be kept to a minimum.

Failure to complete the procedure because of cervical stenosis or inconvenient bleeding is uncommon and occurs in 0–2.5% of cases (Taylor and Cumming, 1979). The tight cervical os is commonly encountered in nullipara or in women who have undergone previous cervical surgery (i.e. cone biopsy, laser or diathermy ablation) or postmenopausal women. Gentle dilatation is occasionally required and can cause pain and uterine cramps, especially during the passage of the hysteroscope through the internal os. Premedication with Gemeprost pessaries (1 mg, 2–3 hours prior to the procedure) to 'soften' the cervix and a paracervical block are useful in facilitating painless hysteroscopy in such difficult cases.

Bleeding from either menstruation or trauma from introduction of the hysteroscope or dilatation can prevent adequate visualization of the uterine cavity. Furthermore, bubbles often form owing to the bleeding and the endocervical glandular secretions. Gentle handling of the flexible hysteroscope in its passage through the cervical canal and uterine cavity can overcome this problem but if the bleeding is brisk then fluid media such as Hyskon or 10% dextrose irrigation as described earlier can provide a clear view of the uterine cavity.

Very rare instances of carbon dioxide embolism and cardiac arrest have been reported but these have occurred with large unmonitored amounts of carbon dioxide following the use of inappropriate insufflators (Crozier *et al.*, 1991). It is highly unlikely for embolism to occur if the correct insufflator is used because flexible hysteroscopy is a very short procedure not requiring more than 200 to 300 ml of carbon dioxide gas. In only a very few cases have anaphylactic reactions due to high molecular weight dextran or lignocaine infiltration been reported to occur. This complication, whilst rare, can be a catastrophic one presenting with acute hypotension, histamine release and bronchospasm. Therefore there must always be resuscitation equipment available including endotracheal intubation and Ambu-bag ventilation and oxygen supply with the full array of emergency drugs, in particular adrenaline (0.5 ml of 1:1000), given subcutaneously.

A mechanical complication of use of fluid or gaseous medium is the rupture of hydrosalpinges and extravasation of the medium but this is usually not associated with any untoward sequelae.

Uterine perforation is rare but can be minimized when the procedure is done under direct vision. Perforation from diagnostic hysteroscopy does not usually produce side-effects and can be treated conservatively. It is more likely to occur when using the rigid hysteroscopes than with the flexible steerable hysteroscopes. However, Gentile and Siegler (1983) described the inadvertent biopsy of the intestine during the procedure!

Postoperative pelvic infection has occasionally been recorded 24 to 48 hours after the diagnostic hysteroscopy and there have been rare reports of peritonitis and septicaemia (Fraser, 1993). Considering the contraindications generally prevents this from occurring, but should it occur then aggressive antibiotic therapy is mandatory.

Some rare complications include vasovagal attacks occurring with distension of the cervix, especially the internal os, or the uterine cavity. The patient may experience faintness, heat and sweating, pallor, brady-cardia and hypotension. This may be aggravated by unfamiliarity with the procedure and anxiety. Oxygen through a face mask and the horizontal or Trendelenburg position can alleviate this situation. Mild sedation or neuroleptanalgesia preoperatively can help the overly anxious patient. Shoulder-tip pain is another rare occurrence following higher rates of carbon dioxide insufflation; it is caused by diaphragmatic irritation as the gas passes through the tubes and intraperitoneally.

17.7 DISCHARGE INFORMATION

All patients should be given relevant discharge information including the symptoms and signs to watch for that may herald postprocedural complications, the next review appointment and any special medications that need to be taken.

It is essential that a friend or relative is present to escort the patient home as troublesome bleeding or fainting spells very rarely can occur, especially if a mild anaesthetic agent has been used. Late complications such as pelvic infection with fever, purulent vaginal discharge or abdominal distension and pain must be explained and the patient clearly instructed on how to get to the emergency service.

However, the vast majority of women are quite well and unaffected by this short and largely painless procedure and are often back to their routine by the next day.

REFERENCES

Crozier, T.A., Luger, A.H., Dravecz, M. *et al.* (1991) Carbon dioxide embolism with cardiac arrest during hysteroscopy. *Iatrogenics*, **1**, 28.

Fraser, I.S. (1993) Personal techniques and results for outpatient diagnostic hysteroscopy. *Gynecol Endosc*, **2** 29–33.

Gentile, G.P. and Siegler, A.M. (1983) Inadvertent intestinal biopsy during laparoscopy and hysteroscopy: a report of two cases. *Fertil Steril*, **36**, 402.

Hill, N.C.W., Broadbent, J.A.M. and Magos, A.L. (1992) The role of outpatient hysteroscopy. *Contemp Rev Obstet Gynaecol*, **4**, 290–314.

Lin, B.L., Iwata, Y., Lin, K.H. and Valle, R.F. (1990) The Fujinon diagnostic fibreoptic hysteroscope; experience with 1,503 patients. *J Reprod Med*, **35**, 685–9.

Pantaleoni, D. (1869) On endoscopic examination of the cavity of the womb. *Medical Press and Circular*, **8**, 26–7.

Rubin, C. (1925) Endometroscopy with the aid of uterine insufflation. *Am J Obstet Gynecol*, **10**(3), 313–17.

Siegler, A.M., Valle, R.F., Lindemann, J.H. and Mencaglia, L. (1990) *Therapeutic Hysteroscopy – Indications and Techniques*, C.V. Mosby, Baltimore.

Taylor, P.J. and Cumming, D.C. (1979) Hysteroscopy in 100 patients. *Fertil Steril*, **31**, 301.

Taylor, P.J. and Gordon, A.G. (1993) *Practical Hysteroscopy*, Blackwell Scientific, Oxford, London.

BIBLIOGRAPHY

Hamou, J.E. (1992) *Hysteroscopy and Microcolpohysteroscopy Text and Atlas*, (transl P.J. Taylor), Appleton & Lange, Norwalk, CT/San Mateo, CA.

Aspects of safety 18

Electrosurgery 18A

C. Paul Wicker

18A.1 INTRODUCTION

Electrosurgery, more commonly known as 'diathermy', has been with us for some time. Endoscopic diathermy is used to cut and/or coagulate tissue in the following situations:

- Sphincterotomy in ERCP.
- Polypectomy.
- 'Hot' biopsy.
- Haemostasis – bleeding ulcer
  - hereditary haemorrhagic telangiectasis
  - angiodysplasia.
- Debulking of tumours and hyperplastic tissue.

In the typical electrosurgical circuit, the surgeon activates the electro-surgical instrument (diathermy pencil, probe or forceps) in contact with the patient's tissues, heat is produced and then the current passes through the patient to the return electrode, which may be in the form of a large plate strapped to the thigh. The current then returns to the electrosurgical generator in order to complete the circuit. Over the years, electrosurgery has been used for a variety of purposes; however, in the surgical sense, it is now used exclusively for the coagulation of bleeding blood vessels, or for the cutting or destruction of tissues (Plate 30). These functions make it the most useful piece of electromedical equipment ever to be invented. Unfortunately, the very features that make it so useful make it extremely dangerous – both to the patient and to the staff who use it.

Although the principles of electrosurgery and endoscopic diathermy are the same, whether used in the surgical or endoscopic setting, there are two main differences that must be mentioned.

Practical Endoscopy Edited by M. Shephard and J. Mason. Published in 1997 by Chapman & Hall, London. ISBN 0 412 54000 2

1. The advantage of using electrosurgery in endoscopy is that lower power levels are required compared with conventional open surgery. This has to be taken into consideration when setting the power levels as high power could lead to extensive tissue damage.
2. It is also important to consider the possibility of capacitive coupling between the electrode and the endoscopic sheath which could lead to burns on the operator's hands or eye region. The use of an S-cord should therefore be considered or, alternatively, the use of the 'Electroshield' active electrode monitor (ValleyLab, 1995).

This chapter is devoted to the explanation of the principles of electrosurgery, its uses and the hazards associated with it.

18A.2   THE ELECTRIC CIRCUIT

A basic knowledge of the electric circuit is essential in order to explain how electrosurgery functions and how its effects are achieved.

An electrical circuit consists of a positive and negative terminal connected by an electrical pathway. Electricity is the movement of electrons past a given point. If the negative terminal is connected to the 'earth', then the system is considered to be 'earthed' or 'grounded'. If the negative terminal is isolated from the earth, then the system itself is 'isolated'. Mains electricity is earthed, whereas the power in a torch battery, having no reference to earth, is isolated. Most modern electrosurgical generators are isolated.

The flow of electrons in the circuit is the 'electric current' and is measured in amps (A). The force that pushes these electrons around the circuit is measured in volts (V). The resistance to the flow of current is measured in ohms (Ω). Power is the energy produced or consumed over a period of time and is measured in watts (W). The first three measurements – volts, amps and ohms – all influence the overall power that is produced or used by an electric circuit.

One other factor must be taken into account in this primer for electrosurgery. If the current flows in one direction around the circuit then it is called 'direct current' (DC). This is the current used by car or torch batteries and also by small appliances, which require 'DC' transformers (e.g. small radios). In contrast to this, alternating current (AC) periodically switches the direction of flow, so that the current first travels one way, and then the other. This process normally happens very fast and the backwards–forwards motion occurs many times per second. This current change shows as a sine waveform on an oscilloscope. In the case of mains electricity the current is switched around 50 times per second (50 Hz). In the case of electrosurgery, this occurs around 500 000 times per second (50 kHz). Medium-wave radio also operates at a similar frequency – 50 kHz–1.6 MHz (1 600 000 times per second).

It is important to release at this stage that the frequency of the waveform has no effect on its power – a current with a power of 50 W would have the same power with a waveform of both 50 Hz or 50 000 Hz.

18A.3   ELECTROSURGICAL CURRENT

It was discovered late in the nineteenth century that high-frequency electric current could be passed through the human body with none of the excitatory effects (electrocution) shown by low-frequency current. It took almost another 30 years, however, before Bovie and Cushing finally produced the first electrosurgical generators that could be used surgically.

18A.3.1   FEATURES OF ELECTROSURGICAL CURRENT

As a result of its very high frequency, electrosurgical current has several features that affect its behaviour.

Radiofrequency current

Electrosurgical current could be likened to radio waves – it has a frequency identical to that of medium-wave radio. This gives it certain properties – capacitance and inductance – that, in effect, make it difficult to limit the current to the wires connecting it to the active and return electrodes. Under certain circumstances, there doesn't need to be a physical connection in order for current to flow.

A surgeon may inadvertently stand on the foot pedal and activate the active electrode (open-keying the active electrode) while it is in the quiver. The active electrode immediately begins to give out radiofrequency current from its tip. This current is looking for a pathway to the return electrode. Because there is no physical pathway, it looks for the next pathway of least resistance. The surgeon, or any other member of staff, act as aerials that attract this radiofrequency current. If they are electrically connected to the patient, then current will flow from the staff member to the patient. If the combination of circumstances (concentrated current over a long enough time) is correct, then a burn will occur.

Capacitive coupling (Figs 18A.7, 18A.8) (LoCicero et al., 1987)

A capacitor is an electrical device, such as a transistor or a resistor, that is composed of two sheets of conductive material separated by a sheet of non-conductive material (e.g. board, plastic, air, wood or rubber). This device is then connected into an electrical circuit. The main feature of a capacitor is that it will appear to 'conduct' alternating current, such as electrosurgical current, despite the fact that there is an insulating material between the two conductive plates. Capacitive coupling is said to occur between the two sheets of conductive material. In the operating theatre, capacitive coupling may occur between the 'earth–**surgeon– glove–patient**–earth', or the 'earth–**operating table–rubber mattress– patient (small contact site)**–earth'. In the first scenario, the surgeon may receive a burn to his finger while coagulating a bleeder using an uninsulated instrument. In the second, the patient may receive a burn via the small contact site to earth.

As current builds up on one side of the capacitor, it has nowhere to go, since it has been stopped by the sheet of non-conductive material. However, it has the effect of causing an opposite charge to build up on the other side of the capacitor, which can complete the circuit. This occurs every time the charge oscillates from positive to negative. Since this happens over 500 000 times per second in electrosurgical current, a charge will be passed around the circuit at 500 000 Hz – radiofrequency current.

Inductance

This refers to the ability of the electrosurgical current to form an electromagnet if the wire is coiled around a conductive material. In the operating theatre this can occur if the return electrode wire is coiled and hung on the operating table, or even placed in close proximity to a conductive material such as the antistatic floor. The circuit here is 'earth–table–electromagnet–patient–contact site–earth'.

At each oscillation of the radiofrequency current, a electromagnet is formed by the conductive material. This magnetic field first flows in one direction, then the other – 500 000 times per second. This magnetic field gives off energy in the form of electrosurgical current. This current may burn the patient as it passes through the small contact site on its way to earth.

18A.3.2   THE PRODUCTION OF HEAT IN TISSUES

Heat is produced when electrosurgical current is passed through human tissues. The degree of heating of the tissues, and the result of this heating, is dependent on three factors – current density in the tissues, the electrical resistance of the tissues and the waveform of the current (Wicker, 1991).

Current density is a product of the power of the current and also the area of tissue through which it is flowing. Hence a given power of current will heat a small area of tissue intensely, or a large area of tissue slowly. Active electrodes are made small in order to increase the heating effect, while return electrodes are made large in order to reduce the heating effect. Current density in tissues can be affected by several factors; for example, pathways of least resistance will encourage 'channelling' of the current, which increases its density. This might happen if, for example, one area of the return electrode conducted current better than another area, or if the current was directed through narrow tracts of tissue such as in the fingers or other extremities.

Electrical resistance in the tissues, properly called 'impedance', can affect the heat produced. High resistance causes an increased heating effect compared with lower resistance. This same effect occurs in the bars of an electric fire, which contain 'resistance wire' that is designed to heat quickly compared with normal flex, which is required to stay cool. When electrosurgical current is applied to tissues, resistance increases as the tissues dry out. Eventually the current will stop flowing as the resistance reaches the point when the current can no longer flow. This point will be reached sooner with waveforms that have a low crest factor (low voltage/current ratio) when compared with waveforms with a high crest factor (high voltage/current ratio) since high resistance requires high voltage in order to make the current flow.

The waveform of the current also affects the degree of heat produced as a result of the penetration of the current into the tissues and the power of the waveform used. High-voltage waveforms penetrate the tissue more than lower voltage waveforms and therefore spread the heating effect more widely. Low-voltage waveforms do not penetrate the tissue as widely and therefore concentrate the heating effect to a smaller area. An increase in power of the waveform will increase the overall heating effect. The electrosurgical generator makes use of these effects by producing three basic waveforms – **coagulate (coag), cut and blend** (Fig. 18A.1) (Wicker, 1991).

With electrosurgical current, an important factor is the 'crest factor'. This factor is a result of the ratio of peak (maximum) volts to the 'root mean square' (average) voltage – a waveform such as coag has a high crest factor when compared with cut. A coag waveform would therefore have a higher peak voltage than a cut waveform of the same power. The crest factor has no influence over power and so a low-power waveform might have a high crest factor and vice versa.

Coag is a high-voltage, low-current (high crest factor) intermittent waveform that heats tissues slowly over a relatively wide area. At low power, this has the effect of causing the tissues to dry out slowly causing coagulation or desiccation, leaving a dry white coagulum. At high

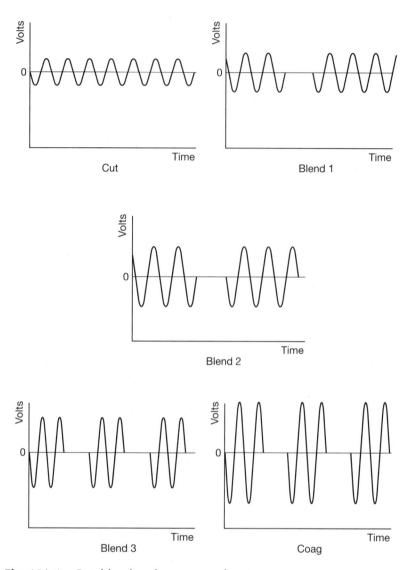

Fig. 18A.1   Cut, blend and coag waveforms

power, the high voltage causes long sparks to form, which cause fulguration or charring of tissue, leaving a black residue.

Cut is a low-voltage, high-current (low crest factor) waveform that heats tissues quickly over a small area. At high power, this intense heating effect has the effect of exploding the cell contents and leaving a hole in the cell matrix – hence the cutting effect (although the electrode is never in direct contact with the tissue). At low power, this waveform produces an excellent desiccating effect since the low voltage cannot produce sparks and the heating of the tissues is much more gentle than is a coag waveform of the same power.

Blend is a hybrid waveform in that it has similarities to both coag and cut. There are usually two or three blend settings, which give various degrees of a cutting or coagulating effect.

18A.4 MONOPOLAR AND BIPOLAR ELECTROSURGERY

Although they are used for different purposes, in effect both these forms are identical apart from the location of the return electrode (Wicker, 1993). In monopolar electrosurgery the return electrode is placed at some distance from the active eletrode, usually in the form of a plate of around 20 cm by 10 cm. In bipolar electrosurgery, the return electrode is incorporated into the same instrument as the active electrode. Normally this would be the two lines of a bipolar forceps. Current flow through the tissues is completely different as a result of the placement of the return electrode; therefore the use of the two types of electrosurgery is different.

Monopolar electrosurgery (Figs 18A.2, 18A.3) (Wicker, 1993) employs a return pathway for the current that is through the patient's body. This makes it inherently dangerous since the possibility for errors is high. Although, in isolated electrosurgery, the current is always trying to return to the return electrode, the features of the high-frequency current can cause problems of leakage of stray currents, which can lead to patient burns (Plate 31).

Bipolar electrosurgery (Fig. 18A.4) (Wicker, 1993) avoids these problems by making the return pathway extremely short – from one tine of

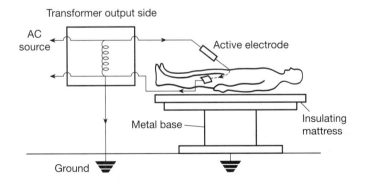

Fig. 18A.2 Grounded monopolar electrosurgery

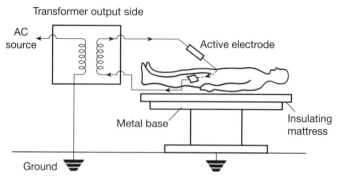

= Direction of RF current flow

Fig. 18A.3   Isolated monopolar electrosurgery

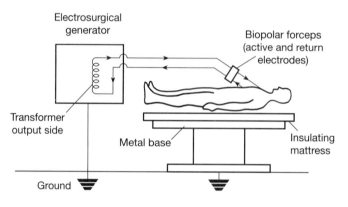

= Direction of RF current flow

Fig. 18A.4   Bipolar electrosurgery

a forceps to the other tine. Since the current never travels through the patient's body, it cannot cause problems and so bipolar current is inherently safer than monopolar. However, because of the proximity of the two tines of the forceps, it is currently impossible to use high-power waveforms with it and so bipolar surgery is useful only for low-power applications such as neurosurgery, ophthalmic surgery and plastic surgery. This situation is changing as technology improves; one company is now producing a bipolar instrument that can produce a high-power current capable of cutting tissue (Valleylab, 1995).

18A.5   EQUIPMENT

18A.5.1   ELECTROSURGICAL GENERATOR

This produces the diathermy current. There are usually two controls:

1. The selector (cut, blend or coag).
2. The intensity – this controls the output levels. There may also be visual and/or audible alarms to warn of poor connection.

Note: The controls should always be set to 'zero' and the unit switched off until ready to be used. Verbal confirmation of the power settings selected should always be given to the operator by the endoscopy assistant before it is used.

18A.5.2   THE ACTIVE CORD (A-CORD)

This carries the electrosurgical current from the power unit to the instrument. There are various types, depending on the make of unit and the manufacturer of the instrument used, so more than one type of active cord may be needed if not all instruments are from the same manufacturer.

18A.5.3   THE RETURN ELECTRODE

This electrode carries the current back to the generator. There are various types:

1. *Reusable*; a metal plate bandaged or stuck to the patient. An electroconductive gel or saline-soaked gauze may be required to ensure good electrical conductivity. The manufacturer's instructions should be followed.
2. *Disposable*; single use, adhesive pads. Follow the manufacturer's instructions.

Whatever the type, the plate should:

1. Have a minimum surface area of 25 cm^2 (to avoid burns).
2. Be placed on the patient's body as close to the operating area as possible (in order to reduce the length of the return pathway and minimize the risk of alternative pathways developing).
3. Not be placed over joints (it may become displaced during movement) or over or close to scar tissue or the site of metal prostheses such as hip joints, orthopaedic plates, etc.
4. Not occlude any radiological screening (avoid the abdomen where there are abdominal X-rays).
5. Avoid excessively hairy, scarred or wet areas.

18A.5.4 FOOT-PEDAL CONTROL

This allows the operator to control the electrosurgery with the foot. Ideally this should be 'shielded' to prevent someone stepping on it accidentally. It should also be waterproof.

18A.5.5 S-CORD SYSTEM

Capacitive coupling may occur between the active electrode and the endoscope sheath. This current can cause burns to anybody who is earthed touching a metal part (e.g. the fibrescope eyepiece and distal tip). This can cause the patient and/or the endoscopist or the assistant to receive an electrical shock. The S-cord effectively 'earths' the fibrescope by transferring any leaked current back to the patient electrode.

18A.5.6 ELECTROSURGICAL INSTRUMENTS

These are manufactured and marketed by a large variety of instrument companies. The main types used are:

1. Polypectomy snare.
2. 'Hot' biopsy forceps.
3. Sphincterotomy knives (papillotomes).
4. Needle knives (needle papillotomes).
5. Electrosurgical probes may also be used to coagulate bleeding blood vessels, or to reduce oesophageal cancers using a combination of cutting/coagulation to reduce the tumour bulk.

All electrosurgical instruments require:

1. A small working surface area at the patient end (for high current density).
2. An insulated shaft (to help prevent current leakage).
3. Insulated handle/connector (to control instrument and attach to active cord; the insulation protects the operator).

18A.5.7 POLICY FOR THE USE OF ELECTROSURGICAL EQUIPMENT

The electrosurgical generator (diathermy machine) is responsible for 3% of all medical negligence claims involving hospital staff. In Scotland during the years 1981–1991 this amounted to 26 cases of accidental patient burning. This is likely to be the tip of the iceberg as many such burns never get reported.

It is therefore imperative that all theatre staff using this equipment are familiar with its use. The first defence against accidental patient burns is a knowledgeable and skilled staff. An example of a policy is given in the boxed text.

Documentation

All endoscopy units should have:

- A copy of the manufacturer's manual for the generator in use in that unit.
- Information regarding the safe use of electrosurgery.
- A copy of recent hazard notices relating to the use of electro-surgery.

General maintenance

- Ensure that the generator is part of the routine maintenance check by the medical physics department.
- Routinely check all electrical cables and the general condition of the control panel, plug and switches. Report any faults or damage immediately.

Before use

- Ensure that the machine is clean and has no obvious faults or damage.
- Check that the generator is functioning correctly as per the manufacturer's handbook.

  As a minimum this should include:

- Check the alarm system prior to the patient's arrival in theatre.
- Ensure that the insulation on the cables is intact.
- If the plate is reusable, ensure that it is clean and in working order.

  Please note: most generators have more than one alarm system (for example, patient voltage monitor, patient plate monitor, patient earthing monitor); make sure that you are aware of how to test for each alarm. The instructions for testing the alarms are in the manufacturer's manuals.

During use

- Ensure that all connections to the generator are made prior to switching it on.

- Shave excess hair prior to applying the plate.
- Make sure that the patient is not touching any earthed metal objects.
- Ensure good contact between the patient and the plate, over an area of good muscle mass.
- Check the plate if the patient is moved during surgery.
- Place the plate as close as possible to the operative site.
- Check all connections if a power increase is called for.
- Check the patient for contact with earth if a power increase is called for.
- Keep active electrode clean during use.
- Always use an insulated quiver.
- Never coil the return electrode cable when it is in use.
- Beware of any modification to existing equipment.
- Make yourself familiar with the equipment in use.

After use

- Always check the patient's skin at the site of the return electrode for signs of damage.
- Wipe foot-pedals with warm water and detergent without immersing them fully in water.
- Keep the active electrode in the quiver until the generator is switched off. (Never lay the active electrode on an earthed surface (for example, a metal trolley) while the generator is switched on as this can lead to patient burns.)
- Never reuse a single-use return electrode.

Conclusion

Constant vigilance is required in order to avoid accidental patient burns. As a minimum, make sure that you are aware of how the generator works and what safety checks the manufacturer recommends prior to its use.

Used by kind permission of the Royal Infirmary of Edinburgh NHS Trust.

18A.6 DANGERS OF ELECTROSURGERY

There are inherent dangers associated with electrosurgery because of its ability to burn or destroy tissue. The main dangers include explosion, mains current (low-frequency) electrocution, interference with other electromedical devices and thermoelectric burns. Of these, thermoelectric burns are the greatest danger to the patient (Wicker, 1991) (Plate 32). These occur as a result of current division, faulty insulation or careless use. It should be remembered that the purpose of electrosurgery is to burn tissues and it is essential that this effect is limited to the active electrode at the desired site. Generally, the most commonly asked questions about the safety of electrosurgery are as in the following text.

18A.6.1 COMMONLY ASKED QUESTIONS ABOUT THE DANGERS OF ELECTROSURGERY

What is electrosurgery?

Electrosurgery refers to the use of radiofrequency electrical current to cut, coagulate or destroy tissue. Unlike cautery, it is the current itself that causes the heating effect; the electrode remains relatively cool.

Why doesn't the patient get electrocuted?

Electrocution happens as a result of neuromuscular stimulation by electric current – this only occurs at low frequency, for example 50 Hz (cycles per second), which is mains electricity. Electrosurgical current is very high frequency, around 500 000 Hz and at these high frequencies there is no effect on muscle or nervous tissue conduction.

Is there a problem with hip or other metal implants?

There is no known problem with accidental burns when the patient plate is placed over the site of an implant. The important considerations are that the site chosen for the return electrode has high conductivity, is free from hair, scars or skin blemishes and is close to the operative site. Electrosurgery near the site of an implant, for example during revision surgery, is unlikely to have any effect on the surrounding tissue, since the implant would serve to dissipate the current over a wider area.

Is there a problem with metal rings?

Rings on the finger pose no problem unless they are in contact with either an earthed object or form part of the return pathway for the current, as they would if touching an earthed object when using an earthed electrosurgical generator. Even if either of these two scenarios were the case, the ring would serve to dissipate the current over a larger area than would otherwise have been the case, thereby reducing the chance of accidental burns. The important consideration here is that the patient does not touch any earthed object, ring or no ring. Please note that, in any event, paper tape is not an insulating tape!

Why does the surgeon or assistant sometimes receive a burn when coagulating a blood vessel?

This frequently happens when the surgeon 'buzzes' a bleeder by touching the end of an artery forceps. As the tissue dries during coagulation, the resistance in this particular pathway increases. The current therefore looks for an easier pathway. The current may blast a hole in the surgeon's (or assistant's) glove causing a burn if the surgeon is electrically connected to either earth (capacitive coupling) or to the patient, thereby forming part of the return pathway. It would be much safer to use insulated instruments to coagulate the blood vessel directly.

Why is it dangerous to 'open key' an electrosurgical instrument?

Open keying is the habit of activating the active electrode before it is touching anything. This has the effect of swamping the room with radiofrequency current, like a radio transmitter. These radio waves are attempting to return to the return electrode attached to the patient. The current can be picked up by anything acting as an aerial (for example, a metal object or even a person) and transmitted to the patient via any small contact sites. Scenario – a surgeon is inadvertently standing on the pedal while the electrosurgical pencil is in its quiver. The assistant, acting like an aerial, picks up on these radio waves, which are flooding the room. His hand is resting on a towel clip that has pierced the drapes and is touching the patient's skin. The radio waves (high-frequency current) travel down the assistant's arm, into the towel clip and back to the return electrode. The result? An accidental burn where the towel clip touches the patient.

Why is it dangerous to use electrosurgery when there is a pacemaker *in situ*?

This is only dangerous if the return pathway incorporates the pacemaker. This might happen if, for example, the surgeon was operating on the right shoulder and the return electrode was on the left side of the patient. Two things might happen – the pacemaker might shut off, leaving the patient in heart block, or the pacemaker might fire rapidly, leading to ventricular fibrillation. Both of these scenarios can be avoided by the use of bipolar electrosurgery, which has a very short return pathway (between the tines of the forceps). If monopolar electrosurgery has to be used, the return electrode should be placed as close as possible to the site of surgery and away from a direct line through the heart.

Why does electrosurgery sometimes affect the ECG reading?

This normally occurs because the ECG electrodes are designed to pick up high-frequency electrical stimuli in the heart's conduction system. Since the electrosurgical current is also high frequency, these signals are also picked up. The danger is not usually to the heart itself, but rather that the ECG electrodes might concentrate these signals over a small area, leading to burns under the ECG electrodes.

Why is a patient not always burned even when he touches an earthed object?

Accidental burns depend on a combination of circumstances that very rarely occur:

- The return electrode must be faulty or improperly applied.
- An alternative pathway for the current exists.
- The current is concentrated over a small area.
- The current intensity is high enough to cause a burn.
- The alternative pathway has a lower resistance than the return electrode.
- The electrosurgery is activated for a long enough time for this alternative pathway to cause a burn.
- The electrosurgical generator has faulty or inadequate monitoring systems.
- The electrosurgery is carried out by an inexperienced operator.

Any one or a combination of the above factors must exist; however, in practice these rarely occur simultaneously.

18A.6.2 INTERFERENCE

All electrosurgery power units radiate radiofrequency (RF) noise when used. This may interfere with:

1. *Pacemakers*; Either the RF noise or sparking whilst 'cutting' can disrupt a pacemaker signal, causing ventricular fibrillation or damaging the pacemaker electronics. The latter may cause the pacemaker to malfunction. The newer types of pacemaker are less prone to this, but care should be exercised in all cases.
2. *Medical equipment*; RF noise from electrocautery units can disrupt the monitor signal or internal electronics of equipment such as cardiac monitors, impairing their accuracy. All types of medical equipment are **potentially** at risk from this, so it is recommended that checks are made before any new equipment is used to see whether it is affected. Most modern medical equipment is double-insulated to minimize this problem.
   Note: Mobile phones may also be affected or cause interference.
3. *Endoscopic photography*; RF noise can affect the automatic exposure control circuits, and often produces visual distortions on video screens.

18A.6.3 CAUSES OF THERMOELECTRIC BURNS

Current division

This occurs when all or a portion of the current travels back to the generator via a pathway other than the return electrode. This in itself will not cause any harm unless the current is concentrated through a small amount of tissue, for example an ECG electrode, a bare-tipped rectal thermometer or when the patient's arm rests against a drip stand or a metal armrest. This effect is most likely to occur in grounded monopolar electrosurgery. In order to prevent this happening the patient should be checked to make sure that he or she is not touching any grounded metal objects, which could provide an alternative pathway to earth (Fig. 18A.5) (Olympus Keymed, n.d.). The return electrode should also be placed correctly on the patient, close to the site of surgery and over an area of good muscle mass. Very hairy skin may need to be shaved prior to applying the plate in order to increase electrical contact. All modern machines have a variety of monitors that alarm and switch the generator off if they detect dangerous conditions arising. These are not necessarily foolproof (Wicker, 1991).

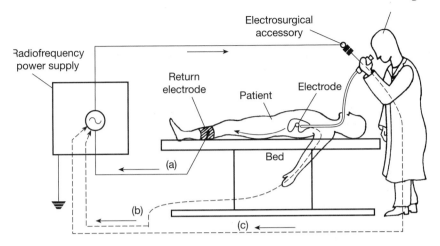

Fig. 18A.5 Leakage currents in endoscopic endosurgery: a = intended current; b,c = unintended currents, which occur when either the operator or the patient is earthed via the operating table or a metallic part of the endoscope

Faulty insulation

This may occur as a result of equipment damage caused by autoclaving or deterioration because of inappropriate storage or handling. Sharp towel clips should not be used to attach the cables to the drapes in case of perforation and contact with the patient's skin.

Careless use

Careless use may include:

- Accidental coagulation of skin edges while coagulating a 'bleeder'.
- Accidental triggering of the footswitch at an inappropriate time.
- Disposing of the active electrode at the end of a case before disconnecting it, which increases the chance of accidental triggering.
- Using inappropriate power levels which increases the probability of sparking to nearby instruments or tissues.

18A.6.4 ENDOSCOPIC SURGERY

The main electrosurgical problems during endoscopy are:

- Capacitive coupling.
- Direct coupling.
- Insulation failure.

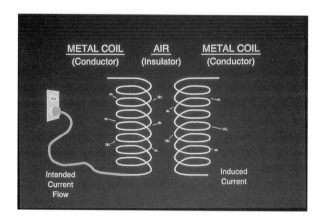

Fig. 18A.6 A capacitor

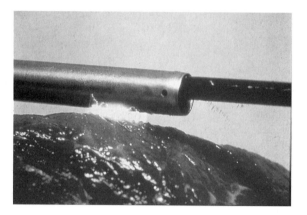

Fig. 18A.7 Capacitive coupling between the active electrode–insulation–metal sleeve, which runs to earth causing a burn (ValleyLab)

Capacitive coupling (Fig. 18A.6) occurs when the electrode couples with the endoscope and the patient's tissues, causing a burn (Fig. 18A.7). This can also cause burns in other places, such as:

• Where the patient touches earth.
• Where the surgeon touches a metal part of the endoscope.

Capacitive coupling increases when longer instruments are used (such as flexible endoscopes) and with higher voltages (such as the coag waveform).

Direct coupling can occur when the insulated electrode is activated when it is in close proximity to or in contact with a metal instrument (Fig. 18A.8). A burn can occur where the patient's tissues touch, or are in close proximity to, the metal instrument. The contact site for the burn may be outside the field of vision.

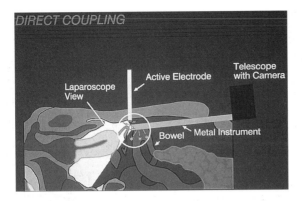

Fig. 18A.8 Direct coupling between a laparoscope and the active electrode, which are in close proximity but not actually touching

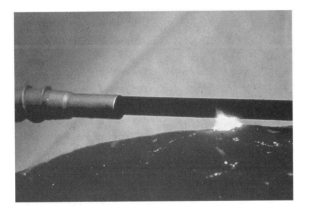

Fig. 18A.9 Insulation failure (ValleyLab)

Insulation failure (Fig. 18A.9) along the length of the endoscope results in current entering the tissues before it reaches the working end of the endoscope. These burns are extremely dangerous because they cannot be visualized when they are occurring. There is also the added danger that the surgeon will ask for increased power because the reduction of current at the tip of the endoscope will falsely indicate that the power is not high enough.

One of the methods used for avoiding burns is the S-cord (scope feedback cord), which takes leakage current from the endoscope back to the negative terminal of the generator (the same as the return electrode) (Fig. 18A.10) (Olympus Keymed, n.d.). Although this system prevents burns in the majority of situations, it can itself encourage burns if there is insulation failure and leakage between the electrode and the outside part of the endoscope that is in contact with the

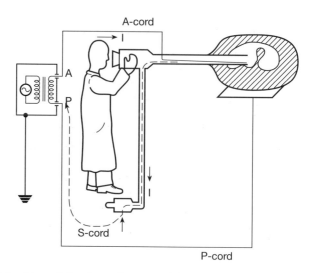

Fig. 18A.10   Use of the S-cord to avoid burns

patient's tissues. The manufacturers of this cord believe, however, that it is safer to use the S-cord because of the other more serious dangers involved in omitting it. This situation appears to have been solved for rigid endoscopes by the invention of the 'Electroshield' (ValleyLab Inc.), which monitors the active electrode and can detect any leakage along the length of the cannula and switch off the generator (ValleyLab, 1995). At present there is no such device for flexible endoscopes.

Combustible gases

Note: Do not perform electrosurgery in presence of combustible gases.

   There are two main instances when combustion may occur:

1. Where anaesthetic gases (e.g. oxygen and nitrous oxide) are present.
2. During colonoscopy where a mannitol bowel preparation has been used. (Bacteria in the gut act on mannitol to produce hydrogen and methane, which can be ignited by a spark.)

   In this instance, the gas in the bowel should be replaced with a non-combustible gas such as carbon dioxide prior to electrocautery.

What are the nursing implications?

When the patient is sedated or under a general anaesthetic he or she is unable to warn staff when burns are taking place. Therefore, it is only constant vigilance by the unit staff that can prevent such burns occurring.

Safety checks should include, but not be limited to the following:

- Check all equipment prior to use.
- Make yourself familiar with the particular generator in use.
- Make sure that the return electrode is attached and working.
- Ensure that the patient is not touching any metal objects which may be grounded (Mayo stands, table fitments, drip stands, etc.).
- Do not use sharp towel clips to attach cables to drapes.
- Always use an insulated quiver to store the active electrode throughout the operation.
- Check the whole system for faults if it does not appear to be working or if the surgeon asks for more power.
- Check the patient's skin when removing the return electrode.
- Encourage staff to learn about the principles, uses and dangers associated with electrosurgery (Wicker, 1991).

18A.6.5   PREOPERATIVE CHECK

- *The endoscope*; provision for attaching S-cord; no protruding metal on insertion tube; no cracks or exposed metal.
- *The instrument*; kinked, frayed or broken wire; breaks in insulation.
- *The patient plate*:
  - Is it in place?
  - Is surface in full contact with patient?
  - Have you avoided hairy or scarred areas?
- *The S-cord and active cord*; check for damage or breaks; use dummy circuit to test connections.
- *The diathermy unit*; use a dummy circuit to check:
  - selection of cut/blend/coag
  - output dial levels
  - footswitch working.

18A.6.6   PROTECTION OF BODY SURFACES

The patient

1. Check patient's body is not in contact with any earthed metal object.
2. Remove any jewellery from patient. The taping of rings, etc. is commonly done, but is not a sure protection because an electrical current can still 'leak' through the tape.

The operator

Note: electrosurgery is potentially very dangerous, and should only be carried out by an experienced operator who has been trained in its use.

1. Rubber gloves should be used at all times.
2. Avoid contact with the patient and endoscopy table/trolley wherever possible during use.
3. Protective rubber eyepiece covers are available, which help prevent flash burns to the operator.
4. Place other metal items such as accessory trolleys, drip stands, etc. as far away from the endoscopy table/trolley as possible.

18A.7   POLICY

These safety checks should be strengthened by a policy that outlines safety procedures and the use of these machines. An example is given in the following text.

18A.7.1   QUALITY ASSURANCE

Topic

Use of electrosurgical equipment

Standard statement

The risk of harm to the patient during the use of electrosurgery will be minimized. (See Table 18A.1 on page 403.)

Practices associated with electrosurgery should be monitored, assessed and changed if necessary using standard setting and auditing (a sample 'audit tool' is given at the end of this chapter).

18A.7.2   MONITORING SYSTEMS

The inherent instability of electrosurgical current makes it mandatory for monitoring systems to be in place in order to guard against the formation of alternative pathways. These monitors have now developed to a high degree, such that it is virtually impossible for accidental burns to occur as a result of faulty equipment. However, it is important to realize that no monitor system can be completely safe; the absence of an alarm may indicate that no problems exist or that the alarm itself may be faulty.

The monitor systems described below may be present either in whole or in part in each generator. Some are specific to certain generators. The boxed statements describe situations that cause the monitors to alarm.

Table 18A.1

Structure	Process	Outcome
A policy is available in the unit regarding the use of electrosurgical equipment	The nurse will be given instruction prior to using the equipment. The nurse will record all accidents that occur with electrosurgery	The patient will be protected from poor practice during the use of electrosurgery. Patient safety will be monitored
Information is available about the safe use of electrosurgery	The nurse will be able to demonstrate a working knowledge of the equipment	Patient safety will be ensured by the appropriate use of the equipment
An inspection programme is carried out by the medical physics department	The nurse will ensure that all equipment has been properly maintained prior to its introduction into theatre	The patient will be protected from faulty equipment
The correct equipment will be clean and available for use when required	The nurse will check all equipment prior to use	Patient safety will be enhanced by the use of appropriate equipment

Used by kind permission of the Royal Infirmary of Edinburgh NHS Trust.

Patient earth monitor

This monitor can detect any abnormal pathways which direct current away from the return electrode. It usually works by measuring the difference between the current leaving the active electrode and that entering the return electrode; any difference indicates that the current is returning via a different pathway.

> **Alarm states**
> - The patient is connected to earth, for example when touching a metal infusion stand on a metal trolley.
> - The cable's insulation has broken.

Patient voltage monitor

This monitor detects when the voltage over the patient's body rises to a dangerous level.

> **Alarm states**
> - Endoscope insulation is damaged.
> - Endoscope lubrication is conducting current.
> - The endoscope is sparking as a result of high voltage outputs.

Plate continuity monitor

This monitor detects whether the return electrode is plugged in to the generator. It doesn't detect whether or not it is attached to the patient or if it is working.

> Alarm states
>
> - The return electrode is disconnected from the circuit.

Return electrode monitor

This monitor uses a dual section plate. A small current is sent from one side of the plate to the other, passing through the patient's skin under the plate. It alarms if the skin resistance between these two plates changes.

> Alarm states
>
> - The return electrode is becoming detached.
> - Tissue resistance is increasing (for example, in a shocked patient when blood supply to the skin is decreasing).
> - The cables are broken.
> - The plate connector is broken.

Active electrode monitor

This monitor is limited to rigid laparoscopes at present. A shield (cover) is slipped over the electrode (there are now a range of electrodes which are readymade with the shield), which is then introduced into the cannula. The shield detects abnormal leakage or capacitance along the length of the (insulated) instrument.

> Alarm states
>
> - The electrode is being keyed next to, or in contact with, another metal instrument.
> - The electrode is being keyed next to, or in contact with, patient's tissues (out of sight of the camera).
> - Insulation failure has occurred along the length of the active electrode.

18A.8   THE FUTURE OF ELECTROSURGERY

There has been a rush of technology recently as minimally invasive surgery has been developed. Although lasers are enjoying popularity at present, electrosurgery continues to provide a cheap and arguably more versatile alternative. Electrosurgery has not been left behind and many improvements in design have been occurring. The improvements lie in three different directions – safety, improved efficiency and wider applications.

18A.8.1   SAFETY FEATURES

The patient plate has been targeted by many manufacturers as the major trouble spot. Improvements in design include plates with integral gels, adhesive and waterproof gels and dual-section plates. There is a move away from plates that need bandages to attach them or gels added to them. Lead plates with saline-soaked socks should now be a thing of the past, as are capacitive plates made from insulating rubber.

Monitoring systems are also improving and it is now possible to detect whether a plate is becoming loose during an operation, whether the patient is touching a grounded object or whether the plate is attached to the patient at all. One company claims that its monitoring system is so good that in nine million cases worldwide there has not been a single case of a faulty return electrode (Valleylab, 1995).

Other improvements include:

- Standardization of colours, symbols and pin systems.
- User-friendly control buttons.
- Disposable accessories designed for specific situations.

18A.8.2   IMPROVEMENTS IN EFFICIENCY

The trend in recent years has been to increase the precision and efficiency of electrosurgical generators. This has been done by looking at the shape of the waveform and adjusting the parameters (e.g. voltage, current, crest factor and power). For example, one of the Eschmann generators produces a square waveform, which is claimed to reduce the sticking of burned and burning tissue to the active electrode (Eschmann Bros and Walsh Ltd, 1995). It should also be possible to devise a waveform that can cut through skin without the danger of unacceptable scarring. At present, high power is required for operations such as prostatectomy; however, shaping the parameters of the waveform could make the current more efficient and therefore less power would be required. Power requirements could be so low that a patient-return electrode would no longer be required since sufficient current would return to the generator via the 'monopolar effect' (capacitance). It will also be possible to shape the waveform so that it will cut tissue selectively; for example, prostatic tissue could be resected leaving the capsule untouched.

18A.9   AUDIT TOOL

An example of a possible auditing tool is given in the boxed section.

TOPIC: THE USE OF ELECTROSURGICAL EQUIPMENT

Criteria

- All equipment is clean.
- No inflammable anaesthetic gases are in use.
- A team member is designated to check the equipment.
- Manuals are kept for equipment in use in theatre.
- Regular maintenance is carried out.
- The wall socket is checked for damage prior to use.
- The plug and lead are checked for damage prior to use.
- The footpedals are checked for damage prior to use.
- The scrub nurse checks the insulation on the instruments prior to use.
- The return electrode is placed on an area free from hair.
- The return electrode is placed on an area free from lesions.
- The return electrode is fastened securely to the patient.
- The return electrode is placed over an area of large muscle mass.
- The return electrode is used as per the manufacturer's instructions.
- The patient is protected from metal contact with earth.
- The return electrode is connected correctly.
- The live electrode is connected correctly.
- The power setting is checked by the surgeon in charge.
- The patient's skin is checked postoperatively.
- Damage to the patient's skin is recorded as per policy.
- Damage to the patient's skin is reported to the hospital administration.
- The ward nurse is informed of any damage to the patient's skin.
- The staff are instructed in the use of electrosurgery.
- The staff are instructed in the dangers of electrosurgery prior to use.

Use of audit tool

The design of this audit tool has been adapted from the National Association of Theatre Nurses' quality assurance document.

Each criterion is audited for an agreed number of patients (1–10). Scores are given for each patient:

- Yes   = 1
- Yes I (incomplete) = ½
- No   = 0
- N/A   = x

Calculations can be interpreted to show:

- **Score per patient, for all criteria.** This indicates the overall assessment per patient during the use of electrosurgery. It could show, for example, that standards were high for most patients; however, one or two scored very badly, indicating a problem at certain times of the day.
- **Overall score for all patients.** This may indicate the overall standard of care for the department for that day. Its value is in looking at the theatre team as a whole rather than looking at individual elements of the team's standards.
- **Score per criterion, for all patients.** This may be useful for identifying single criteria that show either very high standards or room for improvement. It could be useful, for example, when it is known that a problem exists but has to be proved in order to have improvements undertaken. Scores for individual criteria for individual patients can also be taken in this way, which may highlight problems that occur rarely.

EXAMPLE

Results

Criterion: A team member is designated to check the equipment

	1	2	3	4	5	6	7	8	9	10
Yes	1		1							
Yes (incomplete)										
No		0								
N/A										
Score	1	0	1							

Criterion: Manuals are kept for equipment in use in theatre

	1	2	3	4	5	6	7	8	9	10
Yes	1									
Yes (incomplete)		$\frac{1}{2}$								
No		0								
N/A			x							
Score	1	$\frac{1}{2}$	x							

Criterion: Regular maintenance is carried out

	1	2	3	4	5	6	7	8	9	10
Yes	1	1	1							
Yes (incomplete)										
No										
N/A										
Score	1	1	1							

SCORES

Score per patient, for all criteria

	1	2	3	4	5	6	7	8	9	10
Points scored	3	$1\frac{1}{2}$	2							
Applicable	3	3	2							
Final percentages	100 %	50 %	100 %							

Patients 1 and 3 appeared to receive the optimum level of care. There appears to be a problem with patient 2 that would require action and a change in practice.

Overall score for all patients

$$\frac{\text{Sum of all final percentages}}{\text{Number of patients}} = \%$$

$$\frac{250\%}{3} = 83\%$$

This score indicates an overall high level of quality. In the normal situation this final score is a result of the calculation of all the criteria in the audit.

Score per criterion, for all patients

$$\text{Criterion 1} = \frac{2}{3} \times 100 = 66\%$$

$$\text{Criterion 2} = \frac{1\frac{1}{2}}{3} \times 100 = 50\%$$

$$\text{Criterion 3} = \frac{3}{3} \times 100 = 100\%$$

These scores indicate that there are problems with criterion 1 and 2 that bear further investigation. The staff should be commended on the results of criterion 3.

Used by kind permission of the Royal Infirmary of Edinburgh NHS Trust.

18A.10 CONCLUSION

Electrosurgery has shown its resilience to change. The fact that it is one of the most useful electromedical devices to be used in the operating theatre has ensured that it has survived the advent of lasers and minimally invasive surgery. This most useful of devices, however, refuses to allow any complacency when it comes to safety and it is almost inevitable that accidental burns will occur – the only question is when and how severe they will be. Both these factors can be delayed, or perhaps prevented, by the thorough training of all personnel who use electrosurgery and by the constant search for improvements in technology. It is only through constant vigilance that accidental burns may be avoided.

Diathermy machines cause more patient injuries than any other electromedical device in the operating theatre. Most incidents are due to user error.   (Stankevitch, 1980)

The greatest factor in the safe and efficient use of electrosurgery is adequately trained personnel.   (Drew, 1980)

REFERENCES

Drew, R.J. (1980) Quality assurance of electrosurgical devices. *Med Instrument*, (Sept/Oct), 255–6.

Eschmann Bros and Walsh Ltd (1990) *The New TD 411-RS Range* [information leaflet]. Eschmann Bros and Walsh Ltd, London.

LoCicero, J., Frederickson, J.W., Hartz, R. and Michaelis, L., (1987) Pulmonary procedures assisted by optosurgical and electrosurgical devices: comparison of damage potential. *Lasers Surg Med*, 7, 263–72.

Olympus Keymed (n.d.) *Radiofrequency Cutting and Coagulation in Endoscopic Use*. Olympus Keymed, Southend-on-Sea.

Stankevitch, B.A. (1980) 4% of liability claims involve electromedical devices. *Mod Healthcare*, 1(10), 74–6.

ValleyLab Inc (1995) *Surgical Products Guide*. ValleyLab Inc, Boulder, Colorado.

Wicker, C.P. (1991) *Working With Electrosurgery*, National Association of Theatre Nurses, Harrogate.

Wicker, C.P. (1993) *Electrosurgery*, Pentax Medical, South Harrow.

Radiation 18B

Mike Shephard

18B.1 WHAT IS RADIATION?

18B.1.1 BACKGROUND

Radiation was discovered by Professor Wilhelm Conrad Röntgen in 1895 whilst he was working at the University of Wurzburg in Germany. He discovered that a new ray he was experimenting with made a barium platinocyanamide screen fluoresce. He then discovered that this ray could pass through paper, wood and human skin and bones and that the amount of ray that passed through the material depended on its density and the strength of the ray. He managed to produce a picture of the bones of his wife's hand on a photographic plate. As he did not know what these rays were he called them X-rays, and this name has stuck to this day.

18B.1.2 THE NATURE OF X-RAYS

X-rays are **very short wavelength electromagnetic waves**. The electromagnetic spectrum runs from electricity at one end to gamma rays and beyond (Fig. 18B.1). Visible light is included in this spectrum. The reason we cannot see X-rays is that our eyes cannot detect electromagnetic waves of that wavelength.

Because of their very short wavelength, X-rays are able to penetrate solid materials. They were originally produced by 'firing' high-velocity electrons at a 'target' made of tungsten whilst in a vacuum.

Originally, the black and white picture produced on an X-ray film was produced because the X-rays turn the film black but dense material such as bone absorbed the X-rays so the image appeared white on the film. Nowadays, images are produced on the film by the X-ray striking

Practical Endoscopy Edited by M. Shephard and J. Mason. Published in 1997 by Chapman & Hall, London. ISBN 0 412 54000 2

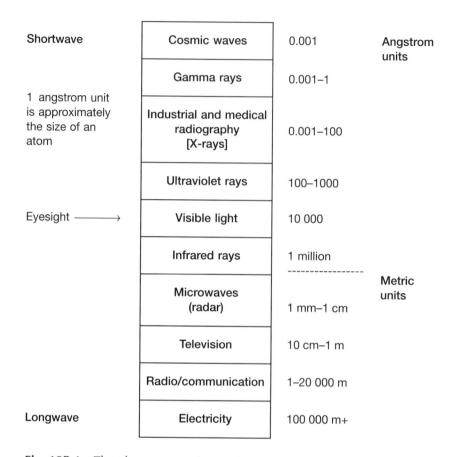

Fig. 18B.1   The electromagnetic spectrum

a fluorescent-coated screen or are recorded digitally, so that a far lower dose of radiation is required.

Contrast media such as Conray and barium work because they have a high density and absorb X-rays, but in doing so outline the particular structure under investigation.

18B.2   THE LAW

All use of X-rays in the United Kingdom is governed by the Ionizing Radiations (Protection of Patients Undergoing Medical Examination or Treatment) Regulations 1985, and the Guidance notes released in 1988. Other countries will have their own sets of regulations, but the principles will be the same.

These require, under normal circumstances:

1. A designated area.
2. A radiation warning sign.
3. Regular checks/maintenance on equipment.
4. Provision of appropriate protective clothing for patients and staff.
5. Monitoring and recording of length of screening.
6. Periodic assessment of finger/eye doses.
7. Appropriate training for all personnel.
8. An appointed radiation protection adviser.
9. Keeping staff and patient doses as low as reasonably practical.

All areas must also have their own radiation policy (local rules), which all staff must be aware of.

18B.3 WHAT IS THE HAZARD?

18B.3.1 HEALTH CONSIDERATIONS

There are **two** main sources of radiation:

1. 'Background' radiation including cosmic rays and radon gas.
2. Medical exposure.

Exposure to radiation can cause:

1. Burns and cataracts.
2. Leukaemia and solid cancers.
3. Genetic mutation.

It is for the last reason that X-rays are avoided if possible during pregnancy, and that X-ray departments enforce the 10- or 28-day rule (local policy dictates which is adopted).

18B.3.2 BACKGROUND RADIATION

Background radiation is largely unavoidable except that certain areas of the world have higher levels of this because of the production of radon gas. In the United Kingdom, Cornwall has the highest level and, whereas the average exposure is 2 mSv per year for the rest of the country, the level for Cornwall is 8 mSv. The majority of people occupationally exposed to radiation get an annual dose of far less than these levels so, put in this context, the risk is very small.

18B.3.3 DIAGNOSTIC RADIOLOGY

Whilst in the X-ray department, the hazard to the patient/operator from radiation comes from two sources (Fig. 18B.2):

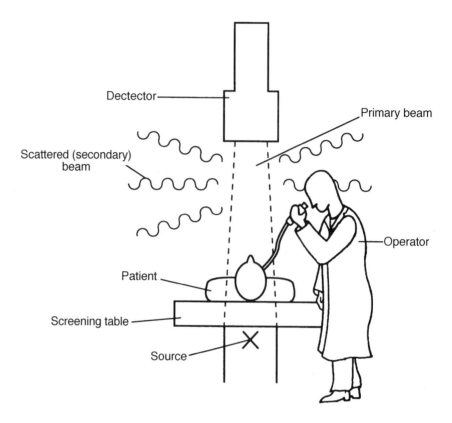

Fig. 18B.2   Primary and secondary radiation sources

1. The main (primary) X-ray beam.
2. Scattered (secondary) radiation.

18B.4   PROTECTION MEASURES

18B.4.1   PROTECTING THE PATIENT

The following methods of protection should be used:

- Use gonad shields and other protective devices.
- Keep exposure time to a minimum.
- Follow 10- or 28-day rule (according to local policy).
- Avoid exposure during pregnancy.
- Keep detector as close to the patient as possible.
- Question whether the investigation/procedure is **really** necessary.

18B.4.2   PROTECTING THE STAFF

In general, there are three ways of protecting staff:

1. *Distance*:
   - Remain close to source **only** when necessary **or** keep as far away as is practicable.
   - Remember the 'inverse square law'.

INVERSE SQUARE LAW

If you **double** the **distance** between yourself and the radiation source, then you **quarter** the **dose received**.

---

2. *Shielding*:
   - Use protective aprons routinely. **Do not** fold/crease them as this damages the protective layer. (Hang them up.)
   - Use other protection if practical (gloves, eye shields, etc.).
   - **Don't** stand side-on to source (many protective aprons have a gap down the side)
   - Keep hands out of primary beam.
3. *Time*:
   - Keep screening to a minimum (avoid protracted procedures if possible, and don't screen unnecessarily).

18B.5   GENERAL

18B.5.1   DOSEMETERS

Dosemeters give an indication of your exposure to radiation but are probably not necessary for endoscopy unit staff unless they spend more than half their working time in the X-ray department on a regular basis. Local policy will dictate whether dosemeters are worn. However, **knowing** that you have a low radiation exposure level can be very reassuring.

18B.5.2   PREGNANCY

Pregnancy is not a contraindication for any member of staff working in the X-ray department, and the decision of whether to work in an X-ray department during pregnancy should be left to the individual concerned, her manager, and/or the hospital.

Lasers 18C

Suresh Nair

18C.1 INTRODUCTION

The development of medical lasers has revolutionized the endoscopic treatment of cancers and gastrointestinal haemorrhage. Nowadays there are many different types of lasers used routinely in medicine covering a wide range of procedures. Each laser has its own method of operation and associated hazards. It is therefore essential that manufacturers' instructions and recommendations are adhered to at all times. The types of laser most commonly used in endoscopy are:

1. Neodymium:yttrium–aluminium–garnet (Nd:YAG).
2. KTP:YAG.
3. Argon.

Carbon dioxide lasers are available but are incompatible with flexible endoscopes. A 'fibre' type CO_2 laser has been introduced but is not widely used.

18C.2 WHAT IS A LASER?

The word 'laser' is an acronym of the process in which high-energy light is created:

Light Amplifications (by) Stimulated Emission (of) Radiation

(In this instance, the term 'radiation' applies to light energy only.)
Laser light is formed when an electron in a lasing medium (usually gas or crystal) is stimulated to produce particles of light. This stimulation is brought about by the application of energy.

Practical Endoscopy Edited by M. Shephard and J. Mason. Published in 1997 by Chapman & Hall, London. ISBN 0 412 54000 2

18C.2.1   THE PROPERTIES OF LASERS

Collimation

Laser light can be thought of as a parallel beam of light that is highly directional. This is called collimation and makes lasers very accurate aiming devices. In theory, the collimated laser light travels into infinity, so safety precautions are required to prevent accidents and injury from the beam.

Coherence

Light travels in waves, and in the case of ordinary light these waves travel randomly in all planes. In a laser light beam, all the waves are in harmony (in phase), so all the particles of laser light leaving the source and travelling in these waveforms will arrive at the target tissue at the same moment. This produces a more concentrated form of energy than that produced by ordinary light, which can be used to coagulate or vaporize tissue (National Association of Theatre Nurses, 1994).

Monochromatic light

Lasers usually produce light of one colour only. The Nd:YAG laser produces a single green band that is not visible to the human eye, so this is usually accompanied by a visible xenon or helium–neon aiming beam. The carbon dioxide laser produces a single band of infrared light. The exception to this rule of monochromatic light is the argon laser, which may have up to 11 different colours. In the surgical argon laser there are two bands, blue and green, both of which are visible to the human eye.

18C.3   LASER SAFETY

18C.3.1   INTRODUCTION

Over the past two decades, numerous texts and articles have appeared in the literature addressing the issues of safety and hazards associated with the use of lasers. Some of these texts have been of a highly technical nature meant for laser technicians and biomedical engineers. A booklet published in 1988 by the American National Standards Institute (ANSI, 1988) specifically deals with the safe use of lasers in medicine and surgery (Kulkaski, 1994). This document may, however, be more appropriate for the laser safety officer of the hospital than for busy clinicians and nursing staff involved in endoscopic laser surgery.

The purpose of this chapter, therefore, is to provide a succinct yet fairly comprehensive account of the potential hazards one can encounter in laser surgery and the safety measures that it would be prudent to adopt to minimize these risks.

18C.3.2 HAZARDS AND SAFETY MEASURES

There are two broad categories of laser mishaps:

Group I thermal injury to patients and personnel from either (a) indirect laser-ignited combustion or (b) direct accidental trauma from unintentional firing, or use in incorrect clinical circumstances.

Group II related to (a) specific types of laser surgery and their morbid sequelae and (b) problems arising from malfunctioning laser and ancillary equipment.

18C.3.3 GROUP I

Thermal injury from indirect laser-ignited combustion

This form of laser surgery mishap has resulted in the greatest number of deaths (Fisher, 1993) and is the most catastrophic of all.

1. *Bronchoscopic laser surgery*; the elastomer endotracheal tubes will burn avidly in the oxygen-rich atmosphere; this can cause severe third-degree burns leading to tracheomalacia or, worse, massive pulmonary oedema and death. The carbonized residue of the polyvinyl chloride tube adheres to the mucosal surfaces, making it difficult to remove.

   During laser surgery in the airway, an all-metal, jet-venturi ventilation system without any combustible material can avoid endotracheal tube fires.

   If using a flexible bronchoscope to do laser surgery (e.g. Nd:YAG laser to coagulate tumours before removal), it is best to pass it through a rigid ventilating bronchoscope. In this way there is no chance of an elastomer endotracheal tube catching fire and the lumen available for ventilation is not compromised. Since the bronchoscope is black, laser energy would be absorbed. However, the surgeon must ensure that the laser fibre-tip is seen beyond the end of the scope as firing the laser with the fibre-end within the working channel can cause the endoscope to catch fire.

2. *Laser surgery at the perineal region or the anus*; it is possible in this circumstance for the methane gas expelled from the patient's rectum to ignite. To avoid this, the lower bowel could be evacuated by an

enema a few hours prior to surgery or a pledget of moist cotton swab could be used to plug the anus.

3. *Sterile drapes or pads*; these can also ignite; this could be prevented by wetting the drapes but this could compromise sterility and is not advisable when electrosurgery is also being performed. Fire-retardant drapes have been manufactured but may not be cost effective enough to be practical. Laser fibre-tips should not be clipped on to the drapes, but instead held in place by the designated stands provided for this purpose by the laser companies.

4. *Preparations used to cleanse the operative area*; these must not contain inflammable solutions such as alcohol, ether or acetone. Even though preparation liquids like Betadine or Hibitane are used, these chemicals can vaporize and produce skin burns if ignited. Before the laser is fired, all areas cleansed with these liquids must be allowed to dry.

In laparoscopic procedures, the preparing solutions may not present so significant a hazard, but it is still prudent to ensure the solutions do not contain combustible agents and that the area is dry before activating the lasers.

A portable fire extinguisher must always be within the operating room in case of laser or electrical fires. It is always wise to have a basin of water near the operator's field to put out non-electrical fires.

Thermal injury from direct accidental trauma from unintentional firing or use in incorrect clinical circumstances

Reflection

Using reflective shiny instruments will cause the laser beam to be deflected to areas other than the intended target. This could cause recognized or unrecognized injury to neighbouring tissues and organs. There could also be deflection of the laser beam to the personnel within the operating room, although the laser is far less likely to be intense enough to cause major injury. Instrumentation must therefore be brushed or coated with a non-reflective finish (Kulkaski, 1994).

Perforation

When doing laser surgery within hollow viscera (e.g. intestines, oeso-phagus, bladder, uterus, bronchus) misdirection of the laser beam or fibre and not being aware of the tissue effects and power density of the particular laser can result in disastrous consequences such as perforat-ing injuries to organs adjacent and beyond the viscera (Fisher, 1993)

Injury to adjacent vascular structures can cause massive haemor-rhage. For example, perforation of the bronchus and unintentional injury to the large vessels can cause a massive haemomediastinum. Similarly, in laser surgery for endometriosis in the pelvis, massive haemorrhage requiring immediate laparotomy can occur from inadvertent perforation of the external and internal iliac vessels. Thermal burns to ureters and bowels that are detected late could result in faecal peritonitis or fistula formation.

Meticulous surgical technique to dissect and display vital structures adequately and judicious use of laser energy are mandatory in the prevention of inadvertent injury. In performing hysteroscopic Nd:YAG laser ablation of the uterine endometrium, the fibre should be dragged towards the operator to avoid perforation of the uterus and inadvertent bowel injury (Garry, 1991).

Spread adjacent to the field of surgery

In performing surgery in areas close to neural tissues and nerves, application of laser beams very precisely and in short pulses minimizes the risk of permanent disability from neural injury. The surgeon must understand that certain lasers (i.e. CO_2 lasers) act very precisely and leave negligible lateral thermal dispersion (Garry, 1991). However, the CO_2 laser may penetrate anything that comes in its path and the skilful use of instruments or water as backstops can prevent unintended laser damage. The Nd:YAG laser has powerful coagulation and hence haemostatic capability but, by the same token, is likely to cause considerable thermal necrosis in depth and via lateral spread that is often not recognized at the time of surgery and may result in later morbid sequelae.

Spread beyond the field of surgery

This includes injury to the eyes of the patient and the personnel (surgeon, nurses, anaesthetist). Appropriately designed eyewear should be made mandatory for all personnel within the operating room including protection for the anaesthetized patient. The eyewear should be of the correct design to screen out the appropriate wavelengths and be of sufficient optical density (Kulkaski, 1994). These specifications must be clearly delineated in the theatre warning signs prominently displayed outside the operating room as well as on the laser regulations laid down for surgeons performing laser surgery. The wavelengths screened and optical density rating must also be distinctly displayed on the goggles.

Designating the laser operating room as a controlled procedure area with the hazard sign (Fig. 18C.1) is necessary to ensure that only appropriately trained and laser-protected authorized personnel move into the area. All windows into the procedure area must have opaque panes to block the passage of the laser beam (Kulkaski, 1994).

Occasionally, the surgeon's hands may come into the line of fire of the laser beam but reflex withdrawal of the affected area from the laser beam usually prevents significant injury from occurring. If, however, the

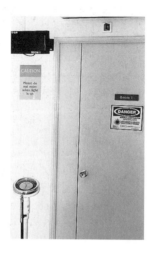

Fig. 18C.1   An example of a laser hazard warning sign posted on to the door to the operating room at an ambulatory day surgery centre

skin of an anaesthetized patient is indirectly lasered, then a serious degree of thermal injury would occur (Fisher, 1993). The exposed skin can be protected by a layer of crumpled aluminium foil (for diffuse reflection) taped in place. To further avoid laser injuries to the eyes and skin, a designated laser safety nurse or technician must always be at the laser machine's controls so that the laser is put on 'standby' mode when not in use or the emergency cut-off switch can be hit to avoid an accident (Kulkaski, 1994).

Use in incorrect clinical circumstances
If the laser is used to ablate a lesion of unknown histopathology this does the patient a great disservice. Biopsies of suspicious lesions must be taken first to determine the severity and extent of the cancer, if any. Laser beam ablation, however, may be used in known cases of malignancy where it is used to clear a lumen obstructed by the tumour (Fisher, 1993).

Using the wrong laser for the incorrect purpose can be detrimental; for example, the CO_2 laser is good for precise cutting, vaporizing or drilling but not for coagulation of tumours or vessels to relieve obstruction or achieve haemostasis, which is better done with the Nd:YAG lasers. A sound knowledge of the physical properties of the various types of lasers available and the variety of tissue effects at different power settings, wavelengths and temporal modes is mandatory before a surgeon can embark on laser surgery. Understanding the complexities of the various delivery systems and their respective optical capabilities (e.g. colposcopic, hysteroscopic and laparoscopic routes) is critical to the efficient and safe use of the laser as a tool for the surgical procedure.

18C.3.4 GROUP II

Morbid sequelae of specific forms of laser surgery

Distension media
There are a multitude of endoscopes that are now available to look into almost any cavity in the body. In certain instances, however, distension media are required to expand the cavity to allow visualization. Be they liquid or gaseous, these media have inherent characteristics and are delivered via special pumps (e.g. laparoflators, hysteroflators) and at designated flow rates and pressures that allow adequate but safe visualization of structures.

Distension medium can cause complications during laser surgery by its introduction into unintended sites (e.g. vessels, to cause gas embolism). If CO_2 gas is introduced into the pleural space or mediastinum it could cause cardiopulmonary embarrassment from a pnemothorax or pnemomediastinum (Fisher, 1993).

During Nd:YAG ablation of the uterine cavity, saline and not CO_2 gas should be used to cool the laser fibre-tip and distend the uterine cavity as carbon dioxide can cause gas embolism. Furthermore, if saline distension is used for prolonged periods at excessive pressure, this will result in intravasation and hypervolaemia due to absorption into the circulatory system and can lead to pulmonary oedema, cardiac failure and, if unchecked, to eventual death (Garry, 1991).

Smoke and vapour
When tissues are heated they undergo desiccation. Thereafter, combustion in oxygen of the dehydrated organic residues produces smoke. Carbon dioxide lasers tend to produce more smoke than do Nd:YAG and KTP (potassium-titany-1-phosphate) lasers.

Smoke produced, for example, by the Co_2 laser comprises mainly particles about 1 µm in size. This is small enough to remain trapped in alveoli and not be exhaled. There has not been any conclusive evidence to show that viable cells exist nor contain replicating DNA or transcripting RNA in the plume of CO_2 lasers vaporizing viral warts or malignant cells (Bellina, Stjernholm and Kurpel, 1982). Furthermore, studies on the infective capacity of viral particles in the CO_2 laser plume from vaporization of papilloma virus warts indicate that infection is highly improbable. Nevertheless, many studies have shown that various deleterious physiological effects on the respiratory tracts occur in animals inhaling the smoke plumes from surgical lasers (Baggish, 1989).

Hence, laser surgeons and personnel must protect themselves from laser plume by appropriate smoke evacuators as the wall-suction is grossly inadequate to cope with CO_2 laser vaporization of lesions in open air. Smoke-evacuators are generally capable of removing smoke particles down to 0.1 µm. In addition, surgical masks that filter down to 0.2 µm are available but must be worn snugly over the nose and mouth to be effective (Fisher, 1993).

Malfunctioning and breakage of equipment, instruments and materials

The breakage of the laser fibre-tips can occur. It usually does not cause any morbid sequelae if they become encapsulated by fibrous tissue but when it is a long segment and lodged between viscera it could cause perforation and peritonitis (Fisher, 1993).

The laser surgeon should know that breakages can occur if the fibre protrudes too far beyond the endoscope or has been improperly stripped, causing distal tip weakness, or is inappropriately used to dissect and probe tissue.

For safe laser surgery using fibre lasers, the surgeon must avoid the above situations and ensure proper stripping using the appropriate stripper provided by the manufacturers.

If the distal end does break off, the video camera must be trained at it and a grasper used to pick up the tip gently without crushing it or 'flicking' it beyond the field of view, never to be found again.

Laser machines can malfunction at critical points of surgery. The hospital must have a laser technician or biomedical engineer who maintains the laser machines and is capable of doing minor repairs and troubleshooting for potential problems. However, if a situation arises where the laser is repeatedly malfunctioning, then surgeons must be resourceful enough in their skills to adopt alternative surgical manoeuvres and energy modalities to complete the surgical task at hand. It is sometimes necessary to abandon the procedure if the procedure cannot be safely completed owing to the absence of alternative or back-up energy modalities.

18C.4 CONCLUSION

Although all the probable hazards cannot be discussed in one short chapter, it is mandatory for surgeons, nurses and laser technicians to have a profound knowledge of the tissue effects of the lasers used and, the potential complications that can occur, and to undergo drills on how to react quickly and effectively to prevent or minimize the detrimental effects of laser energy on the operators and patients (Table 18C.1). To this end a strict training, credentialling and accreditation process is required. Constant upgrading and reviewing of skill levels of surgeons is needed and should be based on the frequency and complexity of usage of the different lasers in relation to the procedures performed and anatomical sites at which they are performed.

Table 18C.1   Audit form – endoscopy (topic: laser)

Code	Observe/ask/records	Question/note
01	Ask staff	What are the different types of laser?
P3	Observe	Does the user connect the equipment correctly and safely?
P1	Records	Is there an induction/in-service programme in operation?
P2	Ask staff	Did you receive instruction in the use of this machine and equipment?
P3	Observe	Is cleaning and checking carried out correctly by skilled personnel?
P3	Ask doctor	Can the user explain the pre-op preparation and checking of equipment?
O3	Observe	Preparation of the environment When the laser is in use: restrict access to area reduce number of personnel use of warning signs and lights carbon dioxide fire extinguisher available use of protective eyewear
P4	Records	Is there a planned maintenance programme?
P5	Records	Security of the laser – laser key holder register Laser log book, used each time the laser is used, record of the operation and patient details
P4	Observe/ask	Are the manufacturer's instructions available? Is there a local policy available?

Each hospital should have a laser surgery documentation file or 'laser log' so that relevant information on type of laser used, delivery systems engaged, energy settings employed, duration of time the laser was applied and the procedures performed can be duly recorded (Kulkaski,

Table 18C.2   Standard statement to ensure safe and correct use of laser equipment (topic: laser; subtopic: patient and staff safety; care group: perioperative patients and endoscopy staff)

Structure	*Process*	*Outcome*
S1 Knowledgeable and skilled endoscopy personnel	P1 Induction programme/in-service training will be carried out by knowledgeable personnel	01 Staff are knowledgeable and skilled in the 'safe' use of laser and aware of the potential hazards when using laser
S2 Approved appropriate equipment manufacturers' instructions available for both the laser and endoscopes	P2 Regular updating of working practice and evaluation for all staff	02 Only the correct equipment will be used The equipment will be clean and safe to use
S3 In-service/induction programme available	P3 Cleaning and checking the use of the equipment is carried out by skilled and knowledgeable personnel only	O3 The patient and staff safety is carried out correctly
S4 Department policy in operation	P4 Regular servicing is carried out according to the instructions of the manufacturer Any faulty equipment is reported	
	P5 Security of the equipment, named key holder and register Record of each time the laser is used; log book	

1994). This is important as it enables credentialling criteria to be laid down and ascertained. Furthermore, should there be any late complication or sequelae there is a record upon which investigations could be conducted to determine the breach in the system. In this way, refresher training could be suggested to prevent its occurrence in the future.

By observing these laser safety standards and handling laser energy with respect, the laser team could help minimize the risk of laser hazards occurring (Table 18C.2). However, it must be done in an efficacious way without undue bureaucracy or voluminous paperwork so that maximum compliance is achieved.

Finally, of paramount importance is the proper and caring counselling of patients for laser surgery. An informative yet simple description of the procedures and possible hazards must be provided to patients. If they understand what preparations they need to make and what to expect on the day of surgery, most of the anxiety and fear inherent in undergoing surgery would be alleviated. This also optimizes requirements for sedation and pain relief to be prescribed to facilitate a successful outcome.

If despite all precautions, an unfortunate accident were to occur, prior and continued communication with the patient and their relatives would ensure that the doctor–patient relationship would still be cordial, close and comforting instead of degenerating into a purely adversarial medicolegal confrontation.

REFERENCES

American National Standards Institute (1988) *American National Standard for the Safe Use of Lasers in Health Care Facilities* (ANSI Z136.3). Laser Institute of America, Toledo.

Baggish, M.S. (1989) Laser smoke: is it hazardous? How should it be managed? Paper presented at Plenary Session, Annual Meeting, American Society of Medical Surgery, Nashville.

Bellina, J.H., Stjernholm, R.L. and Kurpel, J.E. (1982) Analysis of plume emissions after papovavirus irradiation with carbon dioxide laser. *J Reprod Med*, **27**, 268–70.

Fisher, J.C. (1993) Safe use of laser in surgery, in *Laser Surgery in Gynecology*, (ed. V.C. Wright and J.C. Fisher), W.B. Saunders, Philadelphia.

Garry, R. (1991) Safety and hazards of endoscopic laser surgery, in *New Surgical Techniques in Gynaecology*, (ed. C.J.G. Sutton), Parthenon Publishing Group, UK.

Kulkaski, S. (1994) Laser safety, in *Minimal Access Surgery for Nurses and Technicians*, (ed. F.A. Hall), Radcliffe Medical Press, Oxford.

National Association of Theatre Nurses (1994) *Principles of Safe Practice. Laser Safety*. NATN, London.

BIBLIOGRAPHY

Ball, K.A. (1993) Organising and administering an institutional laser program, in *Laser Surgery in Gynecology*, (ed. V.C. Wright and J.C. Fisher), W.B. Saunders, Philadelphia.

Wright, V.C. and Riopelle, M.A. (1993) Credentialling the laser surgeon and laser nurse, in *Laser Surgery in Gynecology*, (ed. V.C. Wright and J.C. Fisher), W.B. Saunders, Philadelphia.

Appendix I
Capital equipment requirements for an endoscopy unit

Major equipment requirements detailed are for a unit with two endoscopy rooms plus a screening room either in the unit or in the radiology department.

ENDOSCOPES

(See Table 1 for specifications.)

UPPER AND LOWER GASTROINTESTINAL

Upper GI endoscopes

6 × standard
2 × paediatric
2 × therapeutic

Lower GI endoscopes

3 × colonoscopes
1 × paediatric colonoscope
3 × flexible sigmoidoscopes

Duodenoscopes

3 × standard (diagnostic)
2 × therapeutic

Practical Endoscopy Edited by M. Shephard and J. Mason. Published in 1997 by Chapman & Hall, London. ISBN 0 412 54000 2

Table 1 Generic endoscope specifications

Application/model	Working length (mm)	Diameter (mm)	Channel (mm)	Comment
Gastroscopes				
Neonatal	900	5–6	2.0	
Paediatric	1000	7–9	2.2	
Standard	1000	9–11	2.8	
Therapeutic	1000	11–13	3.2–6.0	
Special purpose	1000	11–13	Various	• Twin channel for laser
				• Optical zoom for microendoscopy
				• Oblique direction of view for injection therapy
Colonoscopes				
Paediatric	1300	11	2.8	Highly flexible/low radius of curvature to correspond to the geometry of the paediatric bowel
Standard	1300–1700	13	3.2	Handling/torque transmission is a critical performance criterion
Therapeutic	1300–1700	14	4.2	Handling/torque transmission is a critical performance criterion
Special purpose	1300–1700	Various	Various	• Twin channel for laser, ligation and mucosal resection
				• Optical zoom for microendoscopy
				• Small diameter (with adult handling characteristics) for strictures
Bronchoscopes				
Neonatal	550	2	N/A	
Paediatric	550	3	1.0	
Standard	550	5–6	2.0	
Therapeutic	550	6	3.2	Ultrawide channel for laser and 'optical suction' in ITU/bleeders
Duodenoscopes – all side viewing/retro viewing with raiser bridge				
Paediatric	1000	7.5	2.0	
Standard	1200	11	3.2	
Therapeutic	1200	12	4.2	
Sigmoidoscope				
Standard	600	12	3.2	
Flexible cystoscope				
Standard	550	5.3	2.2	
Hysteroscopes				
Therapeutic	290	4.9	2.0	ZIFT and laser
Diagnostic	160	3.6	1.2	

RESPIRATORY (Bronchoscopes)

4 × standard
1 × paediatric
2 × therapeutic (one with 6 mm channel for laser/intensive care unit use)

UROLOGY (Cystoscopes)

4 × standard

GYNAECOLOGY (Hysteroscopes)

2 × diagnostic
2 × therapeutic (if laser/ZIFT used)

SUPPORT EQUIPMENT

ESSENTIAL

- Light-sources: minimum 3 × 300 W xenon light-sources
  plus 1 × 150 W light-source as back-up.
- Video processor and monitor: × 3 (for use with light-sources above), at least two of which should be mounted on mobile trolleys.
- Endoscopy and/or procedure trolleys: the number depending on recovery bays available.
- Diathermy machines: × 2.
- Suction machines: × 2 per procedure room (preferably piped)
  plus: × 1 per mobile trolley
  plus: × 2 portable.
- Automatic disinfectors: minimum × 1 per procedure room. A busy unit may require 2 × double machines.
  plus: 1 × disinfector if radiology dept. used.
- Resuscitation trolley: × 1 per procedure room.
- Anaesthetic machine: 1 or 2 depending on workload.
- Pulse oximeters: × 1 per procedure room
  plus: × 1 per recovery bay
  plus: × 2 portable.
- Oxygen: 1 × outlet per procedure room
  plus: 1 × outlet per recovery bay
  plus: 2 × portable (may be combined with suction).
- Endoscopy records system (microcomputer) × 1

minimum: × 1 terminal per procedure room
plus × 1 other.
- If video system not available for teaching purposes, a minimum of × 2 teaching side-arms (lecturescopes) should be provided.

DESIRABLE

- Video recorder
- Video printer
- Closed-circuit TV/audio link
- YAG laser
- Endoscopic ultrasound

Adapted from: British Society of Gastroenterology (1990) *Provision of Gastrointestinal Endoscopy and Related Services for a District General Hospital*. British Society of Gastroenterology, London.

Appendix 11
Drugs commonly used in endoscopy

ADRENALINE (Ephedrine) 1:10000 injection

Use in endoscopy Arrest of haemorrhage in gastrointestinal and respiratory tract. Prophylactic injection into polyp base prior to polypectomy.

Dose 1. Haemorrhage: 1–2 ml per quadrant around area.
2. Polypectomy: 1–2 ml into base.

Contraindications None. Do not inject intravenously. Use with caution in patients with hyperthyroidism, diabetes mellitus, ischaemic heart disease and hypertension.

Side-effects Anxiety, tremor, tachycardia, arrhythmias, dry mouth, cold extremities.

DIAZEPAM (Diazemuls, Valium, Dizac, Zetran and numerous other preparations)

Use in endoscopy Often used as a sedative, but not as frequently as in the past. In many cases midazolam is used instead of Diazemuls, as it has a shorter action.

Dose 5–15 mg in normal use. Occasionally higher doses required.

Contraindications Respiratory depression, acute pulmonary insufficiency, hypotension.

Caution Muscle weakness, past drug abuse, pregnancy/breast feeding, elderly/debilitated, hepatic/renal impairment, avoid prolonged use.

Practical Endoscopy Edited by M. Shephard and J. Mason. Published in 1997 by Chapman & Hall, London. ISBN 0 412 54000 2

Note: Diazepam is extremely irritant to tissue if accidentally injected outside a vein. To minimize this risk many preparations (e.g. Diazemuls) contain diazepam dissolved in a fatty emulsion to reduce the irritant effect.

Side-effects   Drowsiness/light-headedness for the next day, confusion, ataxia, amnesia.

Occasionally, headache, vertigo, hypotension, salivation changes, gastrointestinal disturbance, libido change, urinary retention, jaundice, blood disorders.

ETHANOLAMINE OLEATE (Ethamolin)

Use in endoscopy   Obliteration of oesophageal varices.

Dose   By slow injections into varix, 1–2 ml per varix.

Contraindications   Known hypersensitivity.

Caution   Extravasation may cause necrosis of tissues.

Side-effects   Allergic reactions (including anaphylaxis). Chest pain, stricture formation.

FLUMAZENIL/FLUMAZEPIL (Anexate, Lanexat, Romazicon)

Use in endoscopy   Used where necessary for the reversal of benzo-diazepine sedation in endoscopic procedures.

Dose   (1) Flumazenil should be administered by slow IV injection or infusion.
(2) Recommended initial dose for an adult: 200 µg IV over 15 s. If after 1 min desired consciousness level has not been obtained, further doses of 100 µg may be administered at 60-second intervals up to a total dose of 1 mg. Usual dose required is 300–600 µg.

Contraindications   Patients with epilepsy who have been receiving benzodiazepine treatment for prolonged periods as it may precipitate attack. May cause symptoms of withdrawal in patients taking long-term benzodiazepine therapy. Pregnant and lactating women, except in emergency.

Side-effects   Nausea, vomiting, flushing, anxiety/agitation if reversal of sedation is too quick, transient increase in blood pressure and heart rate, very rarely convulsions.

GLUCAGON

Use in endoscopy   Relaxes sphincter of Oddi, aiding cannulation during ERCP.

Dose   0.5–1 unit by subcutaneous, intramuscular or intravenous injection. If no response after 15 min then intravenous glucose should be given.

Contraindications   Insulinoma, phaeochromocytoma, glucagonoma.

Side-effects   Nausea, vomiting, diarrhoea, hypokalaemia, rarely hypersensitivity reactions.

GTN SPRAY (glyceryl trinitrate)

Use in endoscopy   Used in ERCP, prior to intubation to bring about relaxation in the sphincter of Oddi, and aiding cannulation of the ampulla.

Dose   Sprayed sublingually – 1 to 2 sprays usually.

Contraindications   Patients with marked anaemia. Patients with head trauma/cerebral haemorrhage. Patients with closed-angle glaucoma.
   Also – caution with hypotensive patients.

GTN is inflammable.

Side-effects   Throbbing headache, flushing, dizziness, postural hypotension, tachycardia.

HYOSCINE BUTYLBROMIDE (Buscopan, Holopon, Hyospasmol, Scopex, Scopoderm)

Use in endoscopy   Used as an antispasmodic agent, which relaxes smooth muscle. Mostly used in ERCP to reduce/stop peristalsis, but can also be used in colonoscopy and occasionally gastroscopy.

Dose   20–40 mg repeated after 30 minutes or as required.

Contraindications   Should not be administered to patients who are hypersensitive to anticholinergic drugs or who are suffering from prostatic enlargement or paralytic ileus.

Side-effects Dry mouth, tachycardia, temporary loss of accommodation, hesitant micturition, constipation. The elderly are particularly susceptible; glaucoma and urinary retention may occur.

Note: It is not uncommon for patients who are given IV anti-cholinergics to develop a tachycardia of 120–150 as a result. It should therefore be used with caution in the already tachycardic patient. The use of a lower (20 mg) dose produces fewer cardiac effects but has a shorter duration.

LIGNOCAINE SOLUTION 4% (Xylocaine, Lidocaine)

Use in endoscopy Topical anaesthesia during bronchoscopy. Cricothyroid injection.

Dose 1–2 ml doses via bronchoscopy to max 20 ml. 4 ml for cricothyroid injection. Solution may be coloured pink to help prevent accidental intravenous injection.

Contraindications Known history of hypersensitivity to local anaesthetics or to other components of the spray solution

Caution Absorption from mucous membranes is relatively high, especially in the bronchial tree. To be used with caution in patients with traumatized mucosa and/or sepsis in the region of the proposed applications – epilepsy, impaired cardiac conduction, shock.

Interaction To be used with caution in patients receiving anti-arrhythmic drugs, such as tocainide, since toxic effects are additive.

Side-effects Rare, allergic reactions (in severe cases anaphylactic shock). Nervousness, dizziness, convulsions, unconsciousness and possible respiratory arrest. Hypotension, myocardial depression, bradycardia and possible cardiac arrest.

LIGNOCAINE SPRAY (Xylocaine, Lidocaine) (10% soln)

Use in endoscopy Anaesthesia of the throat prior to upper gastro-intestinal endoscopy.

Dose No more than 20 applications.

Contraindications Known history of hypersensitivity to local anaesthetics or to other components of the spray solution.

Caution Absorption from wound mucous membranes is relatively high, especially in the bronchial tree. To be used with caution in patients with traumatized mucosa and/or sepsis in the region of the proposed applications – epilepsy, impaired cardiac conduction, brady-cardia, impaired hepatic function and in severe shock.

Interaction To be used with caution in patients receiving anti-arrhythmic drugs, such as tocainide, since toxic effects are additive.

Side-effects Rare, allergic reactions (in severe cases anaphylactic shock). Nervousness, dizziness, convulsions, unconsciousness and pos-sible respiratory arrest. Hypotension, myocardial depression, brady-cardia and possible cardiac arrest.

METOCLOPRAMIDE HYDROCHLORIDE (Maxolon, Octamide, Primperan, Reglan)

Use in endoscopy Nausea and vomiting.

Dose IM 10 mg.

Side-effects Extrapyramidal effects (especially in children and young adults), hyperprolactinaemia, occasionally tardive dyskinesia on pro-longed administration. Also reported: drowsiness, restlessness, diar-rhoea, depression, neuroleptic malignant syndrome, cardiac conduction abnormalities reported following IV administration.

Cautions Hepatic and renal impairment; the elderly; in young adults may mask underlying disorders such as cerebral irritation. May cause acute hypertensive response in phaeochromocytoma; pregnancy and breast feeding.

MIDAZOLAM (Hypnovel, Dormicum, Versed)

Use in endoscopy Sedative with amnesic effects.

Dose 0.5–7.5 mg. Dosages greater than 5 mg are not usually neces-sary.

Contraindications Benzodiazepine sensitivity, pregnancy unless con-sidered essential by the physician, lactating mothers. Use with caution in persons with personality disorders.
  Important: plasma concentration is increased by erythromycin, diltia-zem and verapamil – profound sedation reported. During bolus seda-tion for operative procedures, extreme caution should be exercised in patients with acute pulmonary insufficiency or respiratory depression. Severe hypotension has also been reported.

Side-effects Agitation, restlessness, disorientation, hallucinations, headache, dizziness, hiccoughs.

MORRHUATE SODIUM 5% or 1% (Scleromate)

Use in endoscopy Obliteration of oesophageal varices.

Dose 1–2 ml per varix.

Side-effects Oesophageal ulceration, allergic reactions, stricture, chest pain.

NALOXONE HYDROCHLORIDE (Narcan, Narcanti, Zynox)

Use in endoscopy Used for the complete or partial reversal of opioid depression, including mild to severe respiratory depression.

Dose By intravenous injection, 0.8–2 mg repeated at intervals of 2–3 mins to a max of 10 mg if respiratory function does not improve (then question diagnosis).

Contraindication Use with caution in patients with cardiac irritability (patients with ventricular irritability have developed tachycardia or fibrillation with the administration of naloxone).

Side-effects Occasionally, nausea and vomiting.

PEG SOLUTIONS (Klean-Prep, Go-Lytely)

Products Iso-osmotic bowel preparation. Macrogol 3350 (polyethylene glycol 3350)
Anhydrous sodium sulphate
Sodium bicarbonate
Sodium chloride
Potassium chloride
Cantaim aspartame.

Use in endoscopy Four sachets when reconstituted with water to 4 litres provides an iso-osmotic solution for bowel cleansing before colonoscopy. (**Not to be used in cases of constipation.**)

Dose By mouth 250 ml of prescribed solution every 10–15 min until 4 litres have been consumed or watery stools are free of solid matter.

Note: Not recommended for children.
All 4 litres must be drunk within 4–6 hours.
Some patients cannot tolerate this volume of fluid.

Contraindications   Gastrointestinal obstruction.

PETHIDINE HYDROCHLORIDE (pethidine, Meperidine, Demerol, Alodan, Dolantin(e), Dolosal)

Use in endoscopy   Used as an analgesic for procedures such as colonoscopy and ERCP.

Dose   25–100 mg (50 mg is usually sufficient).

Contraindications   Avoid in raised intracranial pressure or head injury.

Caution   Hypotension, hypothyroidism, asthma (avoid during an attack) and decreased respiratory reserve; pregnancy and breast feeding; may precipitate coma in hepatic impairment; reduce dose in renal impairment, elderly and debilitated.

Side-effects   Nausea, vomiting, constipation, drowsiness – larger doses produce respiratory depression and hypotension, difficulty with micturition, ureteric or biliary spasm, dry mouth, sweating, headache, facial flushing, vertigo, bradycardia, palpitations, postural hypotension, hypothermia, hallucinations, mood changes, miosis, urticaria, pruritus.

PHOSPHATE ENEMA

Use in endoscopy   Administered prior to diagnostic procedures such as proctoscopy, flexible sigmoidoscopy and colonoscopy to evacuate and clean the bowel. More commonly used in flexible sigmoidoscopy when a limited examination of the bowel only is required, thereby reducing the need for total bowel preparation.

Dose   One enema should be administered as required – adult dose. Children under 12 and over 3 years – reduce dose proportionally to the body weight of the child (e.g. a 35 kg (5½ stone) child should receive only half the bottle contents). Not for children under 3.

Contraindications Acute gastrointestinal conditions, inflammatory bowel disease, ulcerative colitis or those with increased colonic absorptive capacity (e.g. Hirschsprung's disease).

Side-effects Prolonged use may lead to irritation of the rectum, very rarely vasovagal attacks occur in elderly patients (fainting).

PROTON PUMP INHIBITORS

Products Omeprazole (Losec, Prilosec, Mopral, Antra, Zoltum)
Lansoprazole (Zoton, Lanzo, Lanzor, Lansox, Agopton)

Use in endoscopy Reflux oesophagitis, peptic ulceration, Zollinger–Ellison syndrome.

Side-effects Diarrhoae, skin rash, headaches. Occasionally, reversible confusional states.

SALBUTAMOL (Ventolin, Astec, Salbuvent, Proventil, Volmax and numerous other preparations)

Use in endoscopy Used for the asthmatic patient or patient with reversible airways obstruction due to bronchospasm. May be used either before or after endoscopy to improve respiratory function.

Dose 2.5 mg to 5 mg.

Cautions Hyperthyroidism, myocardial insufficiency, arrhythmias, hypertension, pregnancy and breast feeding.

Side-effects Fine tremor (usually hands), nervous tension headache, peripheral vasodilatation, palpitations, tachycardia.
Rarely muscle cramps, hypokalaemia after high doses, hypersensitivity reactions including paradoxical bronchospasm, urticaria and angio-oedema reported; slight pain on intramuscular injection.

SODIUM CITRATE (Microlette, Microenema)

Use in endoscopy Bowel prep before flexisigmoidoscopy.

Dose 5 ml single dose. Adults and children over 3 years 5–10 ml per rectum.

Caution   Renal impairment (risk of magnesium accumulation), hepatic impairment, elderly and debilitated patients because of the risk of sodium and water retention in these susceptible individuals.

Contraindications   Acute gastrointestinal conditions.

SODIUM PICOPHOSPHATE (Picolax, Gullalax, Pico-salax, Laxasan, Neopax and numerous other preparations)

Use in endoscopy   Stimulates intestinal mobility. Bowel evacuation before colonoscopy or flexible sigmoidoscopy. Also used in cases of constipation.

Dose   One sachet in water in the morning (before 8 am) and a second in the afternoon (between 2 and 4 pm) of day preceding procedures. Acts within 3 hours of first dose.

Contraindications   Intestinal obstruction. Not to be used in children, unless under very strict observation.

Caution   Patients should be warned that heat is generated on addition to water.

Side-effects   Abdominal cramps are a common side-effect.

SODIUM TETRADECYL SULPHATE (1 and 3% solutions)

Use in endoscopy   Obliteration of oesophageal varices.

Dose   1–2 ml per varix.

Contraindications   Known hypersensitivity.

Side-effects   Allergic reactions including anaphylaxis. Chest pain, stricture formation.
   Note: STD along with other sclerosants causes tissue necrosis if injected outside the vein with resultant ulceration and occasionally further haemorrhage.

THALAMONAL

(Each millilitre contains 50 micrograms fentanyl plus 2.5 mg droperidol.)

Use in endoscopy   Used in bronchoscopy as a sedative and to dry up secretions.

Dose   Up to 2 ml.

Contraindications   Severe depression, obstructive airways disease, respiratory depression. Concurrent administration with monoamine oxidase inhibitors or within 2 weeks of discontinuance of them.

Caution   Significant respiratory depression will occur following the administration of thalamonal in doses in excess of 4 ml (200 µg fentanyl). This may be reversed with naloxone 0.1–0.2 mg IV. Bradycardia, muscular rigidity.

Side-effects   Tolerance and dependence may occur.

VASOPRESSIN

Use in endoscopy   Arrest of acute variceal bleeding.

Dose   IV infusion 20 units in 100 ml 5% dextrose given over 15–20 min.

Contraindications   Severe vascular disease, chronic nephritis.

Cautions   Use with caution in patients with heart failure, asthma, epilepsy and other conditions aggravated by water retention. Pregnancy.

Side-effects   Pallor, nausea, intense vasoconstriction, abdominal cramps, desire to defaecate, hypersensitivity, angina and myocardial ischaemia.
   Note: In life-saving situations the risk of witholding this treatment must be weighed against the benefits.

BIBLIOGRAPHY

British National Formulary (1995) British Medical Association and Royal Pharmaceutical Society, London.
Martindale, The Extra Pharmacopoeia (1996) The Royal Pharmaceutical Society, London.

Index